**National Electronic Library for Health**

*Clinical Evidence* is a key part of the **National electronic Library for Health** and this copy of *Clinical Evidence Concise* has been provided for you to complement the full version available through NeLH.

> **www.nelh.nhs.uk/clinicalevidence**
>
> Published independently by the BMJ Publishing Group, *Clinical Evidence Concise* delivers summaries of evidence on the effects of health care.
>
> - **Save time and effort:** the evidence has been rigorously searched, appraised and summarised for you
>
> - **Keep up to date:** the evidence is constantly changing; no other resource is as comprehensive or as frequent in publishing updates (every month online)
>
> - **Recommend it to your patients:** give them the background to the conditions and treatments so you can make informed decisions together. Online access is free to all in England
>
> - **Use it to suit your needs:** this book provides fast access to the key messages but the evidence detail is easily available on the CD-ROM if you need it

As well as licencing *Clinical Evidence*, NeLH provides The Cochrane Library, National Guidelines and Local Care Pathways databases, and NSF Zones. These combine to deliver a wealth of high quality, evidence-based health resources available to professionals and the public.

Additionally, the unique "Hitting the Headlines" service from the NHS Centre for Reviews and Dissemination appraises the evidence behind the headline news item.

The library also allows open access through the Internet to specialist libraries, including primary care and health management and a database of patient experiences.

For the most part the library is open to all. However, a few resources are restricted to NHS staff only. For example, the library's anatomy resource, which provides three dimensional images built up from body scans that can be rotated and labelled.

## Training & Education

The library provides learning materials that focus on using the resources available. These include *Clinical Evidence* EBM Introductory Workshops and The Cochrane Library tutorials (www.nelh.nhs.uk/training)

We hope you, your colleagues and patients find *Clinical Evidence* and the rest of the NeLH relevant, practical and easy to use. Please give us your feedback by writing to us at CEfeedback@bmjgroup.com or use NeLH feedback.

NeLH is available at **www.nelh.nhs.uk** and *Clinical Evidence* at **www.nelh.nhs.uk/clinicalevidence.**

10 ISSUE

DECEMBER 2003

# clinical
# evidence
## *concise*

The international source of the
best available evidence for
effective health care

BMJ
Publishing
Group

**Editorial Office**
BMJ Publishing Group, BMA House, Tavistock Square, London, WC1H 9JR, United Kingdom.
Tel: +44 (0)20 7387 4499 • Fax: +44 (0)20 7383 6242 • www.bmjpg.com

**Subscription prices for *Clinical Evidence***
*Clinical Evidence* and *Clinical Evidence Concise* (with companion CD-ROM) are both published six monthly (June/December) by the BMJ Publishing Group. The annual subscription rates (for December, Issue 10 and June, Issue 11) are:

**Concise edition**
Personal: £90 • €145 • US$145 • Can$200
Institutional: £190 • €305 • US$305 • Can$420
Student/nurse: £40 • €65 • US$65 • Can$90

**Full edition**
Personal: £100 • €160 • US$160 • Can$220
Institutional: £210 • €335 • US$335 • Can$460
Student/nurse: £45 • €70 • US$70 • Can$100

All individual subscriptions (personal, student, nurse) include online access at no additional cost. Institutional subscriptions are for print editions only. Institutions may purchase online site licences separately. For information on site licences and individual electronic subscriptions please visit the subscription pages of our website www.clinicalevidence.com or email us at CEsubscriptions@bmjgroup.com (UK and ROW) or clinevid@pmds.com (Americas). You may also telephone us or fax us on the following numbers:

**UK and ROW** Tel: +44 (0)20 7383 6270 • Fax: +44 (0)20 7383 6402
**Americas** Tel: +1 800 373 2897/240 646 7000 • Fax: +1 240 646 7005

**Bulk subscriptions for societies and organisations**
The Publishers offer discounts for any society or organisation buying bulk quantities for their members/ specific groups. Please contact Miranda Lonsdale, Sales Manager (UK) at mlonsdale@bmjgroup.com or Maureen Rooney, Sales Manager (USA) at mrooney@bmjgroup.com.

**Contributors**
If you are interested in becoming a contributor to *Clinical Evidence* please contact us at clinicalevidence@bmjgroup.com.

**Rights**
For information on translation rights, please contact Daniel Raymond-Barker at draymond-barker@bmjgroup.com.

British Library Cataloguing in Publication Data. A catalogue record for this book is available from the British Library. ISSN 1475-9225 ISBN 0-7279-1805-2

**Permission to reproduce**
Please contact Alan Thomas at athomas@bmjgroup.com when requesting permission to reprint all or part of any contribution in *Clinical Evidence*.

**Legal Disclaimer**
Care has been taken to confirm the accuracy of the information presented and to describe generally accepted practices. However, the authors, editors, and publishers are not responsible for errors or omissions or for any consequences from application of the information in this book and make no warranty, express or implied, with respect to the contents of the publication.

Categories presented in *Clinical Evidence* indicate a judgement about the strength of the evidence available and the relative importance of benefits and harms. The categories do not indicate whether a particular treatment is generally appropriate or whether it is suitable for individuals.

Printed by William Clowes Ltd, Beccles, Suffolk, UK
Designed by Pete Wilder, The Designers Collective Limited, London, UK

# Team and Advisors

# Acknowledgements

The BMJ Publishing Group thanks the following people and organisations for their advice and support: The Cochrane Collaboration, and especially Iain Chalmers, Mike Clarke, Phil Alderson, Peter Langhorne, and Carol Lefebvre; the National Health Service (NHS) Centre for Reviews and Dissemination, and especially Jos Kleijnen and Julie Glanville; the NHS, and especially Tom Mann, Sir John Patteson, Ron Stamp, Veronica Fraser, Muir Gray, Nick Rosen, and Ben Toth; the British National Formulary, and especially Dinesh Mehta, Eric Connor, and John Martin; Martindale: The Complete Drug Reference, and especially Sean Sweetman; the Health Information Research Unit at McMaster University, and especially Brian Haynes and Ann McKibbon; the United Health Foundation (UHF), and especially Dr Reed Tuckson and Yvette Krantz; Bazian Ltd, and especially Anna Donald and Vivek Muthu; Dr Paul Dieppe, Dr Tonya Fancher, and Professor Richard Kravitz who are working with Clinical Evidence to explore ways of presenting evidence on the usefulness of diagnostic test; previous staff who have contributed to this issue; the clinicians, epidemiologists, and members of patient support groups who have acted as peer reviewers.

The BMJ Publishing Group values the ongoing support it has received from the global medical community for *Clinical Evidence*. In addition to others, we wish to acknowledge the efforts of the UHF and the NHS who have provided educational funding to support the wide dissemination of this valuable resource to many physicians and health professionals in the USA (UHF) and UK (NHS). We are grateful to the clinicians and patients who spare time to take part in focus groups, which are crucial to the development of *Clinical Evidence*. Finally, we would like to acknowledge the readers who have taken the time to send us their comments and suggestions.

# Contents

© BMJ Publishing Group Ltd 2003

*These topics appear on the website but not in this paper edition.

# Welcome to Issue 10

Welcome to Issue 10 of *Clinical Evidence*, the international source of the best available evidence on the effects of common clinical interventions. *Clinical Evidence* summarises the current state of knowledge and uncertainty about the prevention and treatment of clinical conditions, based on thorough searches and appraisal of the literature. It is neither a textbook of medicine nor a set of guidelines. It describes the best available evidence from systematic reviews and RCTs, and if there is no good evidence it says so.

## HOW MUCH DO WE KNOW?

*Clinical Evidence* aims to help people make informed decisions about which treatments to use. It can also show where more research is needed. For clinicians and patients we wish to highlight treatments that work and for which the benefits outweigh the harms, especially those treatments that may currently be underused. We also wish to highlight treatments that do not work or for which the harms outweigh the benefits. For the research community our intention is to highlight gaps in the evidence — where there are currently no good RCTs or no RCTs that look groups of people or at important patient outcomes.

So what can *Clinical Evidence* tell us about the state of our current knowledge? What proportion of commonly used treatments are supported by good evidence, what proportion should not be used or used only with caution, and how big are the gaps in our knowledge? A quick scan of the 1851 treatments covered in Issue 10 shows that 270 (15%) are rated as beneficial, 392 (21%) likely to be beneficial, 139 (7%) as trade off between benefits and harms, 96 (5%) unlikely to be beneficial, 88 (4%) likely to be ineffective or harmful, and 866 (47%), the largest proportion) as unknown effectiveness (see figure 1). Dividing treatments into categories is never easy. It always involves a degree of subjective judgement and is sometimes controversial. We do it because users tell us it is helpful, but judged by its own rules the categorisation is certainly of unknown effectiveness and may well have trade offs between benefits and harms. However, the figures above suggest that the research community has a large task ahead and that most decisions about treatments still rest on the individual judgements of clinicians and patients.

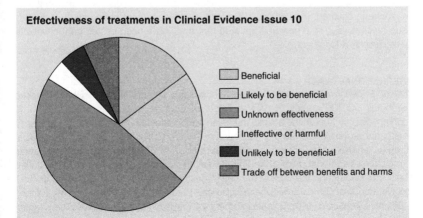

**Effectiveness of treatments in Clinical Evidence Issue 10**

Beneficial
Likely to be beneficial
Unknown effectiveness
Ineffective or harmful
Unlikely to be beneficial
Trade off between benefits and harms

Figure 1

## UPDATING AND EXPANSION

*Clinical Evidence* undergoes a continual process of updating, expansion, and improvement to include new evidence, cover new questions, and respond to user feedback. Each topic is completely updated with a full literature search every 8 months and published on the website as soon as peer review and editing allow, the aim being to minimise the interval between search and publication. The most recent search date for topics included in this issue is June 2003. Figure 2 shows a distribution of the search dates for each topic.

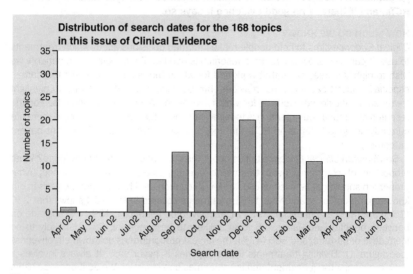

Figure 2

The content of *Clinical Evidence* Issue 10 is a snapshot of all content that was ready for publication in August 2003. Eleven new topics have been added since Issue 9: acute sinusitis, acute bronchitis, otitis externa, acute gout, bipolar disorder, deliberate self harm, domestic violence, hepatitis B, halitosis, sickle cell disease, and migraine headache in children. In addition, 106 topics have been updated and by the time this issue reaches you more new and updated topics will have been posted on the website (www.clinicalevidence.com).

## INTERNATIONAL REACH

*Clinical Evidence* has an international circulation. The UK National Health Service distributes 50 000 copies of *Clinical Evidence Concise* to staff in England. This is accompanied by free online access in England and Wales, which is available not just to healthcare professionals but also to patients. Thanks to the BMA, 14 000 UK medical students receive a copy of the full edition. In the USA 500 000 clinicians receive copies of the concise edition thanks to the United Health Foundation. Also, thanks to the Italian Ministry of Health and the work of the Italian Cochrane Centre, 300 000 Italian doctors receive a copy of *Clinical Evidence Conciso* and CD-ROM,[1] both translated into Italian.

*Clinical Evidence* is also available in other non-English language editions. The Spanish translation (published in collaboration with the Iberoamerican Cochrane Centre and Legis) now comes in all formats: full, concise, CD-ROM, and online.[2] The full text is available in Japanese[3] and Russian[4] (seven broad speciality editions). The concise edition is available in German[5] and French[6] (both with CD-ROM in English).

Finally, *Clinical Evidence* online continues to be available free to people in developing countries as part of an initiative spearheaded by the World Health Organization and the BMJ Publishing Group. Details of those countries that qualify are available from the *Clinical Evidence* website (www.clinicalevidence.com).

## FEEDBACK

If you have any comments on any of the material in *Clinical Evidence*, think that important evidence has been missed, or have suggestions for new topics or questions please let us know. You can contact us at CEfeedback@bmjgroup.com. Many thanks to all of you who have already sent in your comments.

## REFERENCES

1. *Clinical Evidence Conciso: La fonte delle migliori prove de efficacia per la pratica clinica*. Milan, Italy: Centro Cochrane Italiano/Editore Italiano/Editore Zadig, 2003.
2. *Evidencia Clínica*. Barcelona, Spain/Bogotá, Colombia: Asociación Colaboración Cochrane Iberoamerican/Legis, 2003.
3. *Clinical Evidence (Japanese edition)*. Tokyo, Japan: Nikkei Medical, 2002.
4. *Dokazatel'naya meditsina*. Moscow, Russia: Media Sphera Publishing Group, 2003.
5. *Kompendium evidenzbasierte Medizin*. Bern, Switzerland Verlag Hans Huber, 2003.
6. *Décider pour traiter abrégé*. Meudon, France: RanD, 2002.

# A Guide to Clinical Evidence Concise

*Clinical Evidence Concise* is an index of the summary information from each chapter in *Clinical Evidence* Issue 10.

*Clinical Evidence Concise* contains evidence relating to hundreds of therapeutic or preventative interventions, derived from thousands of original studies, and presents it in under 500 pages. For each condition, interventions are categorised according to whether they have been found to be effective or not. The full evidence detail behind these summaries, including clinical questions, figures, tables, and appendices, are featured on the accompanying CD-ROM, along with quantified, referenced, and up to date information about each condition.

Making summaries involves discarding detail, and users of *Clinical Evidence Concise* need to be aware of the limitations of the evidence that is presented. It is not possible to make global statements that are both useful and apply to every patient or clinical context that occur in practice. For example, when stating that we found evidence that a drug is beneficial, we mean that there is evidence that the drug has been shown to deliver more benefits than harms, when assessed in at least one subgroup of people, using at least one outcome at a particular point in time. It does not mean that the drug will be effective in all people given that treatment or that other outcomes will be improved, or even that the same outcome will be improved at a different time after the treatment.

## MEASURE OF TREATMENT EFFECTS
The dilemma is how to present summaries that are useful but not misleading. We have experimented with providing statements with no numerical information at all, with NNTs only, with a batch of absolute and relative risks, or with just the odds ratio. Each measure has its advantages and disadvantages, and not all are available from the included studies. Quantitative results may be misleading in the absence of discussion of their precision, reliability, and applicability. In *Clinical Evidence Concise*, we present non-numerical information only. Detailed quantitative results are presented on the CD-ROM, where we are able to discuss their interpretation in more detail. Your suggestions on improvements are welcome and will be read with interest.

## USING CLINICAL EVIDENCE CONCISE AND COMPANION CD-ROM
*Clinical Evidence Concise* is intended to be used as a first point of call when trying to decide what the options for treatment might be. A detailed exploration of the evidence will require looking up the detail on the CD-ROM, the full print version, or *Clinical Evidence* online. The electronic versions link, whenever possible, to abstracts of the original research in PubMed or published online versions. In this way, *Clinical Evidence* is also designed to act as a pointer, connecting the clinician rapidly to the relevant original evidence.

## INDEX PAGE
Each topic on the CD-ROM contains an index page listing interventions within their assigned categories of whether they have been found to be effective or not. Key messages summarising the evidence for each intervention are listed below the categorisation table. The full evidence detail supporting the categorisation, consisting of the question, a summary statement, benefits, harms, and a comment can be accessed by a hyperlink from the categorisation table. We would value your feedback on the presentation of interventions in future issues.

## CATEGORISATION
We have developed these categories of effectiveness from one of the Cochrane Collaboration's first and most popular products, *A guide to effective care in pregnancy and childbirth*.[1] The categories we now use are explained in the table below.

| TABLE | Categorisation of treatment effects in *Clinical Evidence* | |
|---|---|
| **Beneficial** | Interventions for which effectiveness has been demonstrated by clear evidence from RCTs, and for which expectation of harms is small compared with the benefits. |
| **Likely to be beneficial** | Interventions for which effectiveness is less well established than for those listed under "beneficial". |
| **Trade off between benefits and harms** | Interventions for which clinicians and patients should weigh up the beneficial and harmful effects according to individual circumstances and priorities. |
| **Unknown effectiveness** | Interventions for which there are currently insufficient data or data of inadequate quality. |
| **Unlikely to be beneficial** | Interventions for which lack of effectiveness is less well established than for those listed under "likely to be ineffective or harmful". |
| **Likely to be ineffective or harmful** | Interventions for which ineffectiveness or harmfulness has been demonstrated by clear evidence. |

Fitting interventions into these categories is not always straightforward. For one thing, the categories represent a mix of several hierarchies: the level of benefit (or harm), the level of evidence (RCT or observational data), and the level of certainty around the finding (represented by the confidence interval). Another problem is that much of the evidence that is most relevant to clinical decisions relates to comparisons between different interventions rather than to comparison with placebo or no intervention. Where necessary, we have indicated the comparisons. A third problem is that interventions may have been tested, or found to be effective, in only one group of people, such as those at high risk of an outcome. Again, we have indicated this where possible. But perhaps most difficult of all has been trying to maintain consistency across different topics. We are working on refining the criteria for putting interventions under each category.

## REFERENCES
Full references to the individual studies cited in *Clinical Evidence Concise* are available on the accompanying CD-ROM.

References cited in the definition, incidence/prevalence, aetiology/risk factors, and prognosis sections are listed in the text but are available as hyperlinks from the equivalent section on the CD-ROM.

## TOPIC GLOSSARY
Topics may contain glossary listings; these are available in full on the CD-ROM and can be accessed from the index page of each topic or as hyperlinks from the equivalent section on the CD-ROM. Terms with corresponding CD-ROM definitions will be flagged up with a symbol **G**.

## MAIN GLOSSARY
Words and terms that are used throughout *Clinical Evidence* are listed in the main glossary on the companion CD-ROM.

## TABLES AND FIGURES
The presence of figures and tables on the CD-ROM are flagged up in a similar way to the glossary with the use of **F** for figures and **T** for tables.

## FEEDBACK

We would like feedback from CD-ROM users, in order to improve future releases. Simply follow the guidance on the CD-ROM welcome page. This process should take up just 10 minutes of your time.

The design of *Clinical Evidence Concise* will change progressively over the next few years. We will perform evaluation studies ourselves to measure the relevance of the material to the questions that are being asked in practice, the ease of use, and to check that the message extracted from the summary corresponds closely with that intended. If you have any comments, suggestions, or detect any errors, please let us know at CEfeedback@bmjgroup.com.

For more information on any of our methods or processes, please visit our website at www.clinicalevidence.com.

Please refer to the CD-ROM for more information about *Clinical Evidence*.

## REFERENCES

1. Enkin M, Keirse M, Renfrew M, et al. *A guide to effective care in pregnancy and childbirth*. Oxford: Oxford University Press, 1998.

*Graham Mead, James Woodcock, and Charles Young*

## Effects of treatments for early stage aggressive non-Hodgkin's lymphoma (NHL) in younger adults

### LIKELY TO BE BENEFICIAL

#### Short schedule CHOP plus radiotherapy versus longer schedule CHOP alone

One RCT found that short schedule CHOP🅖 plus radiotherapy significantly improved 5 year survival with the addition of radiotherapy compared with longer schedule CHOP alone. It included many older people. Longer schedule CHOP increased the risk of congestive heart failure and possibly the risk of myelosuppression.

### UNKNOWN EFFECTIVENESS

#### ACVBP versus m-BACOD

One RCT, mostly in people with early stage🅖 disease, found no significant difference in 5 year survival between ACVBP🅖 and m-BACOD🅖.

#### Chemotherapy versus radiotherapy

We found no systematic review or RCTs of chemotherapy compared with radiotherapy.

#### CVP versus BACOP

Subgroup analysis in one RCT found no significant difference in complete remission between CVP🅖 and BACOP🅖.

## Effects of treatments for advanced stage aggressive NHL in younger adults

### LIKELY TO BE BENEFICIAL

#### CHOP versus BCOP

One RCT compared CHOP with BCOP🅖. Subgroup analysis of people with advanced stage🅖 disease found significantly higher complete response with CHOP. Subgroup analysis in people younger than 60 years found similar results but the difference was not significant. However, 20% of people were excluded for poorly defined reasons.

#### CHOP versus HOP

One poorly reported RCT, including people with all grades of NHL, found significantly higher complete response with CHOP with HOP🅖. However, 20% of people were excluded for a variety of reasons.

#### CHOP versus MEV

One RCT, including some older people and people who relapsed after treatment for early stage disease, found weak evidence of a survival benefit with CHOP compared with MEV🅖. Subgroup analysis in people with advanced disease found that more people achieved complete response with CHOP. ▶

# Non-Hodgkin's lymphoma

## CHOP versus MACOP-B

One RCT, including some people aged over 65 years, found no significant difference in 3 year survival between four chemotherapy regimens: CHOP, MACOP-B🄖, m-BACOD🄖, and ProMACE-CytaBOM🄖. It found limited evidence of greater toxicity with MACOP-B and m-BACOD compared with CHOP and ProMACE-CytaBOM. A second RCT, including some people with early disease and some older people, found no significant difference in complete response. Subgroup analysis in younger people found significantly improved 5 year survival with MACOP-B. A third RCT, including people with stage II disease, found no significant difference in complete response. Subgroup analysis from one centre found better quality of life and physical function with MACOP-B compared with CHOP. These two RCTs found a different range of adverse events with CHOP compared with MACOP-B.

## CHOP versus CHOP-B

One RCT in a population of mixed ages found no significant difference in 5 year mortality between CHOP and CHOP-B🄖.

## CHOP versus CHOP-M

One poorly reported RCT in a population of mixed ages and disease stages found similar mortality at 36 months with CHOP and CHOP-M🄖.

## CHOP versus CHOP plus interferon

We found no systematic review or RCTs of CHOP versus CHOP plus interferon.

## CHOP versus CHOP plus monoclonal antibodies

We found one systematic review, which found no RCTs of CHOP versus CHOP plus monoclonal antibodies.

## CHOP versus CHOP/VIA

One RCT, including people with stage II disease, found no significant difference in 3 year survival between CHOP and CHOP/VIA🄖.

## CHOP versus CIOP

One RCT of people with Kiel classification intermediate grade lymphoma, including some people with stage II disease and some people over 65 years of age, found similar overall survival at 42 months with CHOP and CIOP🄖.

## CHOP versus m-BACOD

We found one RCT comparing four different chemotherapy regimens (see CHOP versus MACOP-B above). A second RCT comparing CHOP with m-BACOD, including older adults and with a high withdrawal rate, found no significant difference in mortality at 4 or 5.3 years.

## CHOP versus PACEBOM

One RCT of people with intermediate grade lymphoma, including some people with stage II disease, found no difference in 5 or 8 year mortality in the total population. Subgroup analysis found mortality was lower with PACEBOM🄖 than CHOP in people with stage IV disease at 8 years' follow up, but the difference was not significant.

## CHOP versus ProMACE-CytaBOM

We found one RCT comparing four different chemotherapy regimens (see CHOP v MACOP-B above). A second RCT, including some people with stage II disease and some people over 65 years of age, found longer median survival with CHOP compared with ProMACE-CytaBOM, but significance was not assessed.

▶

**DEFINITION** NHL consists of a complex group of cancers arising mainly from B lymphocytes and occasionally from T lymphocytes (15% of cases). NHL usually develops in lymph nodes but can arise in other tissues almost anywhere in the body. NHL is divided according to histology and stage (spread). **Histology:** Historically histology was divided into aggressive and low grade disease. This chapter focuses on the most common aggressive lymphoma — diffuse large B cell lymphoma in the WHO ❶,[1] and REAL classification systems❻. Interpretation of older studies is complicated by changes in classification systems and diagnostic techniques. We have included studies using older systems if they are primarily in people with the following types of aggressive lymphoma: Working Formulation classification — primarily intermediate grades (grades E–H❶);[2] Kiel classification — centroblastic, immunoblastic, and anaplastic❶;[3] Rappaport classification — diffuse histiocytic, diffuse lymphocytic poorly differentiated, and diffuse mixed (lymphocytic and histiocytic❶).[4] There is no direct correspondence between the terms used in the different classification systems and attempts to generalise results must be treated with caution.[1–4] **Stage:** Historically, NHL has been staged according to disease spread using the Ann Arbor❻ system❶.[5] Ann Arbor stages I and II correspond to early disease, whereas stages III and IV are advanced disease. However, people with bulky disease will usually be treated as having advanced disease even if the stage is only I or II. There is also substantial variation in prognosis within each stage. More recent studies assess stage using a prognostic indicator. We excluded RCTs that were primarily in children (< 16 years old), older people (> 65 years old), people with HIV infection, and people who had received prior treatment except local radiotherapy. We also excluded RCTs of maintenance treatment and RCTs with fewer than 50 people in each arm. In RCTs of mixed populations we have reported subgroup analysis in the population of interest, if available.

**INCIDENCE/ PREVALENCE** NHL occurs more commonly in males than females, and is increasing in incidence in the Western world at about 4% a year. It is the seventh most common cancer in the UK consisting of 8680 new cases in 1998 (3% of cancers) and causing 4500 deaths in 2000.[6]

**AETIOLOGY/ RISK FACTORS** Unknown for most people. Surveys have implicated pesticides and hair dyes. Incidence is higher in people who are immunosuppressed.

**PROGNOSIS** Relates to histological type, stage, age, performance status, and lactate dehydrogenase levels. High grade lymphomas, particularly diffuse large B cell lymphoma and Burkitt's lymphoma, have a high cure rate, with both initial and salvage (high dose) chemotherapy.[7] CHOP is the standard treatment for aggressive❻ NHL and placebo controlled trials would be considered unethical.

Please refer to CD-ROM for full text and references.

# Sickle cell disease

Search date January 2003

*Martin M Meremikwu*

---

## What are the effects of interventions to prevent sickle cell crisis and other acute complications of sickle cell disease? *New*

**BENEFICIAL**

### Penicillin prophylaxis in children under 5 years of age

One systematic review found that penicillin prophylaxis in children younger than 5 years reduced the risk of invasive pneumococcal infections and related deaths.

**LIKELY TO BE BENEFICIAL**

### Hydroxyurea

Two RCTs found that hydroxyurea reduced the risk of acute chest syndrome and the need for blood transfusion in people with sickle cell disease. A non-significant reduction was also found for stroke, hepatic sequestration, and death related to sickle cell disease. Hydroxyurea has been associated with neutropenia, hair loss, skin rash, and gastrointestinal disturbances. We found no evidence on the long term effects of hydroxyurea.

**UNKNOWN EFFECTIVENESS**

### Pneumococcal vaccine

One RCT found insufficient evidence to determine whether polysaccharide pneumococcal vaccine is effective. We found no RCTs of conjugate pneumococcal vaccine in sickle cell disease. Three RCTs found that pneumococcal vaccines caused local reaction and fever but no severe adverse events.

### Malaria chemoprophylaxis

We found no RCTs of malaria chemoprophylaxis in people with sickle cell disease.

### Avoidance of cold environment; limiting physical exercise

We found no RCTs or observational studies of sufficient quality about the effects of this intervention in preventing sickle cell crisis and other life threatening complications.

---

## What are the effects of interventions to treat pain in sickle cell crisis? *New*

**LIKELY TO BE BENEFICIAL**

### Controlled release oral morphine given after an intravenous bolus dose of morphine

One RCT found that controlled release oral morphine was as effective as intravenous morphine after an intravenous loading dose of morphine at onset of treatment.

**TRADE OFF BETWEEN BENEFITS AND HARMS**

### Corticosteroid as adjunct to narcotic analgesics

One RCT found that intravenous methylprednisolone improved pain relief as an adjunct to intravenous morphine, but was associated with a high rate of recurrence of crisis.

▶

◀ **Patient controlled analgesia**

Two small RCTs have found no significant difference between patient controlled analgesia discussing either meperidine or morphine and intermittent parenteral treatment. The incidence of adverse effects was also equal in both regimens.

## UNKNOWN EFFECTIVENESS

### Acupuncture

We found no systematic reviews or RCTs on the effects of acupuncture in sickle cell disease.

### Codeine

We found no systematic reviews or RCTs on the effects of codeine in sickle cell disease.

### Diflunisal

One RCT found no significant difference between oral diflunisal and placebo as an adjunct to meperidine in sickle cell crisis.

### Ketorolac

Four RCTs found insufficient and conflicting evidence on the pain relieving effect of ketorolac in sickle cell crisis.

### Oxygen

Two RCTs found insufficient evidence on the effects of oxygen therapy as an adjunct to analgesics. The RCTs excluded patients with acute chest syndrome.

### Rehydration

We found no systematic reviews or RCTs on the effects of rehydration in sickle cell crisis.

### Aspirin; ibuprofen; paracetamol

We found no RCTs on the effects of these analgesics in sickle cell crisis.

**DEFINITION**     **Sickle cell disease** refers to a group of disorders caused by inheritance of a pair of abnormal haemoglobin genes, including the sickle cell gene. It is characterised by chronic haemolytic anaemia and episodic clinical events called "crises".[1] Vaso-occlusive painful crisis is the most common and occurs when abnormal red cells clog small vessels causing tissue ischaemia. The others are hyper haemolytic crisis (excessive haemolysis), acute chest syndrome**G**, sequestration crisis**G**, and aplastic crisis**G**. Infections such as pneumonia, septicaemia, meningitis, and osteomyelitis are common in people with sickle cell disease. A common variant of sickle cell disease, also characterised by haemolytic anaemia, occurs in people with one sickle and one thalassaemia gene. **Sickle cell trait** occurs in people with one sickle gene and one normal gene. People with sickle cell trait do not have any clinical manifestation of illness. This topic covers people with sickle cell disease with or without thalassaemia.

**INCIDENCE/**     Sickle cell disease is most common among people living in or originating from
**PREVALENCE**   sub-Saharan Africa.[2] The disorder also affects people of Mediterranean, Caribbean, Middle Eastern, and Asian origin. The sickle ceel gene is most common in areas where malaria is endemic: sickle cell trait affects about 10–30% of people in tropical Africa.[3] Sickle cell disease affects and esti- mated 1–2% (120 000) of new borns in Africa[3] and 250 000 newborns worldwide. About 60 000 people in the USA[4] and 10 000 in the UK[5] suffer from the disease

**AETIOLOGY/**     Factors that precipitate or modulate the occurrence of sickle cell crisis are not
**RISK FACTORS** fully understood, but infections, hypoxia, dehydration, acidosis, stress (such as major surgery or childbirth), and cold are believed to play some role. In tropical ▶

# Sickle cell disease

Africa, malaria is the most common cause of anaemic and vaso-occlusive crisis.[3] High levels of fetal haemoglobin🅖 is known to ameliorate the severity and incidence of sickle cell crisis and other complications of the disease.

**PROGNOSIS**   People affected by sickle cell disease are predisposed to bacterial infections, especially to those caused by encapsulated organisms such as *Pneumococcus*, *Haemophilus influenzae*, *Meningococcus*, and *Salmonella* species. Severe bacterial infections such as pneumonia, meningitis, and septicaemia are common causes of morbidity and mortality, especially among young children.[6] About 10% of children with sickle cell anaemia may develop a stroke, and more than half of these may suffer recurrent strokes.[7] Abnormal features of cerebral blood vessels shown by transcranial Doppler scan predict a high risk of stroke in children with sickle cell disease.[8] Frequent episodes of crisis, infections, and organ damage reduce the quality of life of people with sickle cell disease. High rate of painful crisis is an index of clinical severity that correlates with early death. Life expectancy remains low, especially in communities with poor access to health services. In some parts of Africa, about 50% of children with sickle cell disease die before their first birthday.[3] The average life expectancy for men and women with sickle cell disease in the USA is about 42 and 48 years, respectively.[9] Frequent blood transfusions could increase the risk of immune reactions and infections, such as HIV and hepatitis B or C viruses, and Chagas' disease.

Please refer to CD-ROM for full text and references.

Cardiovascular disorders

## What treatments improve outcomes in acute myocardial infarction?

### BENEFICIAL

#### Angiotensin converting enzyme inhibitors

One systematic review in people treated within 14 days of acute myocardial infarction has found that angiotensin converting enzyme inhibitors reduce mortality after 6 weeks compared with placebo. However, a non-systematic review found that angiotensin converting enzyme inhibitors increase persistent hypotension and renal dysfunction at 6 weeks compared with placebo.

#### Aspirin

One systematic review in people with acute myocardial infarction has found that aspirin reduces mortality, reinfarction, and stroke at 1 month compared with placebo.

#### β Blockers

We found evidence from systematic reviews and one subsequent RCT that β blockers reduced mortality compared with no β blockers. One RCT in people receiving thrombolytic treatment found that immediate treatment with metoprolol reduced rates of reinfarction and chest pain at 6 days compared with delayed treatment, but had no significant effect on mortality at 6 days or at 1 year.

#### Primary percutaneous transluminal coronary angioplasty versus thrombolysis (performed in specialist centres)

One systematic review has found that primary percutaneous transluminal coronary angioplasty reduces a combined outcome of death, non-fatal reinfarction, and stroke compared with thrombolysis.

#### Thrombolysis

Two non-systematic reviews in people with acute myocardial infarction and ST elevation or bundle branch block on their initial electrocardiogram found that prompt thrombolytic treatment (within 6 hours and perhaps up to 12 hours and longer after the onset of symptoms) reduces mortality compared with placebo. RCTs comparing different types of thrombolytic agents with each other found no significant difference in mortality. One non-systematic review found that thrombolytic treatment increased the risk of stroke or major bleeding compared with control. The review also found that intracranial haemorrhage is more common in people of advanced age and low body weight; those with hypertension on admission, and those given tissue plasminogen activator rather than another thrombolytic agent. One non-systematic review found conflicting results for intracerebral haemorrhage with bolus treatment compared with infusion of thrombolytic agents.

### LIKELY TO BE BENEFICIAL

#### Nitrates (in the absence of thrombolysis)

One systematic review of the trials conducted in the prethrombolytic era found that nitrates reduced mortality in people with acute myocardial infarction compared with placebo.

▶

# Acute myocardial infarction

UNLIKELY TO BE BENEFICIAL

### Nitrates (in addition to thrombolysis)
Two RCTs in people with acute myocardial infarction (after thrombolysis was introduced) found no significant difference in mortality between nitrates and placebo.

TRADE OFF BETWEEN BENEFITS AND HARMS

### Glycoprotein IIb/IIIa inhibitors
Two large RCTs have found that combined treatment with half dose thrombolysis plus abciximab does not reduce mortality at 1 month compared with full dose thrombolysis in people with acute myocardial infarction, but may prevent non-fatal cardiovascular events. However, the RCTs found that combined treatment with abciximab increased bleeding complications, particularly extracranial haemorrhage. Three RCTs found conflicting evidence about the benefits of adding abciximab to primary coronary angioplasty or stenting in people with acute myocardial infarction, although all found that adding abciximab increased bleeding risk.

LIKELY TO BE INEFFECTIVE OR HARMFUL

### Calcium channel blockers
We found evidence that neither dihydropyridines nor verapamil reduce mortality compared with placebo. One RCT found limited evidence that, in people with left ventricular dysfunction, nifedipine given in the first few days after myocardial infarction may increase mortality compared with placebo.

## Which treatments improve outcomes for cardiogenic shock after acute myocardial infarction?

BENEFICIAL

### Early invasive cardiac revascularisation
One large RCT has found that early invasive cardiac revascularisation⊕ reduces mortality after 6 and 12 months compared with medical treatment alone in people with cardiogenic shock within 48 hours of acute myocardial infarction. A second smaller RCT found similar results, although the difference was not significant.

UNKNOWN EFFECTIVENESS

### Intra-aortic balloon counterpulsation
We found limited evidence from an abstract of an RCT of no significant difference in mortality at 6 months between intra-aortic balloon counterpulsation plus thrombolysis versus thrombolysis alone in people with cardiogenic shock.

### Early cardiac surgery; positive inotropes and vasodilators; pulmonary artery catheterization; ventricular assistance devices and cardiac transplantation
We found no evidence from RCTs about the effects of these interventions.

UNLIKELY TO BE BENEFICIAL

### Thrombolysis
Subgroup analysis of one RCT found no significant difference in mortality after 21 days between thrombolysis and no thrombolysis in people with cardiogenic shock.

# Acute myocardial infarction

**DEFINITION** **Acute myocardial infarction (AMI):** The sudden occlusion of a coronary artery leading to myocardial cell death. **Cardiogenic shock:** Defined clinically as a poor cardiac output plus evidence of tissue hypoxia that is not improved by correcting reduced intravascular volume.[1] When a pulmonary artery catheter is used, cardiogenic shock may be defined as a cardiac index❸ below 2.2 L/minute/m$^2$ despite an elevated pulmonary capillary wedge pressure ($\geq$ 15 mm Hg).[1–3]

**INCIDENCE/** **AMI:** Acute myocardial infarction is one of the most common causes of
**PREVALENCE** mortality worldwide. In 1990, ischaemic heart disease was the world's leading cause of death, accounting for about 6.3 million deaths. The age standardised incidence varies among and within countries.[4] Each year, about 900 000 people in the USA experience AMI, about 225 000 of whom die. About half of these people die within 1 hour of symptoms and before reaching a hospital emergency room.[5] Event rates increase with age for both sexes and are higher in men than in women and in poorer than richer people at all ages. The incidence of death from AMI has fallen in many Western countries over the past 20 years. **Cardiogenic shock:** Cardiogenic shock occurs in about 7% of people admitted to hospital with AMI.[6] Of these, about half have established cardiogenic shock at the time of admission to hospital, and most of the others develop it during the first 24–48 hours after their admission.[7]

**AETIOLOGY/** **AMI:** See aetiology/risk factors under primary prevention, p 28. The immediate
**RISK FACTORS** mechanism of AMI is rupture or erosion of an atheromatous plaque causing thrombosis and occlusion of coronary arteries and myocardial cell death. Factors that may convert a stable plaque into an unstable plaque (the "active plaque") have yet to be fully elucidated. Shear stresses, inflammation, and autoimmunity have been proposed. The changing rates of coronary heart disease in different populations are only partly explained by changes in the standard risk factors for ischaemic heart disease (particularly a fall in blood pressure and smoking). **Cardiogenic shock:** Cardiogenic shock after AMI usually follows a reduction in functional ventricular myocardium, and is caused by left ventricular infarction (79% of people with cardiogenic shock) more often than by right ventricular infarction (3% of people with cardiogenic shock).[8] Cardiogenic shock after AMI may also be caused by cardiac structural defects, such as mitral valve regurgitation due to papillary muscle dysfunction (7% of people with cardiogenic shock), ventricular septal rupture (4% of people with cardiogenic shock), or cardiac tamponade after free cardiac wall rupture (1% of people with cardiogenic shock). Major risk factors for cardiogenic shock after AMI are previous myocardial infarction, diabetes mellitus, advanced age, hypotension, tachycardia or bradycardia, congestive heart failure with Killip class II–III❸, and low left ventricular ejection fraction (ejection fraction < 35%).[7,8]

**PROGNOSIS** **AMI:** May lead to a host of mechanical and cardiac electrical complications, including death, ventricular dysfunction, congestive heart failure, fatal and non-fatal arrhythmias, valvular dysfunction, myocardial rupture, and cardiogenic shock. **Cardiogenic shock:** Mortality rates for people in hospital with cardiogenic shock after AMI vary between 50–80%.[2,3,6,7] Most deaths occur within 48 hours of the onset of shock ❺. People surviving until discharge from hospital have a reasonable long term prognosis (88% survival at 1 year).[10]

Please refer to CD-ROM for full text and references.

# Angina (unstable)

**Search date November 2002**

*Madhu Natarajan*

## What are the effects of treatments?

**BENEFICIAL**

### Aspirin

One systematic review has found that aspirin reduces the risk of death, myocardial infarction, and stroke compared with placebo in people with unstable angina. The evidence suggests no added cardiovascular benefit, and possible added harm, from doses of aspirin over 325 mg daily.

**LIKELY TO BE BENEFICIAL**

### Clopidogrel/ticlopidine

Two RCTs have found that clopidogrel or ticlopidine reduce mortality and myocardial infarction compared with placebo or conventional treatment alone. One RCT found that clopidogrel increased major bleeding, but not haemorrhagic strokes compared with placebo after 6–9 months. Ticlopidine may cause reversible neutropenia. These drugs may be an alternative in people who are intolerant of or allergic to aspirin.

### Direct thrombin inhibitors

One systematic review has found that treatment with direct thrombin inhibitors for 7 days reduces death and myocardial infarction compared with heparin after 30 days.

### Intravenous glycoprotein IIb/IIIa inhibitors

One systematic review found that intravenous glycoprotein IIb/IIIa inhibitors reduced the risk of death or myocardial infarction compared with placebo but increased the risk of major bleeding complications.

### Low molecular weight heparins

One systematic review in people taking aspirin has found that adding low molecular weight heparin reduces the risk of death or myocardial infarction compared with placebo or no treatment and does not significantly increase bleeding complications in the first 7 days after unstable angina. However, it found that longer term treatment with low molecular weight heparin did not significantly reduce death or myocardial infarction compared with placebo. One systematic review found no significant difference between low molecular weight heparin and unfractionated heparin in death or myocardial infarction. Long term low molecular weight heparin increased major bleeding compared with placebo, but not compared with unfractionated heparin.

### Unfractionated heparin added to aspirin

One systematic review has found that adding unfractionated heparin to aspirin for 7 days in people with unstable angina reduced death or myocardial infarction at 1 week. However, a second review found no significant effect after 12 weeks.

**UNKNOWN EFFECTIVENESS**

### β Blockers; nitrates

We found insufficient evidence of effects of these interventions on myocardial infarction or death rates. However, RCTs found that these interventions may reduce frequency and severity of chest pain.

▶

◀ **Routine early invasive treatment**

We found five RCTs that reported on different composite outcomes. Two of these found that early invasive treatment reduced death and other cardiac events compared with conservative treatment at 6 months. However, the remaining three RCTs found no significant difference in death or other cardiac events between early invasive treatment and conservative treatment at 12 months or more.

## UNLIKELY TO BE BENEFICIAL

### Calcium channel blockers

One systematic review found no significant difference between calcium channel blockers and either placebo or standard treatment on mortality or myocardial infarction. Observational studies suggest that short acting dihydropyridine calcium channel blockers may increase mortality.

### Warfarin

One RCT found that adding warfarin to aspirin reduced cardiac events and death after 12 weeks. However, four RCTs found no significant effect after 5 months or more and one RCT found that warfarin was associated with an increase in major bleeding.

## LIKELY TO BE INEFFECTIVE OR HARMFUL

### Oral glycoprotein IIb/IIIa inhibitors

One systematic review found that the oral glycoprotein IIb/IIIa inhibitor sibrafiban did not reduce the combined outcome of death, myocardial infarction, and recurrent ischaemia compared with aspirin. However, it found that oral glycoprotein IIb/IIIa inhibitors with or without aspirin increased bleeding compared with aspirin alone.

**DEFINITION**   Unstable angina is distinguished from stable angina, acute myocardial infarction, and non-cardiac pain by the pattern of symptoms (characteristic pain present at rest or on lower levels of activity), the severity of symptoms (recently increasing intensity, frequency, or duration), and the absence of persistent ST segment elevation on a resting electrocardiogram. Unstable angina includes a variety of different clinical patterns: angina at rest of up to 1 week of duration; angina increasing in severity to moderate or severe pain; non-Q wave myocardial infarction; and post-myocardial infarction angina continuing for longer than 24 hours.

**INCIDENCE/**   In industrialised countries, the annual incidence of unstable angina is about
**PREVALENCE**   6/10 000 people in the general population.

**AETIOLOGY/**   Risk factors are the same as for other manifestations of ischaemic heart
**RISK FACTORS** disease: older age, previous atheromatous cardiovascular disease, diabetes mellitus, smoking cigarettes, hypertension, hypercholesterolaemia, male sex, and a family history of ischaemic heart disease. Unstable angina can also occur in association with other disorders of the circulation, including heart valve disease, arrhythmia, and cardiomyopathy.

**PROGNOSIS**   In people taking aspirin, the incidence of serious adverse outcomes (such as death, acute myocardial infarction, or refractory angina requiring emergency revascularisation) is 5–10% within the first 7 days and about 15% at 30 days. Between 5% and 14% of people with unstable angina die in the year after diagnosis, with about half of these deaths occurring within 4 weeks of diagnosis. No single factor identifies people at higher risk of an adverse event. Risk factors include severity of presentation (e.g. duration of pain, speed of progression, evidence of heart failure), medical history (e.g. previous unstable angina, ▶

# Angina (unstable)

acute myocardial infarction, left ventricular dysfunction), other clinical parameters (e.g. age, diabetes), electrocardiogram changes (e.g. severity of ST segment depression, deep T wave inversion, transient ST segment elevation), biochemical parameters (e.g. troponin concentration), and change in clinical status (e.g. recurrent chest pain, silent ischaemia, haemodynamic instability).

Please refer to CD-ROM for full text and references.

### Search date February 2003

*Gregory Y H Lip and Bethan Freestone*

## What are the effects of interventions to prevent embolism?

### UNKNOWN EFFECTIVENESS

#### Antithrombotic treatment before cardioversion

We found no RCTs of aspirin, heparin, or warfarin as thromboprophylaxis before attempted cardioversion in acute atrial fibrillation.

## What are the effects of interventions for conversion to sinus rhythm?

### TRADE OFF BETWEEN BENEFITS AND HARMS

#### Flecainide *New*

One RCT found that compared with placebo, intravenous flecainide increased the proportion of people who reverted to sinus rhythm within 1 hour and in whom the sinus rhythm was maintained after 6 hours. Flecainide has been associated with serious adverse events such as severe hypotension and torsades de point. Two RCTs found that compared with intravenous amiodarone, oral flecainide increased the proportion of people who reverted to sinus rhythm within 8 hours. We found insufficient evidence to draw any conclusions about comparisons between intravenous flecainide and intravenous amiodarone and flecainide versus quinidine. Two RCTs found no significant difference between flecainide and propafenone. Flecainide and propafenone are not used in people with known or suspected ischaemic heart disease due to possible proarrhythmic effects.

#### Propafenone *New*

One systematic review and subsequent RCTs have found that compared with placebo, propafenone increased the proportion of people converting to sinus rhythm within 1–4 hours. One RCT found no significant difference between intravenous propafenone and amiodarone in the proportion of people converting to sinus rhythm within 1 hour in people with onset of atrial fibrillation of less than 48 hours. Another RCT found that compared with amiodarone, a higher proportion of people converted to sinus rhythm with oral propafenone within 2.5 hours but the difference did not remain significant at 24 hours in people with onset of atrial fibrillation of less than 2 weeks. Two RCTs found no significant difference between flecainide and propafenone. Propafenone and flecainide are not used in people with known or suspected ischaemic heart disease due to possible proarrhythmic effects.

### UNKNOWN EFFECTIVENESS

#### Amiodarone

We found insufficient evidence from three RCTs about the effects of amiodarone as a single agent compared with placebo for conversion to sinus rhythm in people with acute atrial fibrillation. Four small RCTs have found no significant difference between amiodarone versus digoxin in rate of conversion to sinus rhythm at 24–48 hours, although the studies may have lacked power to exclude clinically important differences. We found insufficient evidence from one small RCT to compare amiodarone versus verapamil. We found no RCTs comparing amiodarone with either DC cardioversion or diltiazem.    ▶

Cardiovascular disorders

# Atrial fibrillation (acute)

## DC cardioversion

We found no RCTs of DC cardioversion in acute atrial fibrillation. It may be unethical to conduct RCTs in people with acute atrial fibrillation and haemodynamic compromise.

## Quinidine *New*

We found no RCTs comparing quinidine versus placebo. One small RCT in people with onset of atrial fibrillation of less than 48 hours found that compared with sotalol, quinidine plus digoxin increased the proportion of people converting to sinus rhythm within 12 hours.

## Sotalol *New*

We found no systematic review or RCTs comparing sotalol versus placebo. One small RCT in people with onset of atrial fibrillation of less than 48 hours found that compared with sotalol, quinidine plus digoxin increased the proportion of people converting to sinus rhythm within 12 hours.

### UNLIKELY TO BE BENEFICIAL

## Digoxin

Three RCTs found no significant difference in conversion to sinus rhythm with digoxin versus placebo in people with atrial fibrillation of up to 7 days' duration. Four small RCTs found no significant difference between amiodarone versus digoxin for conversion to sinus rhythm in people with acute atrial fibrillation, although the trials might have lacked power to exclude clincially important differences.

## *What are the effects of interventions to control heart rate?*

### LIKELY TO BE BENEFICIAL

## Digoxin

We found no RCTs only in people with acute atrial fibrillation. Two RCTs found that digoxin versus placebo significantly reduced ventricular rate within 2 hours in people with atrial fibrillation of up to 7 days' duration.

## Diltiazem

One RCT in people with atrial fibrillation or atrial flutter❻ found that intravenous diltiazem (a calcium channel blocker) reduced heart rate over 15 minutes compared with placebo. Another RCT in people with acute atrial fibrillation or atrial flutter found that intravenous diltiazem reduced heart rate within 5 minutes compared with intravenous digoxin.

## Timolol

One small RCT in people with atrial fibrillation of unspecified duration found that intravenous timolol (a β blocker) significantly reduced ventricular rate within 20 minutes compared with placebo.

## Verapamil

Two RCTs found that intravenous verapamil (a calcium channel blocker) reduced heart rate at 10 or 30 minutes compared with placebo in people with atrial fibrillation or atrial flutter. One RCT found no significant difference in rate control or measures of systolic function with intravenous verapamil versus intravenous diltiazem in people with atrial fibrillation or atrial flutter, but verapamil caused hypotension in some people.

◄ **UNKNOWN EFFECTIVENESS**

## Amiodarone

We found no RCTs examining effects of amiodarone alone on heart rate in people with acute atrial fibrillation.

## Sotalol *New*

We found no systematic review or RCTs comparing sotalol with placebo

**DEFINITION**   Acute atrial fibrillation is rapid, irregular, and chaotic atrial activity of less that 48 hours' duration. It includes both the first symptomatic onset of persistent atrial fibrillation**ⓖ** and episodes of paroxysmal atrial fibrillation**ⓖ**. It is sometimes difficult to distinguish episodes of new onset atrial fibrillation from long standing atrial fibrillation that was previously undiagnosed. Atrial fibrillation within 72 hours of onset is sometimes called recent onset atrial fibrillation. By contrast, chronic atrial fibrillation**ⓖ** is a more sustained form of atrial fibrillation, which in turn can be described as paroxysmal, persistent, or permanent atrial fibrillation**ⓖ**. Intermittent atrial fibrillation, with spontaneous recurrences/termination and with sinus rhythm between recurrences is known as paroxysmal atrial fibrillation. More sustained atrial fibrillation, which is considered amenable to cardioversion, is called persistent atrial fibrillation. If cardioversion is considered inappropriate, then the atrial fibrillation is known as "permanent". In this review we have excluded episodes of atrial fibrillation that arise during or soon after cardiac surgery, and we have excluded management of chronic atrial fibrillation.

**INCIDENCE/**   We found limited evidence of the incidence or prevalence of acute atrial
**PREVALENCE**   fibrillation. Extrapolation from the Framingham study[1] suggests an incidence in men of 3/1000 person years at age 55 years, rising to 38/1000 person years at 94 years. In women, the incidence was 2/1000 person years at age 55 years and 32.5/1000 person years at 94 years. The prevalence of atrial fibrillation ranged from 0.5% for people aged 50–59 years to 9% in people aged 80–89 years. Among acute emergency medical admissions in the UK, 3–6% have atrial fibrillation and about 40% were newly diagnosed.[2,3] Among acute hospital admissions in New Zealand, 10% (95% CI 9% to 12%) had documented atrial fibrillation.[4]

**AETIOLOGY/**   Paroxysms of atrial fibrillation are more common in athletes.[5] Age increases the
**RISK FACTORS**   risk of developing acute atrial fibrillation. Men are more likely to develop atrial fibrillation than women (38 years' follow up from the Framingham Study, RR after adjustment for age and known predisposing conditions 1.5).[6] Atrial fibrillation can occur in association with underlying disease (both cardiac and non-cardiac) or can arise in the absence of any other condition. Epidemiological surveys have found that risk factors for the development of acute atrial fibrillation include ischaemic heart disease, hypertension, heart failure, valve disease, diabetes, alcohol abuse, thyroid disorders, and disorders of the lung and pleura.[1] In a UK survey of acute hospital admissions with atrial fibrillation, a history of ischaemic heart disease was present in 33%, heart failure in 24%, hypertension in 26%, and rheumatic heart disease in 7%.[3] In some populations, the acute effects of alcohol explain a large proportion of the incidence of acute atrial fibrillation.

**PROGNOSIS**   We found no evidence about the proportion of people with acute atrial fibrillation who develop more chronic forms of atrial fibrillation (e.g. paroxysmal, persistent, or permanent atrial fibrillation). Observational studies and placebo arms of RCTs have found that more than 50% of people with acute atrial fibrillation revert spontaneously within 24–48 hours, especially if atrial fibrillation is associated with an identifiable precipitant such as alcohol or myocardial infarction. We found little evidence about the effects on mortality and morbidity of acute atrial fibrillation where no underlying cause is found. Acute atrial ▶

# Atrial fibrillation (acute)

fibrillation during myocardial infarction is an independent predictor of both short term and long term mortality.[7] Onset of atrial fibrillation reduces cardiac output by 10–20% irrespective of the underlying ventricular rate[8,9] and can contribute to heart failure. People with acute atrial fibrillation who present with heart failure have worse prognosis. Acute atrial fibrillation is associated with a risk of imminent stroke.[10-13] One case series used transoesophageal echocardiography in people who had developed acute atrial fibrillation within the preceding 48 hours; it found that 15% had atrial thrombi.[14] An ischaemic stroke associated with atrial fibrillation is more likely to be fatal, have a recurrence, and leave a serious functional deficit among survivors, than a stroke not associated with atrial fibrillation.[15]

Please refer to CD-ROM for full text and references.

### Search date January 2003

*Margaret Thorogood, Melvyn Hillsdon, and Carolyn Summerbell*

Cardiovascular disorders

## What are the effects of interventions?

### BENEFICIAL

**Advice from physicians and trained counsellors to quit smoking**

Systematic reviews have found that simple, one off advice from a physician during a routine consultation is associated with 2% of smokers quitting smoking without relapse for 1 year. Advice from trained counsellors who are neither doctors nor nurses also increases quit rates compared with minimal intervention.

**Advice on cholesterol lowering diet**

Systematic reviews have found that advice on cholesterol lowering diet (i.e. advice to lower total fat intake or increase the ratio of polyunsaturated : saturated fatty acid) leads to a small reduction in blood cholesterol concentrations in the long term (≥ 6 months).

**Advice on diet and exercise supported by behavioural therapy for the encouragement of weight loss**

Systematic reviews and subsequent RCTs have found that a combination of advice on diet and exercise supported by behavioural therapy is probably more effective than either diet or exercise advice alone in the treatment of obesity, and might lead to sustained weight loss.

**Advice on reducing sodium intake to reduce blood pressure**

One systematic review has found that, compared with usual care, intensive interventions to reduce sodium intake, unsuited to primary care or population prevention programmes, provide only small reductions in blood pressure. Effects on deaths and cardiovascular events are unclear.

**Bupropion as part of a smoking cessation programme**

One systematic review of antidepressants used as part of a smoking cessation programme has found that bupropion increases quit rates at 1 year.

**Counselling people at high risk of disease to quit smoking**

Systematic reviews and one subsequent RCT have found that antismoking advice improves smoking cessation in people at high risk of smoking related disease.

**Counselling pregnant women to quit smoking**

Two systematic reviews have found that antismoking interventions in pregnant women increase abstinence rates during pregnancy. Interventions without nicotine replacement were as effective as nicotine replacement in healthy non-pregnant women.

**Exercise advice to women over 80 years of age**

One RCT found that exercise advice delivered in the home by physiotherapists increased physical activity and reduced the risk of falling in women over 80 years.

**Nicotine replacement in smokers who smoke at least 10 cigarettes daily**

One systematic review and one subsequent RCT have found that nicotine replacement is an effective additional component of cessation strategies in smokers who smoke at least 10 cigarettes daily. We found no evidence that any method of delivery of nicotine is more effective than others. We found limited evidence from three RCTs with follow up of 2–6 years that the additional benefit of nicotine replacement treatment on quit rates reduced with time.

### Advice from nurses to quit smoking

One systematic review has found that advice to quit smoking increased quitting at 1 year compared with no advice.

### Counselling sedentary people to increase physical activity

We found weak evidence from systematic reviews and subsequent RCTs that counselling sedentary people increases physical activity compared with no intervention. Limited evidence from RCTs suggests that consultation with an exercise specialist rather than a physician may increase physical activity at 1 year. We found limited evidence that interventions delivered by new media can lead to short term changes in physical activity.

### Self help materials for people who want to stop smoking

One systematic review found that self help materials slightly improve smoking cessation compared with no intervention. It found that individually tailored materials were more effective than standard or stage based materials and that telephone counselling increased the effectiveness of postal self help materials.

### Physical exercise to aid smoking cessation

One systematic review found limited evidence that exercise might increase smoking cessation.

### Training health professionals to give advice on smoking cessation (increases frequency of antismoking interventions, but may not improve effectiveness)

One systematic review has found that training professionals increases the frequency of antismoking interventions being offered. It found no good evidence that antismoking interventions are more effective if the health professionals delivering the interventions received training. One RCT found that a structured intervention delivered by trained community pharmacists increased smoking cessation rates compared with usual care delivered by untrained community pharmacists.

### Acupuncture for smoking cessation

One systematic review has found no significant difference between acupuncture and control in smoking cessation rates at 1 year.

### Anxiolytics for smoking cessation

One systematic review found no significant difference in quit rates with anxiolytics compared with control.

*In terms of producing the intended behavioural change.

**DEFINITION**   Cigarette smoking, diet, and level of physical activity are important in the aetiology of many chronic diseases. Individual change in behaviour has the potential to decrease the burden of chronic disease, particularly cardiovascular disease. This topic focuses on the evidence that specific interventions lead to changed behaviour.

**INCIDENCE/**   In the developed world, the decline in smoking has slowed and the prevalence
**PREVALENCE**   of regular smoking is increasing in young people. A sedentary lifestyle is becoming increasingly common and the prevalence of obesity is increasing rapidly.

Please refer to CD-ROM for full text and references.

© BMJ Publishing Group Ltd 2003

## What are the effects of treatments?

### BENEFICIAL

#### Angiotensin converting enzyme inhibitors

Systematic reviews and RCTs have found that angiotensin converting enzyme inhibitors versus placebo significantly reduce ischaemic events, mortality and hospital admission for heart failure. Relative benefits are similar in different groups of people, but absolute benefits are greater in people with severe heart failure. RCTs in people with asymptomatic left ventricular systolic dysfunction have found that angiotensin converting enzyme inhibitors versus placebo significantly delay the onset of symptomatic heart failure and reduce cardiovascular events over 40 months.

#### β Blockers

Systematic reviews have found strong evidence that adding a β blocker to an angiotensin converting enzyme inhibitor significantly decreases mortality and hospital admission. Limited evidence from a subgroup analysis of one RCT found no significant effect on mortality in black people.

#### Digoxin (improves morbidity in people already receiving diuretics and angiotensin converting enzyme inhibitors)

One large RCT in people already receiving diuretics and angiotensin converting enzyme inhibitors found that digoxin versus placebo significantly reduced the number of people admitted to hospital for worsening heart failure at 37 months, but did not significantly reduce mortality.

### LIKELY TO BE BENEFICIAL

#### Angiotensin II receptor blockers

One systematic review has found that angiotensin receptor blockers versus placebo reduced all cause mortality and hospital admission in people with New York Heart Association❻ class II–IV heart failure, although the difference was not significant. It found no significant difference in all cause mortality or hospital admission with angiotensin receptor blockers versus angiotensin converting enzyme inhibitors. It found that angiotensin receptor blockers plus angiotensin converting enzyme inhibitors versus angiotensin converting enzyme inhibitors alone reduced admission for heart failure but did not significantly reduce all cause mortality.

#### Exercise

One systematic review has found that exercise training improved physiological measures compared with control. One included RCT assessed clinical outcomes and found that exercise versus control improved quality of life and reduced cardiac events, mortality, and hospital readmission for heart failure at 12 months. One subsequent RCT found no significant difference for 3 months of supervised aerobic and resistance training followed by 9 months of home based training versus usual care in 6 minute walk distance or quality of life at 12 months.

# Heart failure

◀ **Implantable cardiac defibrillators (in people with heart failure and near fatal arrhythmia)**

One RCT has found good evidence that an implantable cardiac defibrillator reduces mortality in people with heart failure who have experienced a near fatal ventricular arrhythmia.

## Multidisciplinary interventions

One systematic review has found that multidisciplinary programmes significantly reduce admissions to hospital but did not significantly reduce mortality. The review found that telephone contact plus improved coordination of primary care had no significant effect on admission rate. Two included RCTs found that that home-based support versus usual care significantly reduced cardiovascular events at 3–6 years. Subsequent RCTs found that education and nurse led support reduced death and hospital readmission and improved quality of life at 12 weeks to 1 year.

## Prophylactic use of implantable cardiac defibrillators in people at risk of arryhthmia

Two RCTs have found that implantable cardiac defibrillators versus medical treatment reduce mortality in people with heart failure and at high risk of arrhythmia, whereas one RCT found no significant difference in mortality.

## Spironolactone in severe heart failure

One RCT in people with severe heart failure taking diuretics, angiotensin converting enzyme inhibitors, and digoxin has found that adding spironolactone versus placebo significantly reduces mortality after 2 years.

## UNKNOWN EFFECTIVENESS

## Amiodarone

Systematic reviews have found weak evidence suggesting that amiodarone versus placebo may reduce mortality. However, we were not able to draw firm conclusions about effects of amiodarone in people with heart failure.

## Anticoagulation

A preliminary report from one RCT found no significant difference for warfarin versus no antithrombotic treatment or for warfarin versus aspirin for the combined outcome of death, myocardial infarction and stroke after 27 months. However, the study may have lacked power to detect a clinically important difference.

## Antiplatelet agents

A preliminary report from one RCT found no significant difference for aspirin versus no antithrombotic treatment or for aspirin versus warfarin for the combined outcome of death, myocardial infarction and stroke after 27 months. However, the study may have lacked power to detect a clinically important difference.

## Treatments for diastolic heart failure

We found no RCTs in people with diastolic heart failure.

## UNLIKELY TO BE BENEFICIAL

## Calcium channel blockers

One systematic review has found no significant difference in mortality with second generation dihydropyridine calcium channel blockers versus placebo. RCTs comparing other calcium channel blockers versus placebo found no evidence of benefit.

▶

◄ **LIKELY TO BE INEFFECTIVE OR HARMFUL**

## Non-amiodarone antiarrhythmic drugs

Evidence extrapolated from one systematic review in people treated after a myocardial infarction suggests that other antiarrhythmic drugs (apart from β blockers) may increase mortality.

## Positive inotropes (ibopamine, milrinone, vesnarinone)

RCTs found that positive inotropic drugs (other than digoxin) versus placebo significantly increased mortality over 6–11 months.

**DEFINITION**  Heart failure occurs when abnormality of cardiac function causes failure of the heart to pump blood at a rate sufficient for metabolic requirements under normal filling pressure. It is characterised clinically by breathlessness, effort intolerance, fluid retention, and poor survival. It can be caused by systolic or diastolic dysfunction and is associated with neurohormonal changes.[1] Left ventricular systolic dysfunction (LVSD) is defined as a left ventricular ejection fraction below 0.40. It may be symptomatic or asymptomatic. Defining and diagnosing diastolic heart failure can be difficult. Recently proposed criteria include: (1) clinical evidence of heart failure; (2) normal or mildly abnormal left ventricular systolic function; and (3) evidence of abnormal left ventricular relaxation, filling, diastolic distensibility, or diastolic stiffness.[2] However, assessment of some of these criteria is not standardised.

**INCIDENCE/**  Both the incidence and prevalence of heart failure increase with age. Studies
**PREVALENCE**  of heart failure in the USA and Europe found that under 65 years of age the incidence is 1/1000 men a year and 0.4/1000 women a year. Over 65 years, incidence is 11/1000 men a year and 5/1000 women a year. Under 65 years the prevalence of heart failure is 1/1000 men and 1/1000 women; over 65 years the prevalence is 40/1000 men and 30/1000 women.[3] The prevalence of asymptomatic LVSD is 3% in the general population.[4–6] The mean age of people with asymptomatic LVSD is lower than that for symptomatic individuals. Both heart failure and asymptomatic LVSD are more common in men.[4–6] The prevalence of diastolic heart failure in the community is unknown. The prevalence of heart failure with preserved systolic function in people in hospital with clinical heart failure varies from 13–74%.[7,8] Less than 15% of people with heart failure under 65 years have normal systolic function, whereas the prevalence is about 40% in people over 65 years.[7]

**AETIOLOGY/**  Coronary artery disease is the most common cause of heart failure.[3] Other
**RISK FACTORS**  common causes include hypertension and idiopathic dilated congestive cardiomyopathy. After adjustment for hypertension, the presence of left ventricular hypertrophy remains a risk factor for the development of heart failure. Other risk factors include cigarette smoking, hyperlipidaemia, and diabetes mellitus.[4] The common causes of left ventricular diastolic dysfunction are coronary artery disease and systemic hypertension. Other causes are hypertrophic cardiomyopathy, restrictive or infiltrative cardiomyopathies, and valvular heart disease.[8]

**PROGNOSIS**  The prognosis of heart failure is poor, with 5 year mortality ranging from 26–75%.[3] Up to 16% of people are readmitted with heart failure within 6 months of first admission. In the USA, heart failure it is the leading cause of hospital admission among people over 65 years of age.[3] In people with heart failure, a new myocardial infarction increases the risk of death (RR 7.8, 95% CI 6.9 to 8.8). About a third of all deaths in people with heart failure are preceded by a major ischaemic event.[9] Sudden death, mainly caused by ventricular arrhythmias, is responsible for 25–50% of all deaths, and is the most common cause of death in people with heart failure.[10] The presence of asymptomatic LVSD increases an individual's risk of having a cardiovascular event. One large prevention trial found that for a 5% reduction in ejection fraction, the risk ratio for mortality was 1.20 (95% CI 1.13 to 1.29). For hospital admission for heart ▶

# Heart failure

failure, the risk ratio was 1.28 (95% CI 1.18 to 1.38) and the risk ratio of heart failure was 1.20 (95% CI 1.13 to 1.26).[4] The annual mortality of patients with diastolic heart failure varies in observational studies (1.3–17.5%).[7] Reasons for this variation include age, the presence of coronary artery disease, and variation in the partition value used to define abnormal ventricular systolic function. The annual mortality for left ventricular diastolic dysfunction is lower than that found in patients with systolic dysfunction.[11]

---

Please refer to CD-ROM for full text and references.

Search date August 2002

*Bazian Ltd*

*Cardiovascular disorders*

## What are the effects of treatments for chronic peripheral arterial disease?

### BENEFICIAL

**Antiplatelet treatment**

Systematic reviews found that antiplatelet agents versus control treatments significantly reduce the rate of major cardiovascular events over about 2 years. Systematic reviews have found that antiplatelet agents versus placebo or no treatment significantly reduce the risk of arterial occlusion and reduce the risk of revascularisation procedures. The balance of benefits and harms is in favour of treatment for most people with symptomatic peripheral arterial disease, because as a group they are at much greater risk of cardiovascular events.

**Exercise**

Systematic reviews and one subsequent RCT in people with chronic stable claudication have found that regular exercise at least three times weekly versus no exercise significantly improves total walking distance and maximal exercise time after 3–12 months.

### LIKELY TO BE BENEFICIAL

**Bypass surgery (v thrombolysis in people with acute limb ischaemia)**

One systematic review found that surgery versus thrombolysis significantly reduced the number of amputations and the number of people reporting ongoing ischaemic pain, but found no significant difference in mortality after 1 year.

**Percutaneous transluminal angioplasty (transient benefit only)**

Two small RCTs in people with mild to moderate intermittent claudication⊙ found limited evidence that angioplasty versus no angioplasty significantly improved walking distance after 6 months but found no significant difference after 2 or 6 years. Four RCTs in people with femoral to popliteal artery stenoses have found no significant difference with angioplasty alone versus angioplasty plus stent placement in patency rates, occlusion rates, or clinical improvement.

**Smoking cessation (based on consensus of opinion)**

We found no RCTs of smoking cessation in people with peripheral vascular disease. The consensus view is that smoking cessation improves symptoms in people with intermittent claudication. One systematic review has found observational evidence that continued cigarette smoking by people with intermittent claudication is associated with progression of symptoms, poor prognosis after bypass surgery, amputation, and need for reconstructive surgery.

### TRADE OFF BETWEEN BENEFITS AND HARMS

**Cilostazol**

RCTs in people with intermittent claudication have found that cilostazol versus placebo significantly improves initial claudication distance⊙ and absolute claudication distance⊙ measured on a treadmill and significantly reduces the proportion of people with symptoms that do not improve. One RCT with a high withdrawal rate found that pentoxifylline versus cilostazol reduced initial and absolute claudication distance. Adverse effects are common and include headache, diarrhoea and palpitations.

▶

# Peripheral arterial disease

### Bypass surgery (v percutaneous transluminal angioplasty)

One systematic review found that surgery versus percutaneous transluminal angioplasty significantly improved primary blood vessel patency after 12–24 months, but found no significant difference after 4 years. The review found no significant difference in mortality after 12–24 months. Although the consensus view is that bypass surgery is the most effective treatment for people with debilitating symptomatic peripheral arterial disease, we found inadequate evidence from RCTs reporting long term clinical outcomes to confirm this view.

### Pentoxifylline

One systematic review and one subsequent RCT have found insufficient evidence to compare pentoxifylline versus placebo. One RCT found that pentoxifylline reduced absolute claudication distance compared with cilostazol.

**DEFINITION**   Peripheral arterial disease arises when there is significant narrowing of arteries distal to the arch of the aorta. Narrowing can arise from atheroma, arteritis, local thrombus formation, or embolisation from the heart or more central arteries. This topic includes treatment options for people with symptoms of reduced blood flow to the leg that are likely to arise from atheroma. These symptoms range from calf pain on exercise (intermittent claudication), to rest pain, skin ulceration, or ischaemic necrosis (gangrene) in people with critical ischaemia.

**INCIDENCE/**
**PREVALENCE**   Peripheral arterial disease is more common in people aged over 50 years than in younger people, and is more common in men than women. The prevalence of peripheral arterial disease of the legs (assessed by non-invasive tests) is about 3% in people under the age of 60 years, but rises to over 20% in people over 75 years.[1] The overall annual incidence of intermittent claudication is 1.5–2.6/1000 men a year and 1.2–3.6/1000 women a year.[2]

**AETIOLOGY/**
**RISK FACTORS**   Factors associated with the development of peripheral arterial disease include age, gender, cigarette smoking, diabetes mellitus, hypertension, hyperlipidaemia, obesity, and physical inactivity. The strongest association is with smoking (RR 2.0–4.0) and diabetes (RR 2.0–3.0).[3] Acute limb ischaemia⊙ may result from thrombosis arising within a peripheral artery or embolic occlusion.

**PROGNOSIS**   The symptom of intermittent claudication can resolve spontaneously, remain stable over many years, or progress rapidly to critical limb ischaemia⊙. About 15% of people with intermittent claudication eventually develop critical leg ischaemia, which endangers the viability of the limb. The incidence of critical limb ischaemia in Denmark and Italy in 1990 was 0.25–0.45/1000 people a year.[4,5] Coronary heart disease is the major cause of death in people with peripheral arterial disease of the legs. Over 5 years, about 20% of people with intermittent claudication have a non-fatal cardiovascular event (myocardial infarction or stroke).[6] The mortality rate of people with peripheral arterial disease is two to three times higher than that of age and sex matched controls. Overall mortality after the diagnosis of peripheral arterial disease is about 30% after 5 years and 70% after 15 years.[6]

---

Please refer to CD-ROM for full text and references.

*Charles Foster, Michael Murphy, Julian J Nicholas, Michael Pignone, and Bazian Ltd*

---

## What are the effects of interventions in asymptomatic people?

### LIKELY TO BE BENEFICIAL

**Eating more fruit and vegetables**

Observational studies have found limited evidence that eating fruit and vegetables reduces ischaemic heart disease and stroke. The size and nature of effects are uncertain.

**Physical activity**

One RCT and many observational studies have found that moderate to high physical activity reduces coronary heart disease and stroke. They also found that sudden death soon after strenuous exercise was rare, more common in sedentary people, and did not outweigh the benefits.

**Smoking cessation**

We found no direct evidence from RCTs that advice to stop smoking reduces cardiovascular risk compared with no advice. However, we found robust evidence from observational studies that smoking is an important risk factor for overall mortality, coronary heart disease, and stroke, and that smoking cessation should therefore be encouraged. The evidence is strongest for stroke.

### TRADE OFF BETWEEN BENEFITS AND HARMS

**Anticoagulant treatment (warfarin)**

One RCT found that the benefits and harms of oral anticoagulation (to a target international normalised ratio of 1.5) among people without symptoms of cardio-vascular disease were finely balanced, and that net effects were uncertain.

**Aspirin in low risk people**

We found insufficient evidence to identify which asymptomatic individuals would benefit overall and which would be harmed by regular treatment with aspirin. Benefits are likely to outweigh risks in people at higher risk.

### UNKNOWN EFFECTIVENESS

**Antioxidants (other than β carotene and vitamin E)**

We found insufficient evidence on the effects of vitamin C, copper, zinc, manganese, or flavonoids.

### LIKELY TO BE INEFFECTIVE OR HARMFUL

**β Carotene**

Systematic reviews of RCTs found no evidence of benefit from β carotene supplements, and RCTs suggest that they may be harmful.

**Vitamin E**

Systematic reviews of RCTs found no evidence of benefit from vitamin E supplements, and RCTs suggest that they may be harmful

▶

## What are the effects of interventions aimed at lowering blood pressure?

**BENEFICIAL**

### Antihypertensive drug treatments in people with hypertension

Systematic reviews have found that initial treatment with diuretics, angiotensin converting enzyme inhibitors, or β blockers reduce morbidity and mortality compared with placebo, with minimal adverse effects. RCTs found no significant differences in morbidity or mortality among these agents. We found limited evidence from two systematic reviews that diuretics, β blockers, and angiotensin converting enzyme inhibitors reduced coronary heart disease and heart failure more than calcium channel antagonists. However, calcium channel antagonists reduced risk of stroke more than the other agents. One RCT found that a thiazide diuretic reduced cardiovascular events, particularly congestive heart failure, compared with an α blocker. One RCT found that losartan (an angiotensin receptor blocker) reduced cardiovascular events compared with atenolol in people with hypertension and left ventricular hypertrophy.

### Diuretics in high risk people

Systematic reviews have found that diuretics decrease the risk of fatal and non-fatal stroke, cardiac events, and total mortality compared with placebo. The biggest benefit is seen in people with the highest baseline risk. Systematic reviews have found no significant difference in mortality or morbidity between diuretics and β blockers.

**LIKELY TO BE BENEFICIAL**

### Dietary salt restriction

We found no RCTs of the effects of salt restriction on morbidity or mortality. One systematic review has found that a low salt diet may lead to modest reductions in blood pressure compared with a usual diet, with more benefit in people older than 45 years than in younger people❶.

### Fish oil supplementation

We found no RCTs examining the effects of fish oil supplementation on morbidity or mortality in people with primary hypertension. One systematic review has found that fish oil supplementation in large doses of 3 g daily modestly lowers blood pressure.

### Low fat, high fruit and vegetable diet

We found no systematic review and no RCTs examining the effects of low fat, high fruit and vegetable diet on morbidity or mortality of people with raised blood pressure. One RCT found that a low fat, high fruit and vegetable diet modestly reduced blood pressure compared with control diet.

### Physical activity

We found no RCTs in people with primary hypertension examining the effects of exercise on morbidity or mortality. One systematic review has found that aerobic exercise reduces blood pressure compared with no exercise.

### Potassium supplementation

We found no RCTs examining the effects of potassium supplementation on morbidity or mortality in people with primary hypertension. One systematic review has found that a daily potassium supplementation of about 60 mmol (2 g, which is about the amount contained in 5 bananas) reduces blood pressure by small amounts.

### Smoking cessation

Observational studies have found that smoking is a risk factor for cardiovascular disease. We found no direct evidence in people with hypertension that stopping smoking decreases blood pressure.

### Weight loss

We found no RCTs examining the effects of weight loss on morbidity and mortality. One systematic review and additional RCTs have found that modest weight reduction in obese people with hypertension leads to a modest reduction in blood pressure.

## UNKNOWN EFFECTIVENESS

### Calcium supplementation

We found insufficient evidence about effects of calcium supplementation on blood pressure, morbidity, or mortality specifically in people with hypertension. One systematic review in people with and without hypertension found that calcium supplementation may reduce systolic blood pressure by a small amount.

### Magnesium supplementation

We found no RCTs examining the effects of magnesium supplementation on morbidity or mortality in people with hypertension. We found limited and conflicting evidence on the effect of magnesium supplementation on blood pressure in people with hypertension and normal magnesium concentrations.

### Reduced alcohol consumption

We found no RCTs examining the effects of reducing alcohol consumption on morbidity or mortality. One systematic review in moderate drinkers (25–50 drinks/week) found inconclusive evidence regarding effects of alcohol reduction on blood.

## What are the effects of interventions aimed at lowering cholesterol?

## LIKELY TO BE BENEFICIAL

### Cholesterol reduction in high risk people

Systematic reviews have found that reducing cholesterol concentration in asymptomatic people lowers the rate of cardiovascular events. RCTs have found that the magnitude of the benefit is related to an individual's baseline risk of cardiovascular events, and to the degree of cholesterol lowering, rather than to the individual's cholesterol concentration.

### Low fat diet

Systematic reviews and RCTs have found that combined use of cholesterol lowering diet and lipid lowering drugs reduces cholesterol concentration more than lifestyle interventions alone.

**DEFINITION**  Primary prevention in this context is the long term management of people at increased risk but with no evidence of cardiovascular disease. Clinically overt ischaemic vascular disease includes acute myocardial infarction, angina, stroke, and peripheral vascular disease. Many adults have no symptoms or obvious signs of vascular disease, even though they have atheroma and are at ▶

# Primary prevention

increased risk of ischaemic vascular events because of one or more risk factors (see aetiology below). In this topic, we have taken primary prevention to apply to people who have not had clinically overt cardiovascular disease, or people at low risk of ischaemic cardiovascular events. Prevention of cerebrovascular events is discussed in detail elsewhere in *Clinical Evidence* (see stroke prevention topic, p 36).

**INCIDENCE/ PREVALENCE**  According to the World Health Report 1999, ischaemic heart disease was the leading single cause for death in the world, the leading single cause for death in high income countries and second to lower respiratory tract infections in low and middle income countries. In 1998 it was still the leading cause for death, with nearly 7.4 million estimated deaths a year in member states of the World Health Organization. This condition had the eighth highest burden of disease in the low and middle income countries (30.7 million disability adjusted life years).[1]

**AETIOLOGY/ RISK FACTORS**  Identified major risk factors for ischaemic vascular disease include increasing age, male sex, raised low density lipoprotein cholesterol, reduced high density lipoprotein cholesterol, raised blood pressure, smoking, diabetes, family history of cardiovascular disease, obesity, and sedentary lifestyle. For many of these risk factors, observational studies show a continuous gradient of increasing risk of cardiovascular disease with increasing levels of the risk factor, with no obvious threshold level. Although by definition event rates are higher in high risk people, most ischaemic vascular events that occur in the population are in people with intermediate levels of absolute risk because there are many more of them than there are people at high risk; see Appendix 1.[2]

**PROGNOSIS**  A study carried out in Scotland found that about half of people who suffer an acute myocardial infarction die within 28 days, and two thirds of acute myocardial infarctions occur before the person reaches hospital.[3] The benefits of intervention in unselected people with no evidence of cardiovascular disease (primary prevention) are small because in such people the baseline risk is small. However, absolute risk of ischaemic vascular events varies widely, even among people with similar levels of blood pressure or cholesterol. Estimates of absolute risk can be based on simple risk equations or tables; see Appendix 1.[4,5]

Please refer to CD-ROM for full text and references.

# Secondary prevention of ischaemic cardiac events

**Search date November 2002**

*Michael Pignone, Charanjit Rihal, and Bazian Ltd*

## What are the effects of treatments?

### BENEFICIAL

#### Amiodarone in people at high risk of arrhythmic death

Two systematic reviews have found that amiodarone reduces the risk of sudden cardiac death and overall mortality at 1 year compared with placebo in people at high risk of arrhythmic death after myocardial infarction.

#### Angiotensin converting enzyme inhibitors in high risk people without left ventricular dysfunction

One large RCT in high risk people without left ventricular dysfunction found that ramipril reduced the combined outcome of cardiovascular death, stroke, and myocardial infarction compared with placebo after about 5 years.

#### Angiotensin converting enzyme inhibitors in people with left ventricular dysfunction

One systematic review has found that, in people who have had a myocardial infarction and have left ventricular dysfunction, angiotensin converting enzyme inhibitors reduce mortality, admission to hospital for congestive heart failure, and recurrent non-fatal myocardial infarction compared with placebo after 2 years' treatment.

#### Anticoagulants in the absence of antiplatelet treatment

One systematic review and subsequent RCTs have found that high or moderate intensity oral anticoagulants given alone reduce the risk of serious vascular events compared with placebo or no anticoagulants in people with coronary artery disease, but are associated with substantial risk of haemorrhage.

#### Any oral antiplatelet treatment

One systematic review has found that prolonged antiplatelet treatment compared with placebo or no antiplatelet treatment reduces the risk of serious vascular events in people at high risk of ischaemic cardiac events.

#### Aspirin

One systematic review has found that, for prolonged use, aspirin 75–150 mg daily is as effective as higher doses, but found insufficient evidence that doses below 75 mg daily are as effective.

#### β Blockers

Systematic reviews in people after myocardial infarction have found that long term β blockers reduce all cause mortality, coronary mortality, recurrent non-fatal myocardial infarction, and sudden death. One RCT found that about 25% of people suffer adverse effects.

#### Cardiac rehabilitation

One systematic review has found that cardiac rehabilitation including exercise reduces the risk of major cardiac events. One subsequent RCT found no significant difference in quality of life between standard rehabilitation and early return to normal activities, although the study may have lacked power to detect a clinically important difference between groups.

▶

# Secondary prevention of ischaemic cardiac events

### Cholesterol lowering drugs

Systematic reviews and large subsequent RCTs have found that lowering cholesterol in people at high risk of ischaemic coronary events substantially reduces
overall mortality, cardiovascular mortality, and non-fatal cardiovascular events. We
found good evidence from systematic reviews and subsequent RCTs that statins
were the only non-surgical treatment for cholesterol reduction that reduced
mortality. One systematic review has found that the absolute benefits increase as
baseline risk increases, but are not additionally influenced by the person's
absolute blood cholesterol concentration.

### Coronary artery bypass grafting versus medical treatment alone

One systematic review found that coronary artery bypass grafting reduced the risk
of death from coronary artery disease at 5 and 10 years compared with medical
treatment alone. Greater benefit occurred in people with poor left ventricular
function. One subsequent RCT in people with asymptomatic disease found that
revascularisation with coronary artery bypass grafting or coronary percutaneous
transluminal angioplasty reduced mortality at 2 years compared with medical
treatment alone.

### Coronary percutaneous transluminal angioplasty versus medical treatment alone in people with stable coronary artery disease

One systematic review found that coronary percutaneous transluminal angioplasty
improved angina compared with medical treatment alone, but was associated with
a higher rate of coronary artery bypass grafting. The review found higher mortality
and rates of myocardial infarction with percutaneous transluminal angioplasty than
with medical treatment but the difference was not significant. RCTs have found
that percutaneous transluminal angioplasty is associated with increased risk of
emergency coronary artery bypass grafting and myocardial infarction during and
soon after the procedure. One RCT found that percutaneous transluminal angioplasty reduced cardiac events and improved angina severity compared with
medical treatment alone in people over the age of 75 years.

### Intracoronary stents (better than coronary percutaneous transluminal angioplasty alone)

One systematic review found that intracoronary stents reduce the need for repeat
vascularisation compared with coronary percutaneous transluminal angioplasty
alone. It found no significant difference in mortality or myocardial infarction, but
crossover rates from angioplasty to stent were high. RCTs found that intracoronary
stents improved outcomes after 4–9 months compared with percutaneous transluminal angioplasty in people with previous coronary artery bypass grafting, chronic
total occlusions, and for treatment of restenosis after initial percutaneous transluminal angioplasty.

### Exercise without cardiac rehabilitation

One systematic review has found that exercise alone reduces mortality compared
with usual care.

## LIKELY TO BE BENEFICIAL

### Blood pressure lowering in people at high risk of ischaemic coronary events

We found no direct evidence of the effects of blood pressure lowering in people
with established coronary heart disease. Observational studies, and extrapolation
of primary prevention trials of blood pressure reduction, support the lowering of
blood pressure in those at high risk of ischaemic coronary events. The evidence for
benefit is strongest for β blockers, although not specifically in people with

# Secondary prevention of ischaemic cardiac events

hypertension. The optimum target blood pressure in people with hypertention is not clear. Effects of angiotensin converting enzyme inhibitors, calcium channel blockers, and β blockers are discussed separately.

## Coronary artery bypass grafting versus percutaneous revascularisation for multivessel disease (less need for repeat procedures)
One systematic review has found no significant difference between coronary artery bypass grafting and percutaneous transluminal angioplasty in death, myocardial infarction, or quality of life. Percutaneous transluminal angioplasty is less invasive but increased the number of repeat procedures.

## Eating more fish (particularly oily fish)
One RCT has found that advising people with coronary heart disease to eat more fish (particularly oily fish) reduced mortality at 2 years. A second RCT found that fish oil capsules reduced mortality at 3.5 years.

## Mediterranean diet
One RCT has found that advising people with coronary artery disease to eat more bread, fruit, vegetables, and fish, and less meat, and to replace butter and cream with rapeseed margarine reduces mortality at 27 months.

## Psychosocial treatment
RCTs found limited evidence that psychosocial treatments reduced cardiac events or cardiac death compared with no psychosocial treatment in people with coronary heart disease. Two RCTs found that psychological treatments improved quality of life compared with no psychological treatment.

## Smoking cessation
We found no RCTs of the effects of smoking cessation on cardiovascular events in people with coronary heart disease. Moderate quality evidence from epidemiological studies indicates that people with coronary heart disease who stop smoking rapidly reduce their risk of recurrent coronary events or death. Treatment with nicotine patches seems safe in people with coronary heart disease.

## Stress management
One systematic review of mainly poor quality RCTs found that stress management may decrease rates of myocardial infarction or cardiac death in people with coronary heart disease.

## Thienopyridines
One systematic review has found that clopidogrel is at least as safe and effective as aspirin in people at high risk of cardiovascular events.

### UNKNOWN EFFECTIVENESS

## Advice to eat less fat
RCTs found no strong evidence that low fat diets reduced mortality at 2 years.

## Vitamin C
We found insufficient evidence about effects of vitamin C alone.

## Vitamin E
We found no consistent evidence from four RCTs about effects of vitamin E versus placebo or other antioxidants in people with high cardiovascular risk.

### UNLIKELY TO BE BENEFICIAL

## Hormone replacement therapy
Large RCTs found no significant difference between hormone replacement therapy and placebo in major cardiovascular events in postmenopausal women with

established coronary artery disease. Observational studies and one large RCT found that hormone replacement therapy increased risk of breast cancer, venous thromboembolism, and gall bladder disease compared with placebo.

### Oral glycoprotein IIb/IIIa receptor inhibitors

Systematic reviews in people with acute coronary syndromes or undergoing percutaneous coronary interventions have found that oral glycoprotein IIb/IIIa receptor inhibitors (with or without aspirin) increase risk of mortality and bleeding compared with aspirin alone.

### Sotalol

One RCT found limited evidence that sotalol increased mortality within 1 year compared with placebo.

## LIKELY TO BE INEFFECTIVE OR HARMFUL

### Adding anticoagulants to antiplatelet treatment

One systematic review and subsequent RCTs found no consistent evidence that addition of oral anticoagulation at low (INR❸ < 1.5) or moderate (INR 1.5–3.0) intensity to aspirin reduced risk of death or recurrent cardiac events, but found an increased risk of major haemorrhage compared with aspirin alone.

### β Carotene

Four large RCTs of β carotene supplementation in primary prevention found no cardiovascular benefits, and two of the RCTs raised concerns about increased mortality.

### Calcium channel blockers

One systematic review found non-significantly higher mortality with dihydropyridines compared with placebo. One systematic review found no benefit from calcium channel blockers in people after myocardial infarction or with chronic coronary heart disease. Diltiazem and verapamil may reduce rates of reinfarction and refractory angina in people after myocardial infarction who do not have heart failure.

### Class I antiarrhythmic agents

One systematic review has found that class I antiarrhythmic agents given after myocardial infarction increase the risk of cardiovascular mortality and sudden death compared with placebo.

**DEFINITION**    Secondary prevention in this context is the long term management of people with a prior acute myocardial infarction, and of people at high risk of ischaemic cardiac events for other reasons, such as a history of angina or coronary surgical procedures.

**INCIDENCE/**    Coronary artery disease is the leading cause of mortality in developed
**PREVALENCE**    countries and is becoming a major cause of morbidity and mortality in developing countries. There are pronounced international, regional, and temporal differences in death rates. In the USA, the prevalence of overt coronary artery disease approaches 4%.[1]

**AETIOLOGY/**    Most ischaemic cardiac events are associated with atheromatous plaques that
**RISK FACTORS**   can cause acute obstruction of coronary vessels. Atheroma is more likely in elderly people, in those with established coronary artery disease, and in those with risk factors (such as smoking, hypertension, high cholesterol, diabetes mellitus).

▶

# Secondary prevention of ischaemic cardiac events

**PROGNOSIS**  Of people admitted to hospital with acute myocardial infarction, 7–15% die in hospital and another 7–15% die during the following year. People who survive the acute stage of myocardial infarction fall into three prognostic groups, based on their baseline risk❶;[2–4] high (20% of all survivors), moderate (55%), and low (25%) risk. Long term prognosis depends on the degree of left ventricular dysfunction, the presence of residual ischaemia, and the extent of any electrical instability. Further risk stratification procedures include assessment of left ventricular function (by echocardiography or nuclear ventriculography) and of myocardial ischaemia (by non-invasive stress testing).[4–8] Those with low left ventricular ejection fraction, ischaemia, or poor functional status can be assessed further by cardiac catheterisation.[9]

---

Please refer to CD-ROM for full text and references.

Cardiovascular disorders

33

# Stroke management

**Search date September 2002**

*Elizabeth Warburton*

---

## What are the effects of medical treatments for acute ischaemic stroke?

### BENEFICIAL

**Aspirin**

One systematic review in people with ischaemic stroke confirmed by computerised tomography scan has found that aspirin versus placebo within 48 hours of stroke onset significantly reduces death or dependency at 6 months and significantly increases the number of people making a complete recovery. One prospective combined analysis of two large RCTs found indirect evidence that aspirin should not be delayed if a computerised tomography scan is not available within 48 hours and ischaemic stroke is suspected. Subgroup analysis of results from the two large RCTs found no significant difference in further stroke or death with aspirin versus placebo in people who were subsequently found to have haemorrhagic rather than ischaemic stroke.

**Specialised care**

One systematic review has found that specialist stroke rehabilitation units versus conventional (less specialised) care significantly reduces death or dependency after a median follow up of 1 year.

### TRADE OFF BETWEEN BENEFITS AND HARMS

**Thrombolysis**

One systematic review in people with ischaemic stroke (without cerebral haemorrhage) which was excluded by computerised tomography scan) has found that thrombolysis versus placebo significantly reduces the risk of the composite outcome of death or dependency after 1–6 months, but significantly increases the risk of death from intracranial haemorrhage measured in the first 7–10 days.

### UNLIKELY TO BE BENEFICIAL

**Neuroprotective agents (calcium channel antagonists, γ-aminobutyric acid agonists, lubeluzole, glycine antagonists, tirilazad, N-methyl-D-aspartate antagonists)**

RCTs found no evidence that, compared with placebo, calcium channel antagonists, tirilazad, lubeluzole, γ-aminobutyric acid agonists, glycine antagonists, or N-methyl-D-aspartate antagonists☉ significantly improve clinical outcomes. One systematic review found that lubeluzole versus placebo was associated with a significant increase in the risk of having Q-T prolongation to more than 450 ms on electrocardiography.

### LIKELY TO BE INEFFECTIVE OR HARMFUL

**Acute reduction in blood pressure**

One systematic review in people with acute stroke found insufficient evidence about the effects of lowering blood pressure versus placebo on clinical outcome, but RCTs have suggested that people treated with antihypertensive agents may have a worse clinical outcome and increased mortality.

◄ **Immediate systemic anticoagulation**

One systematic review comparing systemic anticoagulants (unfractionated heparin, low molecular weight heparin, heparinoids, oral anticoagulants, or specific thrombin inhibitors) versus usual care without systemic anticoagulants found no significant difference in death or dependence after 3–6 months. One systematic review has found that immediate systemic anticoagulation significantly reduces the risk of deep venous thrombosis and symptomatic pulmonary embolus, but increases the risk of intracranial haemorrhage or extracranial haemorrhage. One RCT in people with acute ischaemic stroke and atrial fibrillation found no significant difference with low molecular weight heparin versus aspirin in recurrent ischaemic stroke within 14 days. One RCT in people within 48 hours of stroke onset found no significant difference with high or low dose tinzaparin versus aspirin in people achieving functional independence at 6 months.

## What are the effects of surgical treatments for intracerebral haematomas?

**UNKNOWN EFFECTIVENESS**

**Evacuation**

We found that the balance between benefits and harms has not been clearly established for the evacuation of supratentorial haematomas. We found no evidence from RCTs on the role of evacuation or ventricular shunting in people with infratentorial haematoma whose consciousness level is declining.

**DEFINITION**     Stroke is characterised by rapidly developing clinical symptoms and signs of focal, and at times global, loss of cerebral function lasting more than 24 hours or leading to death, with no apparent cause other than that of vascular origin.[1] Ischaemic stroke is stroke caused by vascular insufficiency (such as cerebrovascular thromboembolism) rather than haemorrhage.

**INCIDENCE/**     Stroke is the third most common cause of death in most developed coun-
**PREVALENCE**   tries.[2] It is a worldwide problem; about 4.5 million people die from stroke each year. Stroke can occur at any age, but half of all strokes occur in people over 70 years old.[3]

**AETIOLOGY/**     About 80% of all acute strokes are caused by cerebral infarction, usually
**RISK FACTORS** resulting from thrombotic or embolic occlusion of a cerebral artery.[4] The remainder are caused either by intracerebral or subarachnoid haemorrhage.

**PROGNOSIS**     About 10% of all people with acute ischaemic strokes will die within 30 days of stroke onset.[5] Of those who survive the acute event, about 50% will experience some level of disability after 6 months.[6]

Please refer to CD-ROM for full text and references.

Cardiovascular disorders

# Stroke prevention

### Search date January 2003

*Bethan Freestone, Gregory YH Lip, Peter Rothwell, and Cathie Sudlow*

## What are the effects of preventive interventions in people with prior stroke or transient ischaemic attack?

### BENEFICIAL

**Antiplatelet treatment**
One systematic review has found that antiplatelet treatment reduces the risk of serious vascular events in people with prior stroke or transient ischaemic attack compared with placebo or no antiplatelet treatment.

**Blood pressure reduction**
One systematic review and one subsequent RCT found that antihypertensive treatment reduced stroke among people with a prior stroke or transient ischaemic attack, whether or not they were hypertensive.

**Carotid endarterectomy in people with moderately severe (50–69%) symptomatic carotid artery stenosis**
Evidence from a pooled analysis of individual patient data from three RCTs found that carotid endarterectomy reduced stroke and death compared with no endarterectomy in symptomatic people with 50–69% carotid stenosis.

**Carotid endarterectomy in people with severe (> 70%) symptomatic carotid artery stenosis**
Evidence from three RCTs has found that carotid endarterectomy reduces stroke and death compared with no endarterectomy in symptomatic people with more than 70% stenosis, although no benefit was found in people with near-occlusion. Benefit in symptomatic people with more than 70% stenosis is greater than in people with lower grade stenosis.

**Cholesterol reduction**
One large RCT has found that, compared with placebo, simvastatin reduced major vascular events, including stroke, in people with prior stroke or transient ischaemic attack. RCTs found no evidence that non-statin treatments reduced stroke compared with placebo or no treatment.

### LIKELY TO BE BENEFICIAL

**Carotid endarterectomy in people with asymptomatic but severe carotid artery stenosis**
Two systematic reviews found that carotid endarterectomy reduced perioperative stroke, death, and subsequent ipsilateral stroke in people with asymptomatic but severe stenosis. However, because the risk of stroke without surgery in asymptomatic people is relatively low, the benefit from surgery is small.

### UNKNOWN EFFECTIVENESS

**Carotid or vertebral angioplasty**
We found insufficient evidence about the effects of carotid or vertebral percutaneous transluminal angioplasty or stenting compared with medical treatment or carotid endarterectomy in people with a recent carotid or vertebral territory transient ischaemic attack or non-disabling ischaemic stroke who have severe stenosis of the ipsilateral carotid or vertebral artery.

◀ **Different blood pressure lowering regimens (no evidence that any regimen more or less effective than any other)**

> Systematic reviews found no clear evidence of a difference in effectiveness between different antihypertensive drugs. One systematic review found that more intensive treatment reduced stroke and major cardiovascular events, but not mortality, compared with less intensive treatment.

## UNLIKELY TO BE BENEFICIAL

**Alternative antiplatelet agents to aspirin (no evidence that any more or less effective than aspirin)**

> Systematic reviews have found no good evidence that any antiplatelet treatment is superior to aspirin for long term secondary prevention of serious vascular events.

**Carotid endarterectomy in people with moderate (30–49%) symptomatic carotid artery stenosis**

> Evidence from a pooled analysis of individual patient data from three RCTs suggests that carotid endarterectomy is of no benefit in symptomatic people with 30–49% stenosis.

**Carotid endarterectomy in people with symptomatic near-occlusion of the carotid artery**

> We found limited evidence from three RCTs that carotid endarterectomy increases the risk of stroke or death due to surgery in symptomatic people with near occlusion of the ipsilateral carotid artery.

**High dose versus low dose aspirin (no additional benefit but may increase harms)**

> One systematic review and one subsequent RCT have found that low dose aspirin (75–150 mg/day) is as effective as higher doses for preventing serious vascular events. It found insufficient evidence that doses lower than 75 mg daily are as effective. Systematic reviews found no evidence of an association between aspirin dose and risk of intracranial, major extracranial, or gastrointestinal haemorrhage. RCTs found that high dose aspirin (500–1500 mg/day) increased the risk of upper gastrointestinal upset compared with medium dose aspirin (75–325 mg/day).

## LIKELY TO BE INEFFECTIVE OR HARMFUL

**Carotid endarterectomy in people with less than 30% symptomatic carotid artery stenosis**

> Evidence from a pooled analysis of individual patient data from three RCTs suggests that carotid endarterectomy increases the risk of stroke or death due to surgery in symptomatic people with less than 30% carotid stenosis.

**Oral anticoagulation in people with prior cerebrovascular ischaemia and sinus rhythm**

> Systematic reviews found no significant difference between anticoagulation and placebo or antiplatelet treatment for preventing recurrent stroke after presumed ischaemic stroke in people in normal sinus rhythm. Anticoagulants increased the risk of fatal intracranial and extracranial haemorrhage compared with placebo. High intensity anticoagulation increased the risk of major bleeding compared with antiplatelet treatment.

▶

# Stroke prevention

## *What are the effects of preventive interventions in people with atrial fibrillation and prior stroke or transient ischaemic attack?*

### BENEFICIAL

### Aspirin in people with contraindications to anticoagulants

Systematic reviews have found that aspirin reduces the risk of stroke compared with placebo, but found that aspirin is less effective than anticoagulants. These findings support the use of aspirin in people with atrial fibrillation and contraindications to anticoagulants.

### Oral anticoagulation

Systematic reviews have found that adjusted dose warfarin reduces the risk of stroke compared with placebo. Systematic reviews have also found that warfarin reduces the risk of stroke in people with previous stroke or transient ischaemic attack compared with aspirin.

## *What are the effects of preventive interventions in people with atrial fibrillation but no other major risk factors for stroke?*

### LIKELY TO BE BENEFICIAL

### Aspirin in people with contraindications to anticoagulants

One systematic review has found that aspirin reduces the risk of stroke compared with placebo, but another review found no significant difference. These findings support the use of aspirin in people with atrial fibrillation and contraindications to anticoagulants.

### Oral anticoagulation

One systematic review has found that warfarin reduces fatal and non-fatal ischaemic stroke compared with placebo, provided there is a low risk of bleeding and careful monitoring. The people in the review had a mean age of 69 years. One overview in people less than 65 years old has found no significant difference in the annual stroke rate between warfarin and placebo.

**DEFINITION**     Prevention in this context is the long term management of people with a prior stroke or transient ischaemic attack, and of people at high risk of stroke❻ for other reasons such as atrial fibrillation. **Stroke:** See definition under stroke management, p 35. **Transient ischaemic attack:** This is similar to a mild ischaemic stroke except that symptoms last for less than 24 hours.[1]

**INCIDENCE/**     See incidence/prevalence under stroke management, p 35.
**PREVALENCE**
**AETIOLOGY/**     See aetiology under stroke management, p 35. Risk factors for stroke include
**RISK FACTORS** prior stroke or transient ischaemic attack, increasing age, hypertension, diabetes, cigarette smoking, and emboli associated with atrial fibrillation, artificial heart valves, or myocardial infarction. The relation with cholesterol is less clear. One overview of prospective studies among healthy middle aged people found no association between total cholesterol and overall stroke risk.[2] However, one review of prospective observational studies in eastern Asian people found that cholesterol was positively associated with ischaemic stroke but negatively associated with haemorrhagic stroke.[3]

◀ **PROGNOSIS**  People with a history of stroke or transient ischaemic attack are at high risk of all vascular events, such as myocardial infarction, but are at particular risk of subsequent stroke (about 10% in the first year and about 5% each year thereafter); see figure 1❻, and figure 1 in secondary prevention of ischaemic cardiac events.[4,5] People with intermittent atrial fibrillation treated with aspirin should be considered at similar risk of stroke, compared to people with sustained atrial fibrillation treated with aspirin (rate of ischaemic stroke/year: 3.2% with intermittent v 3.3% with sustained).[6]

Please refer to CD-ROM for full text and references.

# Thromboembolism

**Search date November 2002**

*David Fitzmaurice, FD Richard Hobbs, and Richard McManus*

## What are the effects of treatments for proximal deep vein thrombosis?

### TRADE OFF BETWEEN BENEFITS AND HARMS

**Unfractionated and low molecular weight heparin**

Systematic reviews have found that low molecular weight heparin🄖 reduces the incidence of recurrent thromboembolic disease and decreases the risk of major haemorrhage🄖 compared with unfractionated heparin. One systematic review found no significant difference between long term low molecular weight heparin and oral anticoagulation in recurrent thromboembolism, major haemorrhage, or mortality. One systematic review of RCTs found no significant difference in recurrence of thromboembolism between heparin treatment at home and in hospital.

**Warfarin**

We found no RCTs comparing warfarin versus placebo. One RCT found that fewer people had recurrence of proximal deep vein thrombosis within 6 months with combined acenocoumarol (nicoumalone) plus intravenous unfractionated heparin than with acenocoumarol alone; as a result, the trial was stopped. Systematic reviews have found that longer duration of anticoagulation reduces recurrence of deep vein thrombosis compared with shorter duration of anticoagulation. One non-systematic review found limited evidence that longer compared with shorter duration of warfarin was associated with an increased risk of major haemorrhage, but another non-systematic review found no significant difference in major haemorrhage. The absolute risk of recurrent venous thromboembolism decreases with time, but the relative risk reduction with treatment remains constant. Harms of treatment, including major haemorrhage, continue during prolonged treatment. Individuals have different risk profiles and it is likely that the optimal duration of anticoagulation will vary.

### UNKNOWN EFFECTIVENESS

**Compression stockings** *New*

We found no RCTs of standard compression stockings for treating people with proximal deep vein thrombosis. One RCT found that made to measure knee length graduated compression stockings reduced post-thrombotic syndrome over 5–8 years compared with no stockings.

## What are the effects of treatments for isolated calf vein thrombosis?

### TRADE OFF BETWEEN BENEFITS AND HARMS

**Warfarin plus heparin**

One unblinded RCT found no significant difference in recurrent thromboembolism or rates of major haemorrhage between 6 and 12 weeks of anticoagulation. One RCT found that warfarin plus intravenous unfractionated heparin (international normalised ratio🄖 > 2.5–4.2) reduced the rate of proximal extension compared with heparin alone.

## What are the effects of treatments for pulmonary embolism?

### TRADE OFF BETWEEN BENEFITS AND HARMS

#### Oral anticoagulants
We found no direct evidence about the optimum intensity and duration of anticoagulation in people with pulmonary embolism. The best available evidence requires extrapolation of results from studies of people with proximal deep vein thrombosis.

#### Unfractionated and low molecular weight heparin
One small RCT in people with pulmonary embolism found that heparin plus warfarin reduced mortality compared with no anticoagulation at 1 year. One RCT in people with symptomatic pulmonary embolism who did not receive thrombolysis or embolectomy found no significant difference between low molecular weight heparin and unfractionated heparin in mortality or new episodes of thrombo-embolism. Another RCT in people with proximal deep vein thrombosis without clinical signs or symptoms of pulmonary embolism but with high probability lung scan findings found that fixed dose low molecular weight heparin reduced the proportion of people with new episodes of venous thromboembolism compared with intravenous heparin.

### UNLIKELY TO BE BENEFICIAL

#### Thrombolysis
RCTs identified by one systematic review found no significant difference in mortality between thrombolysis plus heparin and heparin alone, and found that thromboly-sis may increase the incidence of intracranial haemorrhage. One small RCT identified by the review found limited evidence that adding thrombolysis to heparin may reduce mortality in people with shock due to massive pulmonary embolism.

---

## What are the effects of computerised decision support on oral anticoagulation management?

### UNKNOWN EFFECTIVENESS

#### Computerised decision support in oral anticoagulation management
We found no RCTs comparing computerised decision support⊖ versus usual management of oral anticoagulation that used clinically important outcomes (major haemorrhage or death). One systematic review and three subsequent RCTs have found that, compared with usual care, computerised decision support in oral anticoagulation increases time spent in the target international normalised ratio range. Another subsequent RCT found no significant difference between compu-terised decision support and standard manual support in the time spent in the target international normalised ratio range. A subsequent RCT of initiation of warfarin found that computerised decision support reduced the mean time taken to reach therapeutic levels of anticoagulation compared with usual care. Most RCTs were small and brief.

DEFINITION   **Venous thromboembolism** is any thromboembolic event occurring within the venous system, including deep vein thrombosis and pulmonary embolism. **Deep vein thrombosis** is a radiologically confirmed partial or total throm-botic occlusion of the deep venous system of the legs sufficient to produce symptoms of pain or swelling. **Proximal deep vein thrombosis** affects the veins above the knee (popliteal, superficial femoral, common femoral, and iliac veins). **Isolated calf vein thrombosis** is confined to the deep veins of the calf and does not affect the veins above the knee. **Pulmonary embolism** ▶

# Thromboembolism

is radiologically confirmed partial or total thromboembolic occlusion of pulmonary arteries, sufficient to cause symptoms of breathlessness, chest pain, or both. **Post-thrombotic syndrome** is oedema, ulceration, and impaired viability of the subcutaneous tissues of the leg occurring after deep vein thrombosis. **Recurrence** refers to symptomatic deterioration because of a further (radiologically confirmed) thrombosis, after a previously confirmed thromboembolic event, where there had been an initial, partial, or total symptomatic improvement. **Extension** refers to a radiologically confirmed new, constant, symptomatic intraluminal filling defect extending from an existing thrombosis.

**INCIDENCE/ PREVALENCE**　We found no reliable study of the incidence/prevalence of deep vein thrombosis or pulmonary embolism in the UK. A prospective Scandinavian study found an annual incidence of 1.6–1.8/1000 people in the general population.[1,2] One postmortem study estimated that 600 000 people develop pulmonary embolism each year in the USA, of whom 60 000 die as a result.[3]

**AETIOLOGY/ RISK FACTORS**　Risk factors for deep vein thrombosis include immobility, surgery (particularly orthopaedic), malignancy, smoking, pregnancy, older age, and inherited or acquired prothrombotic clotting disorders.[4] The oral contraceptive pill is associated with death due to venous thromboembolism (ARI with any combined oral contraception: 1–3/million women a year).[5] The principal cause of pulmonary embolism is a deep vein thrombosis.[4]

**PROGNOSIS**　The annual recurrence rate of symptomatic calf vein thrombosis in people without recent surgery is over 25%.[6,7] Proximal extension develops in 40–50% of people with symptomatic calf vein thrombosis.[8] Proximal deep vein thrombosis may cause fatal or non-fatal pulmonary embolism, recurrent venous thrombosis, and the post-thrombotic syndrome. One case series (462 people) published in 1946 found 5.8% mortality from pulmonary emboli in people in hospital with untreated deep vein thrombosis.[9] One non-systematic review of observational studies found that, in people after recent surgery who have an asymptomatic deep calf vein thrombosis, the rate of fatal pulmonary embolism was 13–15%.[10] The incidence of other complications without treatment is not known. The risk of recurrent venous thrombosis and complications is increased by thrombotic risk factors.[11]

Please refer to CD-ROM for full text and references.

---

## What are effects of treatments in adults with varicose veins?

### LIKELY TO BE BENEFICIAL

### Surgery (v injection sclerotherapy)

We found no RCTs comparing surgery versus no treatment or compression stockings. One RCT found that surgery significantly improved cure of varicose veins compared with injection sclerotherapy at 5 years in people with varicose veins from saphenofemoral, saphenopopliteal, and perforator incompetence. The RCT did not report separately on effects of surgery for each site of venous incompetence.

### UNKNOWN EFFECTIVENESS

### Compression stockings

One crossover RCT found no significant difference in symptoms between compression stockings for 4 weeks versus no treatment in people with varicose veins. However, the study may have lacked power to exclude clinically important effects.

### Injection sclerotherapy

One systematic review has found no RCTs comparing injection sclerotherapy versus no treatment or compression stockings in people with varicose veins. One RCT has found no significant difference between injection sclerotherapy with polidocanol versus sodium tetradecyl sulphate for improving appearance of varicose veins not due to saphenofemoral or saphenopopliteal incompetence at 16 weeks.

**DEFINITION**     Although we found no consistent definition of varicose veins,[1] the term is commonly taken to mean veins that are distended and tortuous. Any vein may become varicose, but the term "varicose veins" conventionally applies to varices of the superficial leg veins. The condition is caused by poorly functioning valves within the lumen of the veins. Blood flows from the deep to the superficial venous systems through these incompetent valves, causing persistent superficial venous hypertension, which leads to varicosity of the superficial veins. Common sites of valvular incompetence include the saphenofemoral and saphenopopliteal junctions and perforating veins connecting the deep and superficial venous systems along the length of the leg. Sites of venous incompetence are determined by clinical examination or, more reliably, by Doppler ultrasound. Symptoms of varicose veins include distress about cosmetic appearance, pain, itch, limb heaviness, and cramps. This review focuses on uncomplicated, symptomatic varicose veins. We have excluded treatments for chronic venous ulceration and other complications. We have also excluded studies that solely examine treatments for small, dilated veins in the skin of the leg, known as thread veins, spider veins, or superficial telangiectasia.

**INCIDENCE/**     One large US cohort study found the annual incidence of varicose veins to be
**PREVALENCE**     2.6% in women and 1.9% in men.[2] Incidence was constant over the age of 40 years. The prevalence of varicose veins in Western populations is about 25–30% among women and 10–20% in men.[3]

**AETIOLOGY/**     One large case control study found that women with two or more pregnancies
**RISK FACTORS**     were at increased risk of varicose veins compared with women with fewer than two pregnancies (RR about 1.2–1.3 after adjustment for age, height, and weight).[2] It found that obesity was also a risk factor, although only among ▶

# Varicose veins

women (RR about 1.3). One narrative systematic review found insufficient evidence about effects of other suggested risk factors, including genetic predisposition; prolonged sitting or standing; tight undergarments; low fibre diet; constipation; deep vein thrombosis; and smoking.[3]

**PROGNOSIS** We found no reliable data about prognosis, nor about the frequency of complications, which include chronic inflammation of affected veins (phlebitis), venous ulceration, and rupture of varices.

---

Please refer to CD-ROM for full text and references.

Search date January 2003

*Ewa Posner*

## What are the effects of treatments for typical absence seizures in children?

### TRADE OFF BETWEEN BENEFITS AND HARMS

#### Ethosuximide*

We found no systematic review or RCTs comparing ethosuximide versus placebo. There is consensus that ethosuximide is beneficial. Ethosuximide is associated with rare but serious adverse effects, including aplastic anaemia, skin reactions, and renal and hepatic impairment. We found no RCTs comparing ethosuximide versus other anticonvulsants (except valproate) in children with typical absence seizures.

#### Lamotrigine

One RCT found that, compared with placebo, lamotrigine increased the proportion of children who remained seizure free. However, lamotrigine is associated with serious skin reactions. We found no RCTs comparing lamotrigine versus other anticonvulsants.

#### Valproate*

We found no RCTs comparing valproate versus placebo. There is consensus that valproate is beneficial. Valproate is associated with rare but serious adverse effects, including behavioural and cognitive abnormalites, liver necrosis, and pancreatitis. Three small RCTs found no significant difference between valproate and ethosuximide. We found no RCTs comparing valproate versus other anti-convulsants (except ethosuximide) in children with typical absence seizures.

*We found no RCT evidence for valproate or ethosuximide versus placebo but there is consensus belief that valproate and ethosuximide are beneficial in typical absence seizures.

### UNKNOWN EFFECTIVENESS

#### Gabapentin

One brief RCT found no significant difference between gabapentin versus placebo in the frequency of typical absence seizures.

**DEFINITION**  Absence seizures are sudden, episodes of unconsciousness lasting a few seconds. Depending on electroencephalogram findings, they are divided into typical and atypical seizures. Typical absence seizures are associated with an electroencephalogram showing regular symmetrical generalised spike and wave complexes with a frequency of 3 Hz. Absence seizures may be the only type of seizures experienced by a child and this then constitutes an epileptic syndrome⊕ called childhood absence epilepsy. In many children, typical absence seizures coexist with other types of seizures. Atypical absence seizures do not show the characteristic electroencephalogram pattern of typical absence seizures; are usually one of many types of seizures in a child with a background of learning disability and severe epilepsy; and tend to be less defined in time.[1] This differentiation into typical versus atypical seizures is important as the natural history and response to treatment varies in the two groups. Interventions for atypical absence seizures are not included in this topic. ▶

# Absence seizures in children

**INCIDENCE/ PREVALENCE**
About 10% of seizures in children with epilepsy are typical absence seizures.[1] Annual incidence has been estimated at 0.7–4.6/100 000 people in the general population and 6–8/100 000 in children aged 0–15 years. Prevalence is 5–50/100 000 people in the general population.[2] Age of onset ranges from 3–13 years with a peak at 6–7 years.

**AETIOLOGY/ RISK FACTORS**
The cause is presumed to be genetic.

**PROGNOSIS**
In childhood absence epilepsy, in which typical absence seizures are the only type of seizures suffered by the child; the seizures cease spontaneously after a few years. In other epileptic syndromes (in which absence seizures may coexist with other types of seizures) prognosis is varied, depending on the syndrome. Absence seizures have significant impact on quality of life. The episode of unconsciousness may occur at any time. Absence seizures usually occur without warning. Affected children need to take precaution to prevent injury during absences. Often school staff are the first to notice the recurrent episodes of absences and treatment is needed because of the impact on learning.

Please refer to CD-ROM for full text and references.

**Search date October 2002**

*Paddy O'Neill and Tony Roberts*

## What are the effects of treatments?

### LIKELY TO BE BENEFICIAL

#### Ibuprofen

One RCT in children aged 1–6 years receiving antibiotic treatment found that ibuprofen versus placebo significantly reduced earache as assessed by parental observation after 2 days.

#### Paracetamol

One RCT in children aged 1–6 years receiving antibiotic treatment found that paracetamol versus placebo significantly reduced earache as assessed by parental observation after 2 days.

### TRADE OFF BETWEEN BENEFITS AND HARMS

#### Antibiotics versus placebo

We found four systematic reviews comparing antibiotics versus placebo in acute otitis media (AOM) but using different inclusion criteria and outcome measures. One review in children aged 4 months to 18 years found a significant reduction in symptoms with a range of antibiotics (cephalosporins, erythromycin, penicillins, trimethoprim–sulfamethoxazole [co-trimoxazole]) versus placebo after 7–14 days of treatment. Another review in children aged less than 2 years found no significant difference in clinical improvement with antibiotics (penicillins, sulphonamides, co-trimoxazole) versus placebo alone or versus placebo with myringotomy❻. A third review in children aged 4 weeks to 18 years found that antibiotics (ampicillin, amoxicillin) versus placebo or observational treatment significantly reduced clinical failure rate within 2–7 days. The final review in children aged 6 months to 15 years found that early use of antibiotics (erythromycin, penicillins) versus placebo significantly reduced the proportion of children still in pain 2–7 days after presentation and reduced the risk of developing contralateral AOM. This review also found that antibiotics increased the risk of vomiting, diarrhoea, or rashes.

#### Choice of antibiotic regimen

One systematic review in children aged 4 months to 18 years found no significant difference between a range of antibiotics in rate of treatment success at 7–14 days or of middle ear effusion at 30 days. Another systematic review in children aged 4 weeks to 18 years found no significant difference between antibiotics in clinical failure rates within 7–14 days. The second review also found that adverse effects, primarily gastrointestinal, were more common with cefixime versus amoxicillin or ampicillin, and were more common with amoxicillin/clavulanate (original formulation) versus azithromycin.

#### Immediate versus delayed antibiotic treatment

One RCT in children aged 6 months to 10 years found that immediate versus delayed antibiotic treatment significantly reduced the number of days of earache, ear discharge, and amount of daily paracetamol used after the first 24 hours of illness but found no difference in daily pain scores. It also found a significant increase in diarrhoea with immediate versus delayed antibiotic treatment.

▶

# Acute otitis media

### Short versus longer courses of antibiotics

One systematic review and two subsequent RCTs have found that 10 day versus 5 day courses of antibiotics significantly reduce treatment failure, relapse, and reinfection at 8–19 days, but found no significant difference at 20–30 days.

## LIKELY TO BE BENEFICIAL

### Myringotomy

One RCT in infants aged 3 months to 1 year found no significant difference in resolution of clinical symptoms with myringotomy only versus antibiotic only or myringotomy plus antibiotic but found higher rates of persistent infection with myringotomy only. A second RCT in children aged 2–12 years found no significant difference in reduction of pain at 24 hours or 7 days with myringotomy versus no treatment. A third RCT in children aged 7 months to 12 years found significantly higher rates of initial treatment failure (resolution of symptoms within 12 hours) for severe episodes of AOM treated by myringotomy and placebo versus antibiotic.

## What are the effects of interventions to prevent recurrence?

## LIKELY TO BE BENEFICIAL

### Xylitol chewing gum or syrup

One RCT found that xylitol syrup or chewing gum versus control significantly reduced the incidence of AOM over 3 months. It found no significant difference with xylitol lozenges versus control gum. More children taking xylitol versus control withdrew because of abdominal pain or other unspecified reasons.

## TRADE OFF BETWEEN BENEFITS AND HARMS

### Long term antibiotic prophylaxis

One systematic review in children and adults has found that long term antibiotic prophylaxis versus placebo significantly reduces recurrence of acute otitis media after 1 month. However, one subsequent RCT in children aged 3 months to 6 years found no significant difference between antibiotic prophylaxis and placebo in preventing recurrence. We found insufficient evidence on which antibiotic to use, for how long, and how many previous episodes of AOM justify starting preventive treatment.

## LIKELY TO BE INEFFECTIVE OR HARMFUL

### Tympanostomy (ventilation tubes)

One small RCT found that tympanostomy**ⓖ** tube insertion versus myringotomy alone or no surgery significantly reduced the mean number of AOM episodes during the first 6-month period after treatment but not during the subsequent 18 months. It also found a trend for more recurrent infections and worse hearing, after tube extrusion, in those treated with tympanostomy.

**DEFINITION** Otitis media is an inflammation in the middle ear. Subcategories include AOM, recurrent AOM, and chronic suppurative otitis media. AOM is the presence of middle ear effusion in conjunction with rapid onset of one or more signs or symptoms of inflammation of the middle ear. Uncomplicated AOM is limited to the middle ear cleft.[1] AOM presents with systemic and local signs, and has a rapid onset. The persistence of an effusion beyond 3 months without signs of infection defines otitis media with effusion (also known as "glue ear"). Chronic suppurative otitis media is characterised by continuing inflammation in the middle ear causing discharge (otorrhoea) through a perforated tympanic membrane.

**INCIDENCE/ PREVALENCE**  AOM is common and has a high morbidity and low mortality in otherwise healthy children. In the UK, about 30% of children under 3 years old visit their general practitioner with AOM each year and 97% receive antimicrobial treatment.[2] By 3 months of age, 10% of children have had an episode of AOM. It is the most common reason for outpatient antimicrobial treatment in the USA.[3]

**AETIOLOGY/ RISK FACTORS**  The most common bacterial causes for AOM in the USA and UK are *Streptococcus pneumoniae*, *Haemophilus influenzae*, and *Moraxella catarrhalis*.[2] Similar pathogens are found in Colombia.[4] The incidence of penicillin resistant *S pneumoniae* has risen, but rates differ between countries. The most important risk factors for AOM are young age and attendance at daycare centres, such as nursery schools. Other risk factors include being white; male sex; a history of enlarged adenoids, tonsillitis, or asthma; multiple previous episodes; bottle feeding; a history of ear infections in parents or siblings; and use of a soother or pacifier. The evidence for an effect of environmental tobacco smoke is controversial.[2]

**PROGNOSIS**  In about 80% of children the condition resolves in about 3 days without antibiotic treatment. Serious complications are rare in otherwise healthy children but include hearing loss, mastoiditis🅖, meningitis, and recurrent attacks.[2] The World Health Organization estimates that each year 51 000 children under the age of 5 years die from complications of otitis media in developing countries.[5]

Please refer to CD-ROM for full text and references.

# Asthma and other wheezing disorders of childhood

**Search date October 2002**

*Duncan Keeley and Michael McKean*

## What are the effects of treatments for acute asthma in children?

### BENEFICIAL

#### Oxygen

An RCT of oxygen versus no oxygen treatment in acute severe asthma would be considered unethical. One prospective cohort study and clinical experience support the need for oxygen in acute asthma.

#### High dose inhaled corticosteroids

We found one systematic review that identified four RCTs comparing high dose inhaled versus oral corticosteroids in children. Three RCTs found no significant difference in hospital admission with nebulised budesonide or dexamethasone versus oral prednisolone in children with mild to moderate asthma. One RCT in children with moderate to severe asthma found that oral prednisolone versus inhaled fluticasone significantly reduced hospital admission and improved lung function at 4 hours. A subsequent RCT in children aged 4–16 years found that nebulised fluticasone versus oral prednisolone significantly improved lung function over 7 days. Another RCT in children aged 5–16 years admitted to hospital with severe asthma found no significant difference with nebulised budesonide versus oral prednisolone in lung function at 24 hours or 24 days after admission.

#### Inhaled ipratropium bromide added to $\beta_2$ agonists (in emergency room)

One systematic review has found that in children aged 18 months to 17 years multiple doses of inhaled ipratropium bromide plus an inhaled $\beta_2$ agonist (fenoterol or salbutamol●) versus the $\beta_2$ agonist alone reduce hospital admissions and improve lung function in children with severe asthma exacerbations. In children with mild to moderate asthma exacerbations, a single dose of inhaled ipratropium bromide plus a $\beta_2$ agonist (fenoterol, salbutamol, or terbutaline) versus a $\beta_2$ agonist alone significantly improves lung function for up to 2 hours, but does not significantly reduce hospital admissions.

#### Metered dose inhaler plus spacer devices for delivery of $\beta_2$ agonists (as effective as nebulisers)

One systematic review in children with acute but not life threatening asthma who were old enough to use a spacer has found no significant difference in hospital admission rates with a metered dose inhaler plus a spacer versus nebulisation for delivering $\beta_2$ agonists (fenoterol, salbutamol, or terbutaline) or $\beta$ agonist (orciprenaline●). Children using metered dose inhaler with spacer may have shorter stays in emergency departments, less hypoxia, and lower pulse rates compared with children receiving $\beta_2$ agonist by nebulisation.

#### Oral corticosteroids

One systematic review has found that oral corticosteroids (prednisone or prednisolone) versus placebo within 45 minutes of an acute asthma attack significantly reduce hospital admission.

LIKELY TO BE BENEFICIAL

## Intravenous theophylline

One systematic review found that in children aged 1–19 years admitted to hospital with severe asthma, intravenous theophylline versus placebo significantly improved lung function and symptom scores 6–8 hours after treatment but found no significant difference in number of bronchodilator treatments required or length of hospital stay. A subsequent RCT found that in children aged 1–17 years admitted to intensive care unit with severe asthma, intravenous theophylline versus control significantly decreased the time to reach clinical asthma score$\bigodot$ of 3 or less but found no significant difference in length of stay in intensive care unit.

UNKNOWN EFFECTIVENESS

## Inhaled ipratropium bromide added to $\beta_2$ agonists (after initial stabilisation)

One RCT in children admitted to hospital with initially stabilised severe asthma found no significant difference in clinical asthma scores during the first 36 hours with nebulised ipratropium bromide versus placebo added to salbutamol and corticosteroid (hydrocortisone or prednisone).

---

## *What are the effects of single agent prophylaxis in childhood asthma?*

BENEFICIAL

## Inhaled corticosteroids

One systematic review has found that inhaled corticosteroids (betamethasone, beclometasone, budesonide, flunisolide, or fluticasone) versus placebo improve symptoms and lung function in children with asthma. Two systematic reviews of studies with long term follow up and a subsequent long term RCT have found no evidence of growth retardation in children with asthma treated with inhaled corticosteroids. Some shorter term studies found reduced growth velocity. One RCT in children aged 6–16 years found no significant difference in improvement of asthma symptoms with inhaled beclometasone versus theophylline, but found less use of bronchodilators and oral corticosteroids with inhaled beclometasone. Small RCTs have found inhaled corticosteroids to be more effective than sodium cromoglicate in improving symptoms and lung function. RCTs in children aged 5–16 years have found that inhaled corticosteroids (beclometasone, budesonide, or fluticasone) versus inhaled long acting $\beta_2$ agonists (salmeterol) or inhaled nedocromil improve symptoms and lung function in children with asthma.

## Inhaled nedocromil

Two RCTs in children aged 6–17 years found that inhaled nedocromil versus placebo significantly reduces asthma symptom scores, asthma severity, broncho-dilator use, and lung function. One large RCT in children aged 5–12 years with mild to moderate asthma found no significant difference with nedocromil versus budesonide versus placebo in lung function, hospital admission rate, or the symptom score on diary cards, but found that budesonide was superior to nedocromil, and that nedocromil was superior to placebo in several measures of asthma symptoms and morbidity.

## Oral montelukast

One RCT in children aged 6–14 years found that oral montelukast versus placebo significantly increased (from baseline) the mean morning forced expiratory volume in 1 second and significantly reduced the total daily $\beta_2$ agonist use but found no ▶

significant difference in daytime asthma symptom score or in nocturnal awakenings with asthma. Another RCT in children aged 2–5 years found that oral montelukast versus placebo significantly improved average daytime symptom scores and reduced the need for rescue oral steroid courses but found no significant difference in average overnight asthma symptom scores. We found no RCTs directly comparing oral montelukast versus inhaled corticosteroids.

## LIKELY TO BE BENEFICIAL

### Inhaled sodium cromoglicate

One systematic review found insufficient evidence for prophylactic treatment with sodium cromoglicate in children aged less than 1 year to 18 years. Several small comparative RCTs have found sodium cromoglicate to be less effective than inhaled corticosteroids in improving symptoms and lung function.

## TRADE OFF BETWEEN BENEFITS AND HARMS

### Inhaled salmeterol

Two RCTs in children aged 4–14 years found that inhaled salmeterol versus placebo significantly improved lung function but found conflicting evidence about a reduced salbutamol use. One RCT comparing inhaled salmeterol versus beclometasone found that salmeterol was associated with a significant deterioration in bronchial reactivity.

### Oral theophylline

One small RCT in children aged 6–15 years found that oral theophylline versus placebo significantly increased mean morning peak expiratory flow rate and significantly reduced the mean number of acute night time attacks and doses of bronchodilator used. Another RCT in children aged 6–16 years found no significant difference in improvement of asthma symptoms with oral theophylline versus inhaled beclometasone, but found greater use of bronchodilators and oral corticosteroids with theophylline over 1 year. Theophylline has serious adverse effects (cardiac arrhythmia, convulsions) if therapeutic blood concentrations are exceeded.

---

## What are the effects of additional treatments in childhood asthma inadequately controlled by standard dose inhaled corticosteroids?

## UNKNOWN EFFECTIVENESS

### Increased dose of inhaled corticosteroid

One RCT in children aged 6–16 years taking inhaled beclometasone comparing the addition of a second dose of inhaled corticosteroid (beclometasone) versus placebo found no significant difference in lung function, symptom scores, exacerbation rates, or bronchial reactivity but found significant reduction of growth velocity at 1 year.

### Long acting $\beta_2$ agonists

One RCT in children aged 6–16 years found that addition of a long acting $\beta_2$ agonist (salmeterol) increased peak expiratory flow rates in the first few months of treatment but found no increase after 1 year. A second short term RCT in children aged 4–16 years also found increased morning peak expiratory flow rates and more symptom free days at 3 months with addition of a long acting $\beta_2$ agonist (salmeterol).

◀ **Oral leukotriene receptor antagonists**

One crossover RCT in children aged 6–14 years with persistent asthma who had been taking inhaled budesonide for at least 6 weeks found that the addition of oral montelukast versus placebo significantly improved lung function and decreased the proportion of days with asthma exacerbations over 4 weeks. These differences were statistically significant but modest in clinical terms.

**Oral theophylline**

One small RCT found that addition of theophylline versus placebo to previous treatment significantly increased the proportion of symptom free days and significantly reduced the use of additional β agonist (orciprenaline) and additional corticosteroid (beclometasone or prednisolone) over 4 weeks.

## What are the effects of treatments for acute wheezing in infants?

**UNKNOWN EFFECTIVENESS**

### Addition of ipratropium bromide to long acting β₂ agonist

One RCT identified by a systematic review in infants aged 3–24 months found that addition of ipratropium bromide to fenoterol versus fenoterol alone significantly reduced the proportion of infants receiving further treatment 45 minutes after initial treatment.

### High dose inhaled corticosteroids

One systematic review found that high dose inhaled corticosteroids versus placebo reduced the requirement for oral corticosteroids but the difference was not statistically significant. The review also found a clear preference for the inhaled corticosteroids by the children's parents over placebo. The clinical importance of these results is unclear.

### Inhaled ipratropium bromide

We found no RCTs comparing inhaled ipratropium bromide versus placebo for treating acute wheeze.

### Oral corticosteroids

One small RCT found no significant difference in daily symptom scores with oral prednisolone versus placebo.

### Short acting β₂ agonists

One RCT in infants aged 3 months to 2 years found that nebulised salbutamol versus placebo significantly improved respiratory rate but found no significant difference in hospital admission. Another RCT that included infants aged less than 18 months to 36 months found no significant difference in change from baseline in clinical symptom scores with nebulised salbutamol versus placebo.

### Short acting β₂ agonists delivered by metered dose inhaler/spacer versus nebuliser

Two RCTs in children aged up to 5 years found no significant difference in hospital admission with delivery of salbutamol through a metered dose inhaler plus spacer versus nebulised salbutamol. Another RCT in infants aged 1–24 months found no significant difference in improvement of symptoms with delivery of terbutaline through a metered dose inhaler plus spacer versus nebulised terbutaline. Nebulised β₂ agonists may cause tachycardia, tremor, and hypokalaemia.

# Asthma and other wheezing disorders of childhood

## What are the effects of prophylaxis in wheezing infants?

### LIKELY TO BE BENEFICIAL

**Oral short acting $\beta_2$ agonist**

One RCT identified by a systematic review in infants aged 3–14 months found that oral salbutamol versus placebo significantly reduced treatment failures.

### TRADE OFF BETWEEN BENEFITS AND HARMS

**Higher dose inhaled corticosteroids**

One RCT in infants aged 6–30 months found that higher prophylactic doses of inhaled corticosteroids (budesonide) versus placebo significantly reduced symptoms and the proportion of children with acute wheezing episodes during a 12 week period but found no significant reduction in the proportion of wheezing episodes per infant. Another RCT in infants aged 11–36 months found that higher prophylactic doses of inhaled corticosteroid (budesonide) significantly reduced the proportion of days requiring oral prednisolone and symptoms of wheezing and sleep disturbance but found no significant improvement for cough. Higher doses of inhaled corticosteroids have the potential for adverse effects.

### UNKNOWN EFFECTIVENESS

**Inhaled ipratropium bromide**

One small RCT identified by a systematic review found no significant difference in relief of symptoms with nebulised ipratropium bromide versus placebo. The study may have lacked power to exclude a clinically important difference between treatments.

**Inhaled short acting $\beta_2$ agonist**

Two RCTs identified by a systematic review in infants aged up to 2 years found no significant improvement in symptoms with inhaled salbutamol versus placebo.

**Lower dose inhaled corticosteroids**

Three RCTs found no clear evidence of effectiveness with lower prophylactic doses of inhaled corticosteroids (budesonide) in children aged 1 week to 6 years with recurrent wheeze.

### UNLIKELY TO BE BENEFICIAL

**Addition of inhaled corticosteroid to short acting $\beta_2$ agonist**

One RCT found no significant improvement in symptoms with addition of inhaled beclometasone versus placebo to inhaled salbutamol.

**DEFINITION**   **Childhood asthma** is characterised by chronic or recurrent cough and wheeze. The diagnosis is confirmed by demonstrating reversible airway obstruction in children old enough to perform peak flow measurements or spirometry. Diagnosing asthma in children requires exclusion of other causes of recurrent respiratory symptoms. **Wheezing in infants** is characterised by a high pitched purring or whistling sound produced predominantly during breathing out and is commonly associated with an acute viral infection such as bronchiolitis (see bronchiolitis, p 56) or asthma. These are not easy to distinguish clinically.

**INCIDENCE/**   **Childhood asthma:** Surveys have found increasing prevalence in children
**PREVALENCE**   diagnosed with asthma. The increase is more than can be explained by an increased readiness to diagnose asthma. One questionnaire study from Aberdeen, Scotland, surveyed 2510 children aged 8–13 years in 1964 and 3403 children in 1989. Over the 25 years, diagnosis of asthma rose from 4% to 10%.[1] The increase in prevalence of childhood asthma from the 1960s to

1980s was accompanied by an increase in hospitals admissions over the same period. In England and Wales this was a sixfold increase.[2] **Wheezing in infants** is common and seems to be increasing though the magnitude of any increase is not clear. One Scottish cross-sectional study (2510 children aged 8–13 years in 1964 and 3403 children in 1989) found that prevalence of wheeze rose from 10% in 1964 to 20% in 1989 and episodes of shortness of breath rose from 5% to 10% over the same period.[1] Difficulties in defining clear groups (phenotypes) and the transient nature of the symptoms, which often resolve spontaneously, have confounded many studies.

**AETIOLOGY/ RISK FACTORS**

**Childhood asthma:** Asthma is more common in children with a personal or family history of atopy; severity and frequency of wheezing episodes and presence of variable airway obstruction or bronchial hyperresponsiveness. Precipitating factors for symptoms and acute episodes include infection, house dust mites, allergens from pet animals, exposure to tobacco smoke, and anxiety. **Wheezing in infants:** Most wheezing episodes in infancy are precipitated by viral respiratory infections.

**PROGNOSIS**

**Childhood asthma:** A British longitudinal study of children born in 1970 found that 29% of 5 year olds wheezing in the past year were still wheezing at the age of 10 years.[3] Another study followed a group of children in Melbourne, Australia from age 7 years (in 1964) into adulthood. The study found a large proportion (73%) of 14 year olds with infrequent symptoms had little or no symptoms by the age of 28 years, whereas two thirds of those 14 year olds with frequent wheezing still had recurrent attacks at the age of 28 years.[4] **Wheezing in infants:** The results of one cohort study (826 infants followed from birth to 6 years) suggests that there may be at least three different prognostic categories for wheezing in infants.[5] The study found one group (14% of total, with risk factors for atopic asthma such as elevated immunoglobulin E levels and maternal history of asthma) were "persistent wheezers" who initially suffered wheeze during viral infections, but the wheezing persisted into school age.[5] A second group (20% of total, with reduced lung function as infants but no early markers of atopy) were "transient wheezers" who also suffered wheeze during viral infections but stopped wheezing after the first 3 years of life. A third group (15% of total) were "late onset wheezers" who did not wheeze when aged under 3 years but had developed wheeze by school age.[5] Another retrospective cohort study found that 14% of children with one attack and 23% of children with four or more attacks in the first year of life had experienced at least one wheezing illness in their past year at age 10 years.[3] Administering inhaled treatments to young children can be difficult. Inconsistencies in results could reflect the effects of the differences in the drugs used, delivery devices used, dosages used, and the differences in the pattern of wheezing illnesses and treatment responses among young children.

Please refer to CD-ROM for full text and references.

Child health

# Bronchiolitis

Search date February 2003

*Juan Manuel Lozano*

---

## What are the effects of preventive interventions?

### BENEFICIAL

**Respiratory syncytial virus immunoglobulins or palivizumab (monoclonal antibody) in children at high risk**

One systematic review has found that, in children born prematurely, in children with bronchopulmonary dysplasia, and in children with a combination of risk factors, prophylactic respiratory syncytial virus immunoglobulin or palivizumab (monoclonal antibody) reduces admission rates to hospital and intensive care units compared with placebo or no prophylaxis.

### UNKNOWN EFFECTIVENESS

**Nursing interventions (cohort segregation⊕, handwashing, gowns, masks, gloves, and goggles) in children admitted to hospital**

We found no RCTs about the effects of these interventions to prevent spread of bronchiolitis to other children.

---

## What are the effects of treatments?

### UNKNOWN EFFECTIVENESS

**Bronchodilators (inhaled salbutamol, inhaled adrenaline [epinephrine])**

Systematic reviews have found that, inhaled bronchodilators achieve short term improvement in overall clinical scores compared with placebo in children treated in hospital, emergency departments, and outpatient clinics. They have found no evidence that bronchodilators reduce admission rates or produce a clinically important improvement in oxygen saturation. Subsequent RCTs found no evidence that nebulised adrenaline, changed short term outcomes during the first 4 days of illness in infants or the duration of hospital stay compared with 0.9% sodium chloride. One small RCT found that nebulised adrenaline reduced the rate of hospital admission compared with salbutamol. However, we were unable to draw reliable conclusions from this small study.

**Corticosteroids**

One systematic review and 10 additional RCTs found limited and conflicting evidence on the effects of corticosteroids compared with placebo.

**Routine broad spectrum antibiotics**

We found no evidence in children with bronchiolitis alone. One unblinded RCT in children with bronchiolitis and uncomplicated pneumonia (crackles on auscultation or consolidation on a chest radiograph) found no significant difference in clinical scores with routine use of antibiotics (ampicillin, penicillin, or erythromycin) compared with placebo. However, the RCT may have lacked power to exclude a clinically important effect.

**Ribavirin**

One systematic review found insufficient evidence that ribavirin reduced mortality, risk of respiratory deterioration, or duration of hospital stay in children admitted to hospital with respiratory syncytial virus bronchiolitis. It found some evidence that ribavirin reduced the duration of mechanical ventilation. Two subsequent RCTs ▶

◀ found no evidence that ribavirin reduced duration of hospital stay, admission rate because of lower respiratory tract symptoms during the first year after the acute episode, or the frequency of recurrent wheezing illness over 1 year of follow up.

**Respiratory syncytial virus immunoglobulins, pooled immunoglobulins, or palivizumab (monoclonal antibody)**
RCTs found insufficient evidence on the effects of immunoglobulin treatment.

**DEFINITION** Bronchiolitis is a virally induced acute bronchiolar inflammation that is associated with signs and symptoms of airway obstruction. Diagnosis is based on clinical findings. Clinical manifestations include fever, rhinitis (inflammation of the nasal mucosa), tachypnoea, expiratory wheezing, cough, rales, use of accessory muscles, apnoea (absence of breathing), dyspnoea (difficulty in breathing), alar flaring (flaring of the nostrils), and retractions (indrawing of the intercostal soft tissues on inspiration). Disease severity🅖 of bronchiolitis may be classified clinically as mild, moderate, or severe.

**INCIDENCE/** Bronchiolitis is the most common lower respiratory tract infection in infants,
**PREVALENCE** occurring in a seasonal pattern with highest incidence in the winter in temperate climates,[1] and in the rainy season in warmer countries. Each year in the USA, about 21% of infants have lower respiratory tract disease and 6–10/1000 infants are admitted to hospital for bronchiolitis (1–2% of children < 12 months of age).[2] The peak rate of admission occurs in infants aged 2–6 months.[3]

**AETIOLOGY/** Respiratory syncytial virus is responsible for bronchiolitis in 70% of cases. This
**RISK FACTORS** figure reaches 80–100% in the winter months. However, in early spring, parainfluenza virus type 3 is often responsible.[1]

**PROGNOSIS** **Morbidity and mortality:** Disease severity is related to the size of the infant, and to the proximity and frequency of contact with infective infants. Children at increased risk of morbidity and mortality are those with congenital heart disease, chronic lung disease, history of premature birth, hypoxia, and age less than 6 weeks.[4] Other factors associated with a prolonged or complicated hospital stay include a history of apnoea or respiratory arrest, pulmonary consolidation seen on a chest radiograph, and (in North America) people of Native American or Inuit race.[5] The risk of death within 2 weeks is high for children with congenital heart disease (3.4%) or chronic lung disease (3.5%) as compared with other groups combined (0.1%).[4] Rates of admission to intensive care units (range 31–36%) and need for mechanical ventilation (range 11–19%) are similar among all high risk groups.[4] The percentage of these children needing oxygen supplementation is also high (range 63–80%).[4] In contrast, rates of intensive care unit admission (15%) and ventilation (8%) in such children are markedly lower.[6] **Long term prognosis:** Information on long term prognosis varies among studies. One small prospective study of two matched cohorts (25 children with bronchiolitis; 25 children without) found no evidence that bronchiolitis requiring outpatient treatment is associated with an increased risk of asthma in the long term.[7] Possible confounding factors include variation in illness severity, smoke exposure, and being in overcrowded environments.[8] We found one prospective study in 50 randomly selected infants admitted with bronchiolitis, followed up by questionnaire for 5 years and a visit in the fifth year. It found a doubling of asthma incidence compared with the general population, although there was large (30%) loss to follow up and no matched control group.[9]

Please refer to CD-ROM for full text and references.

# Cardiorespiratory arrest in children

**Search date October 2002**

*Kate Ackerman and David Creery*

## What are the effects of treatments for non-submersion out of hospital cardiorespiratory arrest?

### LIKELY TO BE BENEFICIAL

**Bag–mask ventilation**

We found no RCTs. One controlled clinical trial in children requiring airway management in the community found no significant difference between endotracheal intubation and bag–mask ventilation in survival or neurological outcome.

**Bystander cardiopulmonary resuscitation**

It is widely accepted that cardiopulmonary resuscitation should be undertaken in children who have arrested. Placebo controlled trials would be considered unethical. One systematic review of observational studies found that children who received bystander cardiopulmonary resuscitation versus no bystander cardiopulmonary resuscitation were more likely to survive to hospital discharge.

**Intubation**

See bag–mask ventilation.

**Airway management and ventilation; direct current cardiac shock (for ventricular fibrillation or pulseless ventricular tachycardia⊕); standard dose intravenous adrenaline (epinephrine)**

Although we found no direct evidence to support their use, widespread consensus based on indirect evidence and extrapolation from adult data holds that these interventions should be universally applied to children who have arrested. Placebo controlled trials would be considered unethical.

### UNKNOWN EFFECTIVENESS

**High dose intravenous adrenaline (epinephrine); intravenous bicarbonate; intravenous calcium; training parents to perform cardiopulmonary resuscitation**

We found no RCTs or prospective cohort studies on the effects of these interventions in children who have arrested in the community.

**DEFINITION**    Non-submersion out of hospital cardiorespiratory arrest in children is a state of pulselessness and apnoea occurring outside of a medical facility and not caused by submersion in water.[1]

**INCIDENCE/**    We found 12 studies (3 prospective, 9 retrospective) reporting the incidence
**PREVALENCE**    of non-submersion out of hospital cardiorespiratory arrest in children⊕.[2–13] Eleven studies reported the incidence in both adults and children, and eight reported the incidence in children.[2–9,11–13] Incidence of arrests in the general population ranged from 2.2–5.7/100 000 people a year (mean 3.1, 95% CI 2.1 to 4.1). Incidence of arrests in children ranged from 6.9–18.0/100 000 children a year (mean 10.6, 95% CI 7.1 to 14.1).[8] One prospective study (300 children) found that about 50% of out of hospital cardiorespiratory arrests occurred in children under 12 months, and about two thirds occurred in children under 18 months.[11]

**AETIOLOGY/**    We found 26 studies reporting the causes of non-submersion pulseless
**RISK FACTORS**    arrests⊕ in a total of 1574 children. The commonest causes of arrest were undetermined causes as in sudden infant death syndrome⊕ (39%), trauma (18%), chronic disease (7%), and pneumonia (4%)⊕.[1,3–12,14–28]

**PROGNOSIS**

We found no systematic review that investigated non-submersion arrests alone. We found 27 studies (5 prospective, 22 retrospective; total of 1754 children) that reported out of hospital arrest.[1-12,14-28] The overall survival rate following out of hospital arrest was 5% (87 children). Nineteen of these studies (1140 children) found that of the 48 surviving children, 12 (25%) had no or mild neurological disability and 36 (75%) had moderate or severe neurological disability. We found one systematic review (search date 1997), which reported outcomes after cardiopulmonary resuscitation for both in hospital and out of hospital arrests in children of any cause, including submersion.[29] Studies were excluded if they did not report survival. The review found evidence from prospective and retrospective observational studies that out of hospital arrest of any cause in children carries a poorer prognosis than arrest within hospital (132/1568 children [8%] survived to hospital discharge after out of hospital arrest v 129/544 children [24%] after in hospital arrests). About half of the survivors were involved in studies that reported neurological outcome. Of these, survival with "good neurological outcome" (i.e. normal or mild neurological deficit) was higher in children who arrested in hospital compared with those who arrested elsewhere (60/77 surviving children [78%] in hospital v 28/68 [41%] elsewhere).[29]

Please refer to CD-ROM for full text and references.

# Constipation in children

Search date April 2003

*Gregory Rubin*

---

## What are the effects of treatments?

### Medical treatment plus toilet training or biofeedback (compared with medical treatment alone)

One small, short term RCT in children with encopresis found that adding toilet training or biofeedback to medical treatment (enemas and osmotic or stimulant laxatives) reduced soiling compared with medical treatment alone.

### Cisapride

Two RCTs in people aged 2–18 years found that cisapride improved stool frequency and symptoms of constipation after 8–12 weeks of treatment in an outpatient setting compared with placebo. We found no evidence from primary care settings. Use of cisapride has been restricted in some countries because of adverse cardiac effects.

### Biofeedback training

One systematic review found no significant difference between biofeedback plus conventional treatment and conventional treatment alone in persisting defecation problems at 12 months.

### Increased dietary fibre

We found no RCTs in children on the effects of increasing dietary fibre.

### Osmotic laxatives

We found no RCTs that compared osmotic laxatives with placebo in children. Two small RCTs found no significant difference in stool frequency or consistency between lactulose and lactitol after 2–4 weeks in children aged 8 months to 16 years. One of these RCTs found that lactulose increased abdominal pain and flatulence compared with lactitol. One small, short term RCT in children with encopresis found that adding toilet training or biofeedback to stimulant or osmotic laxatives reduced soiling compared with medical treatment alone.

### Stimulant laxatives

One systematic review found no reliable RCTs comparing stimulant laxatives versus placebo or other treatments in children. One small, short term RCT found that adding toilet training or biofeedback to stimulant or osmotic laxatives reduced soiling compared with medical treatment alone.

**DEFINITION** Constipation is characterised by infrequent bowel evacuations; hard, small faeces; or difficult or painful defecation. The frequency of bowel evacuation varies from person to person.[1] Encopresis is defined as involuntary bowel movements in inappropriate places at least once a month for 3 months or more, in children aged 4 years and older.[2]

**INCIDENCE/ PREVALENCE** Constipation with or without encopresis is common in children. It accounts for 3% of consultations to paediatric outpatient clinics and 25% of paediatric gastroenterology consultations in the USA.[3] Encopresis has been reported in 2% of children at school entry. The peak incidence is at 2–4 years of age. ▶

**AETIOLOGY/ RISK FACTORS**  No cause is discovered in 90–95% of children with constipation. Low fibre intake and a family history of constipation may be associated factors.[4] Psycho-social factors are often suspected, although most children with constipation are developmentally normal.[3] Chronic constipation can lead to progressive faecal retention, distension of the rectum, and loss of sensory and motor function. Organic causes for constipation are uncommon, but include Hirschsprung's disease (1/5000 births; male to female ratio of 4 : 1; constipation invariably present from birth), cystic fibrosis, anorectal physiological abnormalities, anal fissures, constipating drugs, dehydrating metabolic conditions, and other forms of malabsorption.[3]

**PROGNOSIS**  Childhood constipation can be difficult to treat and often requires prolonged support, explanation, and medical treatment. In one long term follow up study of children presenting under the age of 5 years, 50% recovered within 1 year and 65–70% recovered within 2 years; the remainder required laxatives for daily bowel movements or continued to soil for years.[3] It is not known what proportion continue to have problems into adult life, although adults presenting with megarectum or megacolon often have a history of bowel problems from childhood.

Please refer to CD-ROM for full text and references.

# Depression in children and adolescents

**Search date September 2002**

*Philip Hazell*

---

## What are the effects of treatments?

### BENEFICIAL

#### Cognitive therapy (in mild to moderate depression)

One systematic review in children and adolescents with mild to moderate depression has found that cognitive behavioural therapy◉ significantly improves symptoms compared with non-specific support.

### LIKELY TO BE BENEFICIAL

#### Interpersonal therapy in adolescents (in mild to moderate depression)

Two RCTs found that interpersonal therapy◉ versus clinical monitoring or waiting list control significantly increased recovery rate over 12 weeks in adolescents with mild to moderate depression.

### TRADE OFF BETWEEN BENEFITS AND HARMS

#### Selective serotonin reuptake inhibitors

One RCT found no significant difference, one RCT found equivocal results (statistically significant differences on some depression measures but not others), and one RCT found a significant improvement in depressive symptoms with fluoxetine versus placebo after 8–9 weeks. One RCT found that, in adolescents with major depression, paroxetine versus placebo significantly improved remission after 8 weeks. We found no RCTs on other selective serotonin reuptake inhibitors. Selective serotonin reuptake inhibitors are frequently associated with dizziness, lightheadedness, drowsiness, poor concentration, nausea, headache, and fatigue if treatment is reduced or stopped.

### UNKNOWN EFFECTIVENESS

#### Cognitive therapy (depressed adolescents with depressed parent)

One RCT in depressed adolescents with depressed parents found no significant difference in recovery from depression with cognitive behavioural therapy plus usual care versus usual care alone over 2 years.

#### Electroconvulsive therapy

We found no RCTs on electroconvulsive therapy in children and adolescents with depression.

#### Intravenous clomipramine (adolescents)

One small RCT found that in non-suicidal adolescents, intravenous clomipramine versus placebo significantly reduced depression scores at 6 days. However, the trial was too small and brief for us to draw reliable conclusions.

#### Lithium

One RCT found no significant difference with lithium versus placebo in global assessment or depression scores after 6 weeks in children with depression and family history of bipolar affective disorder. Lithium was associated with adverse effects.

#### Long term effects of treatments

We found no systematic review or RCTs examining long term outcomes of interventions for depression in children and adolescents.

◀ **Monoamine oxidase inhibitors**

One RCT found insufficient evidence to compare moclobemide versus placebo in children aged 9–15 years with major depression. We found no RCTs on non-reversible monoamine oxidase inhibitors in children or adolescents.

## St John's Wort

We found no RCTs on St John's Wort (*Hypericum perforatum*) in children or adolescents with depression.

## Venlafaxine

One RCT found no significant difference with venlafaxine versus placebo in improvement of depressive symptoms in children and adolescents with major depression after 6 weeks.

## Family therapy; group treatments other than cognitive behavioural therapy

We found insufficient evidence in children and adolescents about the effects of these interventions.

### UNLIKELY TO BE BENEFICIAL

## Oral tricyclic antidepressants (adolescents)

One systematic review found no significant difference with oral tricyclic antidepressants (amitriptyline, desipramine, imipramine, nortriptyline) versus placebo in depression scores in adolescents and children with depression. Subgroup analyses found that oral tricyclic antidepressants versus placebo significantly reduced symptoms in adolescents but not in children. The review also found that oral tricyclic antidepressants were associated with adverse effects.

### LIKELY TO BE INEFFECTIVE OR HARMFUL

## Oral tricyclic antidepressants (children)

Subgroup analyses in one systematic review found no significant difference with oral tricyclic antidepressants (amitriptyline, desipramine, imipramine, nortriptyline) versus placebo in children with depression. The review also found that oral tricyclic antidepressants were associated with adverse effects.

**DEFINITION**   Compared with adult depression, depression in children (6–12 years) and adolescents (13–18 years) may have a more insidious onset, may be characterised more by irritability than sadness, and occurs more often in association with other conditions such as anxiety, conduct disorder, hyperkinesis, and learning problems.[1]

**INCIDENCE/**   Estimates of prevalence of depression among children and adolescents in the
**PREVALENCE**   community range from 2–6%.[2,3] Prevalence tends to increase with age, with a sharp rise around onset of puberty. Pre-adolescent boys and girls are affected equally by the condition, but depression is seen more frequently among adolescent girls than boys.[4]

**AETIOLOGY/**   The aetiology is uncertain, but may include genetic vulnerability,[5] childhood
**RISK FACTORS** events and current psychosocial adversity.[4]

**PROGNOSIS**   In children and adolescents, the recurrence rate following a first depressive episodes in childhood or adolescence is 70% by 5 years, which is similar to the recurrence rate in adults. It is not clear if this is related to severity of depression.[4] Young people experiencing a moderate to severe depressive ▶

# Depression in children and adolescents

episode may be more likely than adults to have a manic episode within the next few years.[4,6] Trials of treatment for child and adolescent depression have found high rates of spontaneous remission (as much as two thirds of people in some inpatient studies).

**Please refer to CD-ROM for full text and references.**

### Search date February 2003

*Jacqueline Dalby-Payne and Elizabeth Elliott*

Child health

---

## What are the effects of treatments?

**BENEFICIAL**

### Oral rehydration solutions (as effective as iv fluids)

One systematic review and two additional RCTs in children with mild to moderate dehydration in developed countries found no significant difference between oral rehydration solutions versus intravenous fluids in duration of diarrhoea, time spent in hospital, or weight gain at discharge. One small RCT in children with mild to moderate dehydration managed in the emergency department found that oral rehydration reduced length of stay in the department but did not significantly reduce admission to hospital compared with intravenous fluids. One RCT in children with severe dehydration in a developing country found that oral rehydration solutions reduced the duration of diarrhoea and increased weight gain at discharge, and was associated with fewer adverse effects compared with intravenous fluids.

**LIKELY TO BE BENEFICIAL**

### Lactose-free feeds (for duration of diarrhoea)

We found evidence from one systematic review and subsequent RCTs that lactose-free feeds versus feeds containing lactose reduce the duration of diarrhoea in children with mild to severe dehydration.

### Loperamide (reduces duration of diarrhoea, but adverse effects are unclear)

Two RCTs found that, in children with mild to moderate dehydration, loperamide versus placebo significantly reduces the duration of diarrhoea. Another RCT found no significant difference with loperamide versus placebo in the duration of diarrhoea. We found insufficient evidence about adverse effects.

**UNKNOWN EFFECTIVENESS**

### Clear fluids for rehydration (other than oral rehydration solutions)

We found no systematic review or RCTs on "clear fluids" (water, carbonated drinks, and translucent fruit juices) versus oral rehydration solutions for treatment of mild to moderate dehydration caused by acute gastroenteritis.

**DEFINITION**  Acute gastroenteritis is characterised by rapid onset of diarrhoea with or without vomiting, nausea, fever, and abdominal pain.[1] In children, the symptoms and signs can be non-specific.[2] Diarrhoea is defined as the frequent passage of unformed liquid stools.[3]

**INCIDENCE/ PREVALENCE**  Worldwide, about 3 billion–5 billion cases of acute gastroenteritis occur in children under 5 years of age each year.[4] In the UK, acute gastroenteritis accounts for 204/1000 general practitioner consultations each year in children under 5 years of age.[5] Gastroenteritis leads to hospital admission in 7/1000 children under 5 years of age a year in the UK[5] and 13/1000 in the USA.[6] In Australia, gastroenteritis accounts for 6% of all hospital admissions in children under 15 years of age.[7]

# Gastroenteritis in children

**AETIOLOGY/ RISK FACTORS**    In developed countries, acute gastroenteritis is predominantly caused by viruses (87%), of which rotavirus is most common;[8–11] bacteria cause most of the remaining cases, predominantly *Campylobacter*, *Salmonella*, *Shigella*, and *Escherichia coli*. In developing countries, bacterial pathogens are more frequent, although rotavirus is also a major cause of gastroenteritis.

**PROGNOSIS**    Acute gastroenteritis is usually self limiting but if untreated can result in morbidity and mortality secondary to water and electrolyte losses. Acute diarrhoea causes 4 million deaths a year in children under 5 years of age in Asia (excluding China), Africa, and Latin America, and over 80% of deaths occur in children under 2 years of age.[12] Although death is uncommon in developed countries, dehydration secondary to gastroenteritis is a significant cause of morbidity and need for hospital admission.[6,7,13]

Please refer to CD-ROM for full text and references.

# Gastro-oesophageal reflux in children

### Search date January 2003

*Yadlapalli Kumar and Rajini Sarvananthan*

## What are the effects of treatments?

### LIKELY TO BE BENEFICIAL

**Sodium alginate**

Two RCTs in infants and in children under 2 years old found that sodium alginate reduced the frequency of regurgitation at 8–14 days compared with placebo.

### UNKNOWN EFFECTIVENESS

**Domperidone**

We found insufficient evidence from one small RCT about effects of domeperidone in children with gastro-oesophageal reflux.

**Feed thickeners**

One systematic review of feed thickeners in newborn infants found no RCTs. One small RCT in older infants aged 1–16 weeks found no significant difference between carob flour and placebo thickening after 1 week, although the study may have lacked power to detect a clinically important difference.

**$H_2$ antagonists**

We found insufficient evidence from two small RCTs about effects of $H_2$ antagonists in children with gastro-oesophageal reflux. Neither RCT reported clinically meaningful results.

**Metoclopramide**

We found insufficient evidence from three small RCTs about the clinical effects of metoclopramide compared with placebo or other treatments.

**Positioning (left lateral or prone)**

We found insufficient evidence about clinical effects. Small crossover RCTs in children aged under 6 months found limited evidence that prone or left lateral positioning improved oesophageal pH variables compared with supine positioning. Both prone and left lateral positions may be associated with a higher risk of sudden infant death syndrome compared with supine positioning.

**Proton pump inhibitors**

We found no RCTs about proton pump inhibitors for gastro-oesophageal reflux in children.

**Surgery**

We found no RCTs about surgery for gastro-oesophageal reflux in children.

### LIKELY TO BE INEFFECTIVE OR HARMFUL

**Cisapride**

One systematic review found no significant difference between cisapride and placebo in the proportion of children with improved symptoms at the end of treatment. Cisapride has been withdrawn or restricted in several countries because of an association with heart rhythm abnormalities.

**DEFINITION**    Gastro-oesophageal reflux disease is the passive transfer of gastric contents into the oesophagus due to transient or chronic relaxation of the lower oesophageal sphincter.[1] A survey of 69 children (median age 16 months) with gastro-oesophageal reflux disease attending a tertiary referral centre found ▶

# Gastro-oesophageal reflux in children

that presenting symptoms were recurrent vomiting (72%), epigastric and abdominal pain (36%), feeding difficulties (29%), failure to thrive (28%), and irritability (19%).[2] However, results may not be generalisable to younger children or children presenting in primary care, who make up the majority of cases. Over 90% of children with gastro-oesophageal reflux disease have vomiting before 6 weeks of age.[1]

**INCIDENCE/ PREVALENCE**  Gastro-oesophageal regurgitation is considered a problem if it is frequent, persistent, and is associated with other symptoms such as increased crying, discomfort with regurgitation, and frequent back arching.[1,3] A cross-sectional survey of parents of 948 infants attending 19 primary care paediatric practices found that regurgitation of at least one episode a day was reported in 51% of infants aged 0–3 months. "Problematic" regurgitation occurred in significantly fewer infants (14% v 51%; P < 0.001).[3] Peak regurgitation reported as "problematic" was reported in 23% of infants aged 6 months.[3]

**AETIOLOGY/ RISK FACTORS**  Risk factors for gastro-oesophageal reflux disease include immaturity of the lower oesophageal sphincter, chronic relaxation of the sphincter, increased abdominal pressure, gastric distension, hiatus hernia, and oesophageal dys-motility.[1] Premature infants and children with severe neurodevelopmental problems or congenital oesophageal anomalies are particularly at risk.[1]

**PROGNOSIS**  Regurgitation is considered benign, and most cases resolve spontaneously by 12–18 months of age.[4] In a cross-sectional survey of 948 parents, the peak age for reporting four or more episodes of regurgitation was at 5 months of age (23%), which decreased to 7% at 7 months (P < 0.001). One cohort study found that those infants with frequent spilling🌀 in the first 2 years of life (90 days or more in the first 2 years) were more likely to have symptoms of gastro-oesophageal reflux at 9 years of age than those with no spilling (RR 2.3, 95% CI 1.3 to 4.0).[5] The prevalence of "problematic" regurgitation also reduced from 23% in infants aged 6 months to 3.25% in infants aged 10–12 months.[3] Rare complications of gastro-oesophageal reflux disease include oesophagitis with haematemesis and anaemia, respiratory problems (such as cough, apnoea, and recurrent wheeze), and failure to thrive.[1] A small comparative study (40 children) suggested that, when compared with healthy children, infants with gastro-oesophageal reflux disease had slower development of feeding skills and had problems affecting behaviour, swallowing, food intake, and mother–child interaction.[6]

Please refer to CD-ROM for full text and references.

Search date January 2003

*Teresa Kilgour and Sally Wade*

*Child health*

## What are the effects of treatments?

### LIKELY TO BE BENEFICIAL

#### Whey hydrolysate milk
One RCT found limited evidence that replacing cows' milk formula with whey hydrolysate formula☺ reduced crying recorded in a parental diary.

### TRADE OFF BETWEEN BENEFITS AND HARMS

#### Dicycloverine
Two systematic reviews of RCTs of variable quality found limited evidence that dicycloverine☺ reduced crying in infants with colic compared with placebo. RCTs found that dicycloverine increased drowsiness, constipation, and loose stools compared with placebo, but the difference did not reach significance. Case reports of harms in infants have included breathing difficulties, seizures, syncope, asphyxia, muscular hypotonia, and coma.

### UNKNOWN EFFECTIVENESS

#### Car ride simulation device
One RCT comparing a car ride simulation device plus non-specific reassurance, counselling mothers about specific management techniques plus non-specific reassurance, and non-specific reassurance alone, found no significant difference among groups in maternal anxiety or hours of infant crying over 2 weeks.

#### Casein hydrolysate milk
Two RCTs found insufficient evidence about the effects of replacing cows' milk formula with casein hydrolysate hypoallergenic formula☺.

#### Cranial osteopathy
We found no RCTs about the effects of cranial osteopathy☺ in infants with colic.

#### Focused counselling
One RCT comparing counselling mothers about specific management techniques (responding to crying with gentle soothing motion, avoiding over stimulation, using a pacifier, and prophylactic carrying) plus non-specific reassurance☺, a car ride simulation device plus non-specific reassurance, and non-specific reassurance alone, found no significant difference among groups in maternal anxiety or hours of infant crying over 2 weeks. Another small RCT found that focused counselling decreased duration and extent of crying compared with substitution of soya or cows' milk with casein hydrolysate formula.

#### Herbal tea
One small RCT found that herbal tea (containing extracts of camomile, vervain, liquorice, fennel, and balm mint in a sucrose solution) improved symptoms of colic rated by parents at 7 days compared with sucrose solution alone. However, we were unable to draw reliable conclusions from this small study.

#### Infant massage
One RCT found no significant difference between massage and a crib vibrator in colic related crying or parental rating of symptoms of infantile colic, but it may have lacked power to detect a clinically important difference.  ▶

# Infantile colic

**Low lactose (lactase treated) milk**

Four small crossover RCTs found insufficient evidence on the effects of low lactose (lactase treated) milk in infants with colic.

**Reduction of stimulation of the infant**

One RCT found limited evidence that advice to reduce stimulation (by not patting, lifting, or jiggling the baby, or by reducing auditory stimulation) reduced crying after 7 days in infants under 12 weeks of age compared with an empathetic interview. However, we were unable to draw reliable conclusions from this small study.

**Soya based infant feeds**

One small RCT found that soya based infant feeds☉ reduced the duration of crying in infants with colic compared with standard cows' milk formula. However, we were unable to draw reliable conclusions from this small study.

**Spinal manipulation**

Two RCTs found insufficient evidence about the effects of spinal manipulation☉.

**Sucrose solution**

One small crossover RCT found limited evidence that sucrose solution improved symptoms of colic as rated by parents after 12 days compared with placebo. However, we were unable to draw reliable conclusions from this small study.

## UNLIKELY TO BE BENEFICIAL

**Increased carrying**

One RCT found no significant difference in daily crying time between carrying the infant, even when not crying, for at least an additional 3 hours a day and a general advice group (to carry, check baby's nappy, feed, offer pacifier, place baby near mother, or use background stimulation such as music). The "advice to carry" group carried their babies for 4.5 hours daily compared with 2.6 hours daily in the general advice group.

**Simethicone (activated dimeticone)**

One RCT found no significant difference between simethicone (activated dimeticone) and placebo in colic rated by carers. Another RCT found no significant difference between simethicone and placebo in improvement as rated by parental interview, 24 hour diary, or behavioural observation. Another poor quality RCT found that simethicone reduced the number of crying attacks on days 4–7 of treatment compared with placebo.

**DEFINITION**    Infantile colic is defined as excessive crying in an otherwise healthy baby. The crying typically starts in the first few weeks of life and ends by 4–5 months. Excessive crying is defined as crying that lasts at least 3 hours a day, for 3 days a week, for at least 3 weeks.[1] Due to the natural course of infantile colic it can be difficult to interpret trials which do not include a placebo or no treatment group for comparison.

**INCIDENCE/**    Infantile colic causes 1/6 (17%) families to consult a health professional. One
**PREVALENCE**    systematic review of 15 community based studies found a wide variation in prevalence, which depended on study design and method of recording.[2] Two prospective studies identified by the review yielded prevalence rates of 5% and 19%.[2] One RCT (89 breast and formula fed infants) found that, at 2 weeks of age, the prevalence of crying more than 3 hours a day was 43% among formula fed infants and 16% among breastfed infants. The prevalence at 6 weeks was 12% (formula fed) and 31% (breast fed).[3]

◄ **AETIOLOGY/** The cause of infantile colic is unclear and, despite its name, might not have an
**RISK FACTORS** abdominal cause. It may reflect part of the normal distribution of infantile crying. Other possible explanations are painful intestinal contractions, lactose intolerance, gas, or parental misinterpretation of normal crying.[1]

**PROGNOSIS** Infantile colic improves with time. One study found that 29% of infants aged 1–3 months cried for more than 3 hours a day, but by 4–6 months of age the prevalence had fallen to 7–11%.[4]

Please refer to CD-ROM for full text and references.

# Measles

**Search date December 2002**

*Bazian Ltd*

---

## What are the effects of preventive interventions?

BENEFICIAL

### Live combined measles, mumps, and rubella (MMR) vaccine; live monovalent measles vaccine

Large cohort studies, large time series, and population surveillance data from different countries have all found that combined MMR🔾 and live monovalent measles vaccination programmes reduce the risk of measles infection to near zero, especially in populations in which vaccine coverage🔾 is high.

We found no RCTs comparing the effects of MMR versus no vaccination or placebo on measles infection rates. Such trials are likely to be considered unethical because of the large body of whole-population evidence finding benefit from vaccination.

Unlike live monovalent measles vaccine🔾, MMR additionally protects against mumps and rubella, which themselves cause serious complications (mumps causes orchitis, pancreatitis, infertility, meningoencephalitis, deafness, and congenital fetal abnormalities; rubella causes deafness, blindness, heart defects, liver, spleen and brain damage, and stillbirth).

One systematic review, one RCT, one large population based survey, and one population based study found no evidence that MMR was associated with acute developmental regression🔾. Large time series studies have consistently found no evidence that MMR or live monovalent measles vaccine was associated with autism.

One large, long term population surveillance study and one population based case control study found no evidence that either MMR or monovalent measles vaccine was associated with inflammatory bowel disease. One large cohort study and two population based case control studies found no association between monovalent measles vaccine and inflammatory bowel disease.

One systematic review and one additional RCT found that MMR and monovalent measles vaccine were associated with a small and similar risk of self limiting fever within 3 weeks of vaccination compared with 100% risk of acute fever in people with measles.

**DEFINITION**  Measles is an infectious disease caused by a ribonucleic acid paramyxoma-virus. The illness is characterised by an incubation period of 10–12 days; a prodromal period of 2–4 days with upper respiratory tract symptoms; Koplik's spots on mucosal membranes and high fever; followed by further fever, and a widespread maculopapular rash that persists for 5–6 days.[1]

**INCIDENCE/**  Measles incidence varies widely according to vaccination coverage. World-
**PREVALENCE**  wide, there are an estimated 30 million cases of measles each year,[2] but an incidence of only 0–10/100 000 people in countries with widespread vaccination programmes, such as the USA, UK, Mexico, India, China, Brazil, and Australia.[3] In the USA, before licensing of effective vaccines, more than 90% of people were infected by the age of 15 years. After licensing in 1963, incidence fell by about 98%.[1] Mean annual incidence in Finland was 366/100 000 in 1970,[4] but declined to about zero by the late 1990s.[5] Similarly, annual incidence declined to about zero in Chile, the English speaking Caribbean, and Cuba during the 1990s when vaccination programmes were introduced.[6,7]

**AETIOLOGY/ RISK FACTORS** Measles is highly contagious. The virus is spread through airborne droplets that persist for up to 2 hours in closed areas following the presence of an infected person. Measles is highly contagious. As with other infectious diseases, risk factors include overcrowding, low herd immunity🌀, and immunosuppression. People with immunosuppression, children younger than 5 years of age, and adults older than 20 years of age have a higher risk of severe complications and death, although these also occur in healthy people (see prognosis below).[1] Newborn babies have a lower risk of measles than older infants, owing to the persistence of protective maternal antibodies, although in recent US outbreaks, maternal antibody protection was lower than expected.[1]

**PROGNOSIS** The World Health Organization estimated that in the year 2000, measles caused 777 000 deaths and 27.5 million disability adjusted life years.[8] **Disease in healthy people:** In developed countries, most prognostic data come from the pre-vaccination era and from subsequent outbreaks in non-vaccinated populations. In the USA, about 30% of reported measles cases involve complications of the disease. From 1989–1991 in the USA, measles resurgence among young children (< 5 years) who had not been immunised led to 55 622 cases with more than 11 000 hospital admissions and 125 deaths.[1] Measles complications include diarrhoea (8%), otitis media (7%), pneumonia (6%), death (0.1–0.2%), acute encephalitis (about 0.1% followed by death in 15% and permanent neurological damage in about 25%), seizures (with or without fever in 0.6–0.7%), idiopathic thrombocytopenia (1/6000 reported cases), and subacute scerlosing panencephalitis causing degeneration of the central nervous system and death 7 years after measles infection (range 1 month to 27 years; 0.5–1.0/100 000 reported cases).[1,9] Measles during pregnancy results in higher risk of premature labour, spontaneous abortion, and low birth weight infants. An association with birth defects remains uncertain.[1] **Disease in malnourished or immunocompromised people:** In malnourished or immunocompromised people, particularly those with vitamin A deficiency, measles case fatality can be as high as 25%. Worldwide, measles is a major cause of blindness and causes 5% of deaths in young children (< 5 years).[1,10]

Please refer to CD-ROM for full text and references.

# Migraine headache in children

Search date January 2003

*Nick Barnes, Guy Millman, and Elizabeth James*

---

## What are the effects of treatment for acute attacks of migraine headache in children? New

### UNKNOWN EFFECTIVENESS

**Antiemetics; codeine phosphate; non-steroidal anti-inflammatory drugs; paracetamol; 5HT$_1$ antagonists**

We found insufficient evidence to compare these interventions with each other or with placebo in children with migraine headache.

---

## What are the effects of prophylaxis for migraine in children? New

### LIKELY TO BE BENEFICIAL

**Stress management**

We found limited evidence from one small RCT that self administered stress management❻ improved headache severity and frequency compared with no stress management.

**β blockers**

We found conflicting evidence from small RCTs about effects of β blockers compared with placebo in children with migraine headache

**Dietary manipulation❻; pizotifen; progressive muscle relaxation❻; thermal biofeedback❻**

We found insufficient evidence about effects of these interventions to prevent migraine in children.

**DEFINITION**     Migraine is defined by the International Headache Society (IHS) as a recurrent headache that occurs with or without aura❻ and lasts 2–48 hours.[1] It is usually unilateral in nature, pulsating in quality, of moderate or severe intensity, and is aggravated by routine physical activity. Nausea, vomiting, photophobia, and phonophobia are common accompanying symptoms❶. This topic focuses on children younger than 18 years. Diagnostic criteria for children are broader than criteria for adults, allowing for a broader range of duration and a broader localisation of the pain❶.[2] Diagnosis is difficult in young children, because the condition is defined by subjective symptoms. Studies that do not explicitly use criteria that are congruent with IHS diagnostic criteria (or revised IHS criteria in children under 15 years of age) have been excluded from this topic.

**INCIDENCE/**     Migraine occurs in 3–10% of children,[3–7] and currently affects 50/1000
**PREVALENCE**  school age children in the UK and an estimated 7.8 million children in the European Union.[8] Studies in developed countries suggest that migraine is the most common diagnosis among children presenting with headache to a medical practitioner. It is rarely diagnosed in children under 2 years of age because of the symptom based definition, but increases steadily with age thereafter.[1,9,10] It affects boys and girls similarly before puberty, but after puberty girls are more likely to suffer from migraine.[4,6,10] See incidence/prevalence of migraine headache, p 290.

**AETIOLOGY/ RISK FACTORS**   The cause of migraine headaches is unknown. We found few reliable data identifying risk factors or quantifying their effects in children. Suggested risk factors include stress, foods, menses, and exercise in genetically predisposed children and adolescents.[10,11]

**PROGNOSIS**   We found no reliable data about prognosis of childhood migraine headache diagnosed by IHS criteria. It has been suggested that more than half the children will have spontaneous remission after puberty.[10] It is believed that migraine that develops during adolescence tends to continue in adult life, although attacks tend to be less frequent and severe in later life.[12] We found one longitudinal study from Sweden (73 children with "pronounced" migraine and mean age onset 6 years) with over 40 years follow up, which predated the IHS criteria for migraine headache.[13] It found that migraine headaches had ceased before the age of 25 years in 23% of people. However, By the age of 50 years, more than 50% of people continued to have migraine headaches. We found no prospective data examining long term risks in children with migraine.

Please refer to CD-ROM for full text and references.

Child health

# Nosebleeds in children

**Search date June 2003**

*Gerald McGarry*

---

## What are the effects of treatments for recurrent idiopathic epistaxis in children?

### LIKELY TO BE BENEFICIAL

**Antiseptic cream**
One RCT found that chlorhexidine/neomycin cream reduced nosebleeds compared with no treatment at 8 weeks.

### UNKNOWN EFFECTIVENESS

**Antiseptic cream versus cautery**
One small RCT found no significant difference in nosebleeds between chlorhexidine/neomycin cream and silver nitrate cautery at 8 weeks. However, the study may have lacked power to detect clinically important differences between treatments. Some children found the smell and taste of the antiseptic cream unpleasant. All children found cautery painful, despite the use of local anaesthesia.

**Cautery plus antiseptic cream**
One small RCT found insufficient evidence about the effects of silver nitrate cautery plus chlorhexidine/neomycin cream compared with chlorhexidine/neomycin cream alone.

**Cautery versus no treatment**
We found no RCTs about the effects of this intervention.

| | |
|---|---|
| **DEFINITION** | Recurrent idiopathic epistaxis is recurrent, self limiting, nasal bleeding in children for which no specific cause is identified. There is no consensus on the frequency or severity of recurrences. |
| **INCIDENCE/ PREVALENCE** | A cross sectional study of 1218 children (aged 11–14 years) found that 9% had frequent episodes of epistaxis.[1] It is likely that only the most severe episodes are considered for treatment. |
| **AETIOLOGY/ RISK FACTORS** | In children, most epistaxis occurs from the anterior part of the septum in the region of Little's area.[2] Initiating factors include local inflammation, mucosal drying, and local trauma (including nose picking).[2] Epistaxis caused by other specific local (e.g. tumours) or systemic factors (e.g. clotting disorders) is not considered here. |
| **PROGNOSIS** | Recurrent epistaxis is less common in adolescents over 14 years and many children "grow out" of this problem. |

---

Please refer to CD-ROM for full text and references.

# Reducing pain during blood sampling in infants

Search date May 2003

*Deborah Pritchard*

## What are the effects of interventions to reduce pain related distress during heel puncture?

### LIKELY TO BE BENEFICIAL

**Holding (skin to skin) versus swaddling in term infants**

RCTs found that holding reduced crying during heel puncture compared with swaddling in term infants.

**Oral glucose**

RCTs found that oral glucose reduced pain responses (particularly the duration of crying) in preterm and term infants compared with water or no treatment.

**Oral sucrose**

Systematic reviews and additional RCTs found good evidence in preterm infants and limited evidence in term infants that oral sucrose reduced pain responses (particularly the duration of crying) compared with water or no treatment. One RCT found that sucrose did not appear to increase the benefit of holding. Three RCTs in term infants found that sucrose plus pacifier was more effective than pacifier alone, although one RCT in preterm infants found no significant difference in pain score between a pacifier⊙ dipped in sucrose and pacifier alone. One RCT found insufficient evidence about the effects of oral sucrose compared with lidocaine–prilocaine emulsion in term infants undergoing heel puncture.

**Other sweeteners**

RCTs have found that other sweeteners (hydrogenated glucose⊙ or an artificial sweetener, 10 parts cyclamate and 1 part saccharin) reduce pain scores and the percentage of time spent crying in term infants compared with water.

**Pacifiers**

RCTs in term and preterm infants have found that pacifiers given before heel puncture reduce pain responses compared with no treatment.

**Positioning (tucking arms and legs) in preterm infants**

One RCT found limited evidence that pain responses were reduced by tucking the arms and legs into a mid-line flexed position during heel puncture.

**Rocking**

We found limited evidence that rocking reduces pain related stress compared with placebo.

### UNKNOWN EFFECTIVENESS

**Multiple doses of sweet solution**

One small RCT found no significant difference with multiple versus single doses of sucrose in pain scores for heel puncture.

**Swaddling**

One small RCT found no significant difference in pain responses from swaddling compared with no swaddling.

# Reducing pain during blood sampling in infants

## UNLIKELY TO BE BENEFICIAL

### Breast milk or breast feeding

RCTs found no evidence that breast milk or breast feeding during heel puncture reduced pain responses or crying in neonates compared with water.

### Prone position

One RCT found no significant difference in pain score between prone position and either side or supine position during heel puncture.

### Topical anaesthetics

Systematic reviews and additional RCTs found no evidence of reduced pain responses, particularly crying, following heel puncture with topical anaesthetic (lidocaine, lidocaine–prilocaine emulsion, or tetracaine [amethocaine]) compared with placebo.

### Warming

Two RCTs in term infants found no benefit of warming before heel puncture.

---

## What are the effects of interventions to reduce pain related distress during venepuncture?

## LIKELY TO BE BENEFICIAL

### Breast feeding *New*

One RCT found that breast feeding during venepuncture reduced pain responses compared with oral water or being held. The RCT found no significant difference in pain response between breast feeding and oral glucose.

### Oral glucose

RCTs have found that oral glucose reduces pain responses (particularly the duration of crying) in term and preterm infants compared with water or no treatment. One RCT found no significant difference in pain scores between sucrose and glucose.

### Oral sucrose

RCTs have found that oral sucrose reduces pain responses (particularly the duration of crying) in term and preterm infants compared with water or no treatment. One RCT found no significant difference in pain between sucrose and glucose.

### Pacifiers

One RCT found that pacifiers reduced pain responses compared with water or no treatment in term infants undergoing venepuncture.

### Topical anaesthetics

Four RCTs found limited evidence that lidocaine–prilocaine emulsion reduced pain responses to venepuncture compared with placebo. Two RCTs found that tetra-caine (amethocaine) gel reduced pain and crying during venepuncture compared with placebo.

## UNKNOWN EFFECTIVENESS

### Other sweeteners

We found no RCTs of other sweeteners for venepuncture.

**DEFINITION**     Methods of sampling blood in infants include heel puncture, venepuncture, and arterial puncture. Heel puncture involves lancing of the lateral aspect of the infant's heel, squeezing the heel, and collecting the pooled capillary blood. Venepuncture involves aspirating blood through a needle from a peripheral vein. Arterial blood sampling is not discussed in this review. RCTs in this review were performed in a hospital care setting and the evidence relates to preterm and ill infants who have multiple blood tests, rather than infants undergoing heel puncture tests for routine screening. The results therefore cannot be applied to routine screening heel puncture tests in healthy infants.

**INCIDENCE/**     Almost every infant in the developed world undergoes heel puncture to screen
**PREVALENCE**   for metabolic disorders (e.g. phenylketonuria). Many infants have repeated heel punctures or venepunctures to monitor blood glucose or haemoglobin. Preterm or ill neonates may undergo 1–21 heel punctures or venepunctures per day.[1–3] These punctures are likely to be painful. Heel punctures comprise 61–87% and venepunctures comprise 8–13% of the invasive procedures performed on ill infants. Analgesics are rarely given specifically for blood sampling procedures, but 5–19% of infants receive analgesia for other indications.[2,3] In one study, comfort measures were provided during 63% of venepunctures and 75% of heel punctures.[3]

**AETIOLOGY/**     Blood sampling in infants can be difficult to perform, particularly in preterm or
**RISK FACTORS** ill infants. Young infants may have increased sensitivity and more prolonged responses to pain than older age groups.[4] Factors that may affect the infant's pain responses include postconceptional age, previous pain experience, and procedural technique.

**PROGNOSIS**     Pain caused by blood sampling is associated with acute behavioural and physiological deterioration.[4] Experience of pain during heel puncture seems to heighten pain responses during subsequent blood sampling.[5] Other adverse effects of blood sampling include bleeding, bruising, haematoma, and infection.

---

Please refer to CD-ROM for full text and references.

# Sudden infant death syndrome

**Search date March 2003**

*David Creery and Angelo Mikrogianakis*

---

## What are the effects of interventions to reduce the risk of sudden infant death syndrome?

### BENEFICIAL

**Advice to avoid prone sleeping**

Several observational studies found that campaigns involving advice to encourage non-prone sleeping positions❻ were followed by a reduced incidence of sudden infant death syndrome. RCTs are unlikely to be conducted.

### LIKELY TO BE BENEFICIAL

**Advice to avoid tobacco smoke exposure**

Several observational studies found limited evidence that campaigns to reduce several risk factors for sudden infant death, which included tobacco smoke exposure, were followed by a reduced incidence of sudden infant death syndrome. RCTs are unlikely to be conducted.

### UNKNOWN EFFECTIVENESS

**Advice to avoid bed sharing**

One observational study found that a campaign to reduce several risk factors for sudden infant death, which included advice to avoid bed sharing, was followed by a reduced incidence of sudden infant death syndrome. RCTs are unlikely to be conducted.

**Advice to avoid over heating or over wrapping**

Three observational studies found limited evidence that campaigns to reduce several risk factors for sudden infant death, which included over wrapping❻, were followed by a reduced incidence of sudden infant death syndrome. RCTs are unlikely to be conducted.

**Advice to avoid soft sleeping surfaces**

We found no evidence on the effects of avoiding soft sleeping surfaces in the prevention of sudden infant death syndrome.

**Advice to breastfeed**

One non-systematic review of observational studies and three additional observational studies found that campaigns to reduce several risk factors for sudden infant death, which included advice to breastfeed, were followed by a reduced incidence of sudden infant death syndrome. In some countries, however, incidence had begun to fall before the national advice campaigns. RCTs are unlikely to be conducted.

**Advice to promote soother use**

We found insufficient evidence on soother use in the prevention of sudden infant death syndrome.

**DEFINITION**      Sudden infant death syndrome (SIDS) is the sudden death of an infant aged under 1 year that remains unexplained after review of the clinical history, examination of the scene of death, and postmortem.

**INCIDENCE/**      The incidence of SIDS has varied over time and among nations (incidence per
**PREVALENCE**    1000 live births of SIDS in 1996: Netherlands 0.3, Japan 0.4, Canada 0.5, England and Wales 0.7, USA 0.8, and Australia 0.9).[1]

**AETIOLOGY/ RISK FACTORS**   By definition, the cause of SIDS is not known. Observational studies have found an association between SIDS and several risk factors including prone sleeping position,[2,3] prenatal or postnatal exposure to tobacco smoke,[4] soft sleeping surfaces,[5,6] hyperthermia/over wrapping❶,[7,8] bed sharing (particularly with mothers who smoke),[9,10] lack of breastfeeding,[11,12] and soother❺ use.[7,13]

**PROGNOSIS**   Although by definition prognosis is not applicable for an affected infant, the incidence of SIDS is increased in the siblings of that infant.[14,15]

Please refer to CD-ROM for full text and references.

# Urinary tract infection in children

**Search date September 2002**

*James Larcombe*

---

## What are the effects of treatment of acute infection?

### Antibiotics versus placebo

Placebo controlled trials of antibiotics for symptomatic acute urinary tract infection (UTI) in children are considered unethical.

### LIKELY TO BE BENEFICIAL

### Oral versus initial intravenous antibiotics

One RCT found no significant difference between oral cephalosporins alone and initial intravenous plus continued oral cephalosporins in duration of fever, reinfection, renal scarring, or extent of scarring in children aged 2 years or younger with first confirmed UTI. The RCT found weak evidence that in children with grades III–IV❻ reflux, renal scarring at 6 months may be more common with oral versus initial intravenous treatment.

### UNKNOWN EFFECTIVENESS

### Immediate empirical versus delayed antibiotic treatment

We found no RCTs on the effects of giving early empirical treatment versus awaiting the results of microscopy or culture in acute urinary tract infection in children. Retrospective analysis of one RCT found no significant difference in risk of renal scarring with antibiotic (cephalosporins) treatment within 24 hours versus 24 hours after the onset of fever in children under 2 years with urinary tract infections.

### UNLIKELY TO BE BENEFICIAL

### Longer (7–14 days) versus shorter (2–4 days) courses of oral antibiotics

One systematic review found no significant difference for longer (7–14 days) versus shorter courses (2–4 days) of the same antibiotic in cure rate at 7 days after treatment in children with no history of renal tract abnormality and judged not to have acute pyelonephritis❻.

### Longer versus short courses of initial intravenous antibiotics

Two RCTs found no significant difference between long (7–10 days) and short (3 days) course of initial cephalosporins in renal scarring in children with acute pyelonephritis❻.

### LIKELY TO BE INEFFECTIVE OR HARMFUL

### Prolonged delay in treatment (> 7 days)

We found no RCTs. Five retrospective studies found that medium to long term delays (4 days to 7 years) in treatment may be associated with an increased risk of renal scarring.

### Single dose versus longer course (10 days) of oral amoxicillin

One systematic review has found that longer (10 days) versus single dose amoxicillin increases cure rate at 3–30 days after the start of treatment.

**Child health**

◀ *What are the effects of preventive interventions?*

### LIKELY TO BE BENEFICIAL

#### Immunotherapy

One systematic review in premature and low birth weight neonates has found that intravenous immunoglobulins⊕ reduce serious infections, including UTIs, compared with placebo. One RCT in children with recurrent urinary tract infection found that adding pidotimod (an immunotherapeutic agent) reduced recurrence compared with adding placebo to antibiotic treatment.

#### Prophylactic antibiotics

One systematic review and an additional RCT found limited evidence that prophylactic antibiotics (co-trimoxazole, nitrofurantoin) reduced UTI recurrence in children compared with placebo or no treatment. One RCT found that nitrofurantoin significantly reduced recurrence of UTI over 6 months compared with trimethoprim. It also found that more children discontinued treatment with nitrofurantoin because of adverse effects. We found no RCTs evaluating the optimum duration of prophylactic antibiotics.

### UNKNOWN EFFECTIVENESS

#### Surgical correction of moderate to severe bilateral vesicouretic reflux (grades III–IV) with bilateral nephropathy

One small RCT found a steady, but not significant, decline in glomerular filtration rate over 10 years with medical treatment versus surgery in children with moderate to severe bilateral vesicoureteric reflux.

### UNLIKELY TO BE BENEFICIAL

#### Surgical correction of minor functional anomalies

We found no RCTs. One observational study suggested that children with minor anomalies do not develop renal scarring and therefore may not benefit from surgery.

#### Surgical correction of moderate to severe vesicoureteric reflux with adequate glomerular filtration rate (similar benefits to medical management)

One systematic review and one subsequent RCT found that, although surgery abolished reflux, there was no significant difference between surgical and medical management (prophylactic antibiotic treatment) in preventing recurrence or complications from urinary tract infection after 6 months to 5 years in children with moderate to severe vesicoureteric reflux.

**DEFINITION**   UTI is defined by the presence of a pure growth of more than $10^5$ colony forming units of bacteria per millilitre. Lower counts of bacteria may be clinically important, especially in boys and in specimens obtained by urinary catheter. Any growth of typical urinary pathogens is considered clinically important if obtained by suprapubic aspiration. In practice, three age ranges are usually considered on the basis of differential risk and different approaches to management: children under 1 year; young children (1–4, 5, or 7 years, depending on the information source); and older children (up to 12–16 years). Recurrent UTI is defined as a further infection by a new organism. Relapsing UTI is defined as a further infection with the same organism. ▶

# Urinary tract infection in children

**INCIDENCE/ PREVALENCE** Boys are more susceptible before the age of 3 months; thereafter the incidence is substantially higher in girls. Estimates of the true incidence of UTI depend on rates of diagnosis and investigation. At least 8% of girls and 2% of boys will have a UTI in childhood.[1]

**AETIOLOGY/ RISK FACTORS** The normal urinary tract is sterile. Contamination by bowel flora may result in urinary infection if a virulent organism is involved or if the child is immunosuppressed. In neonates, infection may originate from other sources. *Escherichia coli* accounts for about three quarters of all pathogens. *Proteus* is more common in boys (about 30% of infections). Obstructive anomalies are found in 0–4% and vesicoureteric reflux in 8–40% of children being investigated for their first UTI.[2] Although vesicoureteric reflux is a major risk factor for adverse outcome, other as yet unidentified triggers may also need to be present.

**PROGNOSIS** After first infection, about half of girls have a further infection in the first year and three quarters within 2 years.[3] We found no figures for boys, but a review suggests that recurrences are common under 1 year of age, but rare subsequently.[4] Renal scarring occurs in 5–15% of children within 1–2 years of their first UTI, although 32–70% of these scars are noted at the time of initial assessment.[2] The incidence of renal scarring rises with each episode of infection in childhood.[5] Retrospective analysis of an RCT comparing oral versus intravenous antibiotics found that new renal scarring after a first UTI was more common in children with vesicoureteric reflux than in children without reflux (logistic regression model: AR of scarring 16/107 [15%] with reflux v 10/165 [6%] without reflux; RR 2.47, 95% CI 1.17 to 5.24).[6] A study (287 children with severe vesicoureteric reflux treated either medically or surgically for any UTI) evaluated the risk of renal scarring with serial DMSA scintigraphy❻ over 5 years. It found that younger children (< 2 years) were at greater risk of renal scarring than older children regardless of treatment for the infection (AR for deterioration in DMSA scan over 5 years 21/86 [24%] for younger children v 27/201 [13%] for older children; RR 1.82, 95% CI 1.09 to 3.03).[7] Renal scarring is associated with future complications: poor renal growth, recurrent adult pyelonephritis, impaired glomerular function, early hypertension, and end stage renal failure.[8–11] A combination of recurrent UTI, severe vesicoureteric reflux, and the presence of renal scarring at first presentation is associated with the worst prognosis. One prospective observational study assessed the persistence of scarring on DMSA scans in children with a first UTI.[12] Grading of scars was as follows: mild (< 25% kidney affected), moderate (25–50% kidney), and severe (> 50% kidney). The study found that vesicoureteric reflux was associated with more persistent scarring at 6 months (in children with severe scarring on initial scan, 7/8 [88%] with reflux had a persisting lesion v 1/7 [14%] without reflux; RR 6.13, 95% CI 0.98 to 38.00; in children with mild to moderate scarring on initial scan, 3/8 [38%] with reflux had persisting lesions v 5/31 [16%] without reflux; RR 2.70, 95% CI 0.81 to 9.10).[12] The study also found that vesicoureteric reflux was associated with a higher risk of pyelonephritis on the initial scan (RR for pyelonephritis with reflux v without 1.62, 95% CI 1.14 to 2.31).

Please refer to CD-ROM for full text and references.

### Search date September 2002

*Marion Jonas and John Scholefield*

## What are the effects of treatments for chronic anal fissure?

### BENEFICIAL

#### Internal anal sphincterotomy

One systematic review found no significant difference with internal anal sphincterotomy❻ versus anal stretch in persistence of fissures, and that both procedures healed 70–95% of fissures. It found no significant difference with open versus closed internal sphincterotomy in persistence of fissures. Three RCTs have found that sphincterotomy significantly improved fissure healing compared with topical glyceryl trinitrate (GTN) after 6 weeks to 1 year.

### LIKELY TO BE BENEFICIAL

#### Anal advancement flap (as effective as internal anal sphincterotomy)

One RCT found no significant difference with lateral internal anal sphincterotomy versus anal advancement flap❻ in patient satisfaction or fissure healing.

#### Botulinum A toxin-haemagglutinin complex (botulinum A toxin-hc)

One small RCT found that botulinum A toxin-hc❻ versus placebo increased fissure healing after 2 months. One small RCT found that botulinum A toxin-hc versus topical GTN 0.2% significantly increased fissure healing rates after 2 months. Two RCTs found no significant difference with high dose versus low dose botulinum A toxin-hc in healing rates after 2–3 months.

#### Topical glyceral trinitrate (GTN)

Two RCTs found that topical GTN❻ versus placebo significantly increased fissure healing after 8 weeks. Two further RCTs found no significant difference in fissure healing after 4 weeks of treatment, although they may have lacked power to detect a clinically important benefit. Three RCTs have found that sphincterotomy significantly improved fissure healing compared with topical GTN after 6 weeks to 1 year. One systematic review found that botulinum A toxin-hc versus GTN significantly increased fissure healing after 2 months. One RCT found no significant difference with glyceryl trinitrate ointment versus a glyceryl trinitrate patch in fissure healing after 8 weeks. One RCT found no significant difference between topical GTN versus topical diltiazem in healing at 8 weeks.

### TRADE OFF BETWEEN BENEFITS AND HARMS

#### Anal stretch

One systematic review found no significant difference with internal anal sphincterotomy versus anal stretch❻ in persistence of fissures, and that both procedures healed 70–95% of fissures. Anal stretch versus internal anal sphincterotomy significantly increased rates of flatus incontinence.

### UNKNOWN EFFECTIVENESS

#### Botulinum A toxin-haemagglutinin complex (botulinum A toxin-hc) plus nitrates

We found no RCTs comparing botulinum toxin A-hc plus nitrates versus placebo. One small RCT in people with anal fissures that had failed to heal with topical nitrates found that botulinum A toxin-hc plus topical isosorbide dinitrate three times daily versus botulinum A toxin-hc alone significantly increased fissure healing at 6 weeks but found no significant difference at 8 or 12 weeks.

Digestive system disorders

# Anal fissure

### Diltiazem

We found no placebo controlled RCTs. One small RCT found no significant difference with oral diltiazem versus topical diltiazem in fissure healing after 8 weeks. One small RCT found no significant difference in healing rate between topical diltiazem versus topical GTN at 8 weeks.

### Indoramin

One RCT found no significant difference with oral indoramin versus placebo in fissure healing after 6 weeks, but may have been too smal to detect a clinically important difference.

**DEFINITION**     Anal fissure is a split or tear in the lining of the distal anal canal. It is a very painful condition often associated with fresh blood loss from the anus and perianal itching. **Acute anal fissures** have sharply demarcated, fresh mucosal edges, and often with granulation tissue at the base. **Chronic anal fissures** margins are indurated, there is less granulation tissue, and muscle fibres of the internal anal sphincter may be seen at the base. Fissures persisting for longer than 6 weeks are generally defined as chronic.

**INCIDENCE/**     Anal fissures are common in all age groups, but we found no evidence to
**PREVALENCE**     quantify the incidence.

**AETIOLOGY/**     Low intake of dietary fibre may be a risk factor for the development of acute anal
**RISK FACTORS**     fissures.[1] People with anal fissure often have raised resting anal canal pressures with anal spasm.[2,3] Men and women are equally affected by anal fissures, and up to 11% of women develop anal fissures after childbirth.[4]

**PROGNOSIS**     Placebo controlled studies found that 70–90% of untreated "chronic" fissures did not heal during the study.[5,6]

---

Please refer to CD-ROM for full text and references.

Search date February 2003

*John Simpson and William Speake*

Digestive system disorders

## What are the effects of treatments?

**BENEFICIAL**

### Adjuvant antibiotics

One systematic review and one subsequent RCT in children and adults with simple⊙ or complicated appendicitis⊙ undergoing appendicectomy have found that prophylactic antibiotics reduce wound infections and intra-abdominal abscesses compared with no antibiotics. Subgroup analysis from the systematic review has found that antibiotics reduce the number of wound infections in children with complicated appendicitis compared with no antibiotics. Subgroup analysis from the systematic review also found no significant difference in the number of wound infections between antibiotics and no antibiotics in children with simple appendicitis. One subsequent RCT in children with simple appendicitis found no significant difference with antibiotic prophylaxis compared with no antibiotic prophylaxis in wound infections, but the RCT may have been too small to exclude a clinically important difference.

**LIKELY TO BE BENEFICIAL**

### Laparoscopic surgery versus open surgery (in children)

One systematic review has found that, in children, laparoscopic surgery reduced the number of wound infections and the length of hospital stay compared with open surgery, but found no significant difference in postoperative pain, time to mobilisation, or proportion of intra-abdominal abscesses.

**TRADE OFF BETWEEN BENEFITS AND HARMS**

### Antibiotics versus surgery

We found no RCTs comparing antibiotics with placebo or no treatment. One small RCT in adults with suspected appendicitis found that conservative treatment with antibiotics reduced pain and morphine consumption for the first 10 days compared with appendicectomy. However, the RCT found that 35% of people were readmitted within 1 year with acute appendicitis after conservative management with antibiotics and subsequently had an appendicectomy.

### Laparoscopic surgery versus open surgery (in adults)

One systematic review has found that laparoscopic surgery in adults reduces the number of wound infections, pain on the first postoperative day, duration of hospital stay, and time taken to return to work compared with open surgery. However, laparoscopic surgery increased postoperative intra-abdominal abscesses compared with open surgery.

**UNKNOWN EFFECTIVENESS**

### Open surgery versus no treatment

We found no RCTs comparing surgery with no surgery.

### Stump inversion at open appendicectomy

One RCT found no significant difference between stump inversion and simple ligation in wound infection, length of hospital stay, or intra-abdominal abscesses. Another RCT found that stump inversion increased wound infections compared with simple ligation, but found no significant difference between groups for intra-abdominal abscesses or length of hospital stay. ▶

# Appendicitis

**DEFINITION**  Acute appendicitis is acute inflammation of the vermiform appendix.

**INCIDENCE/ PREVALENCE**  The incidence of acute appendicitis is falling, although the reason for this is unclear. The reported lifetime risk of appendicitis in the USA is 8.7% in men and 6.7% in women,[1] and there are about 60 000 cases reported annually in England and Wales. Appendicitis is the most common surgical emergency requiring operation.

**AETIOLOGY/ RISK FACTORS**  The cause of appendicitis is uncertain although various theories exist. Most relate to luminal obstruction, which prevents escape of secretions and inevitably leads to a rise in intraluminal pressure within the appendix. This can lead to subsequent mucosal ischaemia, and the stasis provides an ideal environment for bacterial overgrowth. Potential causes of the obstruction are faecoliths, often because of constipation, lymphoid hyperplasia, or caecal carcinoma.[2]

**PROGNOSIS**  The prognosis of untreated appendicitis is unknown, although spontaneous resolution has been reported in at least 1/13 (8%) episodes.[3] The recurrence of appendicitis after conservative management,[3,4] and recurrent abdominal symptoms in certain people,[5] suggests that chronic appendicitis and recurrent acute or subacute appendicitis may also exist.[6] The standard treatment for acute appendicitis is appendicectomy. RCTs comparing treatment with no treatment would be regarded as unethical. The mortality from acute appendicitis is less than 0.3%, rising to 1.7% after perforation.[7] The most common complication of appendicectomy is wound infection, occurring in between 5 and 33% of cases.[8] Intra-abdominal abscess formation occurs less frequently in 2% of appendicectomies.[9] A perforated appendix in childhood does not appear to have subsequent negative consequences on female fertility.[10]

Please refer to CD-ROM for full text and references.

### Search date October 2002

*John Simpson and Robin Spiller*

## What are the effects of treatments for uncomplicated diverticular disease?

### LIKELY TO BE BENEFICIAL

#### Rifaximin (plus glucomannan v glucomannan alone)

One RCT found that oral rifaximin⊕ plus glucomannan versus glucomannan plus placebo significantly increases the proportion of people with uncomplicated diverticular disease⊕ who are symptom free after 12 months of treatment.

### UNKNOWN EFFECTIVENESS

#### Bran and ispaghula husk

Two small RCTs found no consistent effect of bran or ispaghula husk versus placebo on symptom relief after 12–16 weeks.

#### Elective surgery

We found no RCTs of elective open or laparoscopic colonic resection.

#### Lactulose

One RCT found no significant difference with lactulose versus a high fibre diet in the number of people who considered themselves to be "much improved" after 12 weeks.

#### Methylcellulose

One small RCT found no significant difference with methylcellulose versus placebo in mean symptom score after 3 months.

## What are the effects of treatments to prevent complications of diverticular disease?

### UNKNOWN EFFECTIVENESS

#### Increased fibre intake

We found no RCTs of advice to consume a high fibre diet or of dietary fibre supplementation.

### TRADE OFF BETWEEN BENEFITS AND HARMS

#### Mesalazine (after an attack of acute diverticulitis) *New*

One RCT found that mesalazine reduced symptomatic recurrence compared with no treatment in people previously treated for an episode of acute diverticulitis⊕, but associated with abdominal pain.

## What are the effects of treatments for acute diverticulitis?

### UNKNOWN EFFECTIVENESS

#### Medical treatment

We found no RCTs of medical treatment versus placebo. One RCT comparing intravenous cefoxitin versus intravenous gentamicin plus intravenous clindamycin found no significant difference in rates of clinical cure. Observational studies in people with acute diverticulitis have found low mortality rates with medical treatment, but found that recurrence rates may be high.

# Colonic diverticular disease

◀ **Surgery (for diverticulitis complicated by generalised peritonitis)**
We found no RCTs of surgery versus no surgery or versus medical treatment. One RCT comparing acute resection versus no acute resection (involving a transverse colostomy) of the sigmoid colon found no significant difference in mortality. A second RCT comparing primary versus secondary sigmoid colonic resection found no significant difference in mortality, but found that primary resection significantly reduced rates of postoperative peritonitis and emergency reoperation.

**DEFINITION**  Colonic diverticula are mucosal out pouchings through the large bowel wall. They are often accompanied by structural changes (elastosis of the taenia coli, muscular thickening, and mucosal folding). They are usually multiple and occur most frequently in the sigmoid colon.

**INCIDENCE/** In the UK, the incidence of diverticulosis❸ increases with age; about 5% of
**PREVALENCE** people are affected in their fifth decade of life and about 50% by their ninth decade.[1] Diverticulosis is common in developed countries, although there is a lower prevalence of diverticulosis in Western vegetarians consuming a diet high in roughage.[2] Diverticulosis is almost unknown in rural Africa and Asia.[3]

**AETIOLOGY/** There is an association between low fibre diets and diverticulosis of the colon.[3]
**RISK FACTORS** Prospective observational studies have found that both physical activity and a high fibre diet are associated with a lower risk of developing diverticular disease.[4,5] One case control study found an association between the ingestion of non-steroidal anti-inflammatory drugs and the development of severe diverticula complications, including pericolic abscess, generalised peritonitis, bleeding, and fistula formation.[6] People in Japan, Singapore, and Thailand develop diverticula that mainly affect the right side of the colon.[7]

**PROGNOSIS**  Symptoms will develop in 10–25% of people with diverticula at some point in their lives.[1] It is unclear why some people develop symptoms and some do not. Even after successful medical treatment of acute diverticulitis almost two thirds of people suffer recurrent pain in the lower abdomen.[8] Recurrent diverticulitis is observed in 7–42% of people with diverticular disease, and after recovery from the initial attack the calculated yearly risk of suffering a further episode is 3%.[9] About half of recurrences occur within 1 year of the initial episode and 90% occur within 5 years.[10] Complications of diverticular disease (perforation, obstruction, haemorrhage, and fistula formation) are each seen in about 5% of people with colonic diverticula when followed up for 10–30 years.[11] Intra-abdominal abscess formation may also occur.

Please refer to CD-ROM for full text and references.

Digestive system disorders

---

## What are the effects of treatments?

### BENEFICIAL

#### Adjuvant chemotherapy

Three systematic reviews and one subsequent RCT have found that adjuvant chemotherapy reduces mortality compared with surgery alone in people with Dukes'❻ A, B, and C colorectal cancer. One RCT found that adding levamisole to adjuvant fluorouracil did not significantly reduce mortality or recurrence compared with adjuvant fluorouracil alone in people with Dukes' A, B, and C colorectal cancer. One RCT found that mortality and recurrence rates were similar with adjuvant fluorouracil plus high or low dose folinic acid in people with Dukes' A, B, and C colorectal cancer.

### UNKNOWN EFFECTIVENESS

#### Routine intensive follow up

One systematic review and one subsequent RCT have found that intensive follow up increases survival compared with less intensive follow up in people treated surgically with curative intent.

### TRADE OFF BETWEEN BENEFITS AND HARMS

#### Preoperative radiotherapy

Two systematic reviews and two subsequent RCTs found that adding preoperative radiotherapy to surgery is at least as effective as surgery alone for mortality and recurrence in people with rectal cancer. One RCT found no significant difference in mortality between preoperative and postoperative radiotherapy but preoperative radiotherapy reduced local tumour recurrence. One systematic review has found that preoperative radiotherapy increases early postoperative morbidity.

#### Total mesorectal excision

We found no RCTs of total mesorectal excision❻ in people with rectal cancer. Observational studies suggest that total mesorectal excision may reduce the rate of local recurrence compared with conventional surgery.

**DEFINITION**  Colorectal cancer is a malignant neoplasm arising from the lining (mucosa) of the large intestine (colon and rectum). Nearly two thirds of colorectal cancers occur in the rectum or sigmoid colon. Colorectal cancer may be categorised as A, B, or C Dukes'.

**INCIDENCE/**  Colorectal cancer is the third most common malignancy in the developed
**PREVALENCE**  world. It accounts for about 20 000 deaths each year in the UK and 60 000 deaths each year in the USA. Although the incidence of, and mortality from, colorectal cancer has changed little over the past 40 years, the incidence of the disease has fallen recently in both the UK and the USA.[1,2] In the UK, about a quarter of people with colorectal cancer present as emergencies with either intestinal obstruction or perforation.[3,4]

**AETIOLOGY/**  Colon cancer affects almost equal proportions of men and women, most
**RISK FACTORS**  commonly between the ages of 60 and 80 years. Rectal cancer is more common in men.[1] The pathogenesis of colorectal cancer involves genetic and environmental factors. The most important environmental factor is probably diet.[5]

▶

# Colorectal cancer

**PROGNOSIS**  Overall 5 year survival is about 50% and has not changed over the past 40 years. Disease specific mortality in both USA and UK cancer registries is decreasing but the reasons for this are unclear.[1,2] Surgery is undertaken with curative intent in over 80% of people, but about half experience cancer recurrence.

---

Please refer to CD-ROM for full text and references.

# Gastro-oesophageal reflux disease

### Search date November 2002

*Paul Moayyedi, Brendan Delaney, and David Forman*

## What are the effects of interventions in the initial treatment of gastro-oesophageal reflux disease (GORD) associated with oesophagitis?

### BENEFICIAL

#### H₂ receptor antagonists

One systematic review in people with oesophagitis found that $H_2$ receptor antagonists significantly increased healing compared with placebo, but reduced healing compared with proton pump inhibitors.

#### Proton pump inhibitors

One systematic review has found that proton pump inhibitors increased incidence of healing compared with placebo or $H_2$ receptor antagonists. One systematic review found that esomeprazole significantly increased healing at 4 weeks compared with omeprazole. RCTs have found no significant difference in clinical benefit among other proton pump inhibitors.

### UNKNOWN EFFECTIVENESS

#### Antacids/alginates

Two RCTs found limited evidence that antacids versus placebo reduced symptom scores at 4–8 weeks, but found no significant difference in endoscopic healing. We found limited evidence on the effects of antacids versus $H_2$ receptor antagonists in people with oesophagitis. The first RCT found no significant difference between antacids versus cimetidine on endoscopic healing at 8 weeks. The second RCT found that antacids were significantly less effective for healing compared with ranitidine at 12 weeks.

#### Lifestyle advice

RCTs found insufficient evidence on the effects of lifestyle measures for the treatment of reflux oesophagitis.

### LIKELY TO BE INEFFECTIVE OR HARMFUL

#### Motility stimulants

One RCT found that cisapride significantly increased endoscopic healing compared with placebo at 12 weeks. The use of cisapride has been restricted in some countries because of concerns about heart rhythm abnormalities. We found no RCTs of domperidone or metoclopramide.

## What are the effects of interventions in the maintenance treatment of GORD associated with oasophagitis?

### BENEFICIAL

#### Proton pump inhibitors

RCTs have found that proton pump inhibitors compared with placebo or $H_2$ receptor antagonists increase remission rates in people with healed reflux oesophagitis at 6–18 months. RCTs have found that proton pump inhibitors compared with placebo or $H_2$ receptor antagonists increase remission rates in people with healed reflux oesophagitis at 6–18 months. One systematic review has found that standard dose lansoprazole (30 mg/day) was as effective as omeprazole (20 mg/ ▶

Digestive system disorders

day) for maintaining healing at 12 months. However, it found that lower dose lansoprazole (15 mg/day) was less effective than higher dose lansoprazole (30 mg/day), omeprazole, or esomeprazole for maintaining healing for up to 12 months.

## TRADE OFF BETWEEN BENEFITS AND HARMS

### Laparoscopic surgery

One systematic review found no fully published RCTs comparing laparoscopic surgery versus medical treatment for maintenance treatment in people with GORD and oesophagitis. Two RCTs found no significant difference between open and laparasopic fundoplication for remission at 3 months to 2 years. One RCT found that complication rates were lower with laparoscopic versus open surgery.

### Open surgery

RCTs have found that open Nissen fundoplication compared with medical treatment improved the endoscopic grade of oesophagitis in people with chronic GORD and oesophagitis at between 3 and 38 months. However, longer term follow up from one of those RCTs found no significant difference in endoscopic appearance between surgery and medical treatment at 10 years. Two RCTs found no significant difference between open and laparascopic fundoplication for remission at 3 months to 2 years. One RCT found that mortality was higher with open surgery compared with medical treatment. One RCT found that complication rates were higher with open versus laparoscopic surgery.

## UNKNOWN EFFECTIVENESS

### Antacids/alginates

We found no RCTs on the effects of antacids/alginates on long term management of reflux oesophagitis.

### H₂ receptor antagonists

One RCT found no significant difference between ranitidine versus placebo for relapse of oesophagitis at 6 months in people with previously healed reflux oesophagitis. RCTs have found that $H_2$ receptor antagonists are less effective than proton pump inhibitors for maintaining remission up to 12 months.

### Lifestyle advice

We found no RCTs on the effects of lifestyle advice on long term management of reflux oesophagitis.

## LIKELY TO BE INEFFECTIVE OR HARMFUL

### Motility stimulants

We found limited evidence on the effects of cisapride compared with placebo. Three RCTs found that cisapride compared with placebo improved maintenance of healing at 6–12 months. Two further RCTs found no evidence of a difference. However, they might have lacked power to detect a clinically important effect. We found no RCTs comparing other prokinetics versus placebo or each other in people with GORD and oesophagitis. The use of cisapride has been restricted in some countries because of concerns about effects on heart rhythms.

**DEFINITION**  GORD is defined as reflux of gastroduodenal contents into the oesophagus causing symptoms that are sufficient to interfere with quality of life.[1] People with GORD often have symptoms of heartburn and acid regurgitation.[2] GORD can be classified according to results of upper gastrointestinal endoscopy. An ▶

endoscopy showing mucosal breaks in the distal oesophagus indicate the presence of oesophagitis, which is graded in severity from grade A (mucosal breaks of < 5 mm in the oesophagus) to grade D (circumferential breaks in the oesophageal mucosa).[1,3] Alternatively, severity may be graded according to the Savary–Miller classification (grade I: linear, non-confluent erosions to grade IV: severe ulceration or stricture).

**INCIDENCE/ PREVALENCE** Surveys from Europe and the USA suggest that 20–25% of the population have symptoms of GORD, and 7% have heartburn daily.[4,5] In primary care settings, about 25–40% of people with GORD have oesophagitis on endoscopy, but most have endoscopy negative reflux disease.[6]

**AETIOLOGY/ RISK FACTORS** We found no evidence of clear predictive factors for GORD. Obesity is reported to be a risk factor for GORD but epidemiological data are conflicting.[7,8] Smoking and alcohol are also thought to predispose to GORD, but observational data are limited.[8,9] It has been suggested that some foods, such as coffee, mints, dietary fat, onions, citrus fruits, or tomatoes, may predispose to GORD.[10] However, we found insufficient data on the role of these factors. We found limited evidence that drugs that relax the lower oesophageal sphincter, such as calcium channel blockers, may promote GORD.[11] Twin studies suggest that there may be a genetic predisposition to GORD.[9]

**PROGNOSIS** GORD is a chronic condition, with about 80% of people relapsing once medication is discontinued.[12] Many people therefore require long term medical treatment or surgery. Endoscopy negative reflux disease remains stable, with a minority of people developing oesophagitis over time.[13] However, people with severe oesophagitis may develop complications such as oesophageal stricture and Barrett's oesophagus.[1]

Please refer to CD-ROM for full text and references.

# *Helicobacter pylori* infection

**Search date December 2002**

*Brendan Delaney, Paul Moayyedi, and David Forman*

*Digestive system disorders*

---

## *What are the effects of treatments?*

### *H pylori* eradication for healing and preventing recurrence of duodenal ulcer

Systematic reviews and one subsequent RCT have found that *H pylori* eradication increases ulcer healing at 6 weeks and reduces 1 year recurrence compared with acid suppression or antisecretory treatment❶. One systematic review found that *H pylori* eradication compared with ulcer healing alone, or compared with ulcer treatment plus subsequent acid suppression maintenance treatment reduced the risk of rebleeding.

### *H pylori* eradication for healing and preventing recurrence of gastric ulcer

One systematic review found no good evidence on endoscopic healing of gastric ulcers. One systematic review has found that *H pylori* eradication treatment compared with antisecretory treatment reduces recurrent ulcers at 1 year. Observational evidence identified by the review found that eradication treatment heals 83% of gastric ulcers within 6 weeks of starting treatment. We found no RCTs of *H pylori* eradication treatment on preventing complications of gastric ulcers.

### *H pylori* eradication for non-ulcer dyspepsia

One systematic review in people with non-ulcer dyspepsia has found that *H pylori* eradication significantly reduces dyspeptic symptoms compared with placebo at 3–12 months.

### *H pylori* eradication rather than empirical acid suppression for uninvestigated dyspepsia

One RCT found that *H pylori* eradication increased relief from dyspeptic symptoms compared with placebo after 1 year.

### *H pylori* eradication rather than endoscopy in people with uninvestigated dyspepsia not at risk of malignancy

One RCT has found that *H pylori* eradication increased relief from dyspeptic symptoms after 1 year compared with placebo. One systematic review and one subsequent RCT have found no significant difference between *H pylori* testing plus eradication compared with management based on initial endoscopy in dyspepsia after 1 year. The review found that H pylori testing plus eradication reduced the need for requiring endoscopy compared with endoscopy based management.

### Three day quadruple regimen (*v* 1 week triple regimen)

One RCT comparing a 3 day quadruple regimen versus a 1 week triple regimen found no significant difference in *H pylori* eradication at 6 weeks, but found that people taking the 3 day quadruple regimen experienced fewer days of adverse effects.

### Triple regimen (*v* dual regimen)

We found no systematic review or RCTs of the effects of dual regimen❶ compared with triple regimens❶ on dyspeptic symptom scores, proportion of subjects with symptoms, quality of life, or mortality. One systematic review has found that dual versus triple regimens eradicate *H pylori* from fewer people.

◀ **Two week triple regimen (v 1 week triple regimen)**

One systematic review found that 14 days treatment with proton pump inhibitor based treatment increased *H pylori* cure rates compared with 7 days treatment.

### UNKNOWN EFFECTIVENESS

#### *H pylori* eradication for gastric B cell lymphoma

We found no RCTs of *H pylori* eradication treatment in people with B cell gastric lymphoma❻. Observational studies found limited evidence that 60–93% of people with localised, low grade B cell lymphoma respond to *H pylori* eradication treatment possibly avoiding, or delaying the need for radical surgery, radiotherapy, or chemotherapy.

#### *H pylori* eradication for prevention of gastric cancer (adenocarcinoma)

We found no RCTs of *H pylori* eradication in people at risk of gastric cancer. One RCT in people with gastric atrophy or intestinal metaplasia found that *H pylori* eradication increased the regression of high risk lesions compared with no eradication. We found consistent evidence from observational studies of an association between *H pylori* infection and increased risk of distal gastric adeno-carcinoma.

#### One triple regimen versus another

We found no systematic review or RCTs of the effects of different triple regimens on symptoms, quality of life, or mortality. One systematic review has found that clarithromycin 500 mg twice daily versus clarithromycin 250 mg twice daily plus a proton pump inhibitor❻ plus amoxicillin significantly increases *H pylori* eradication, but found no significant difference between clarithromycin 500 mg twice daily compared with clarithromycin 250 mg twice daily plus a proton pump inhibitor plus metronidazole in *H pylori* eradication rates. Another systematic review has found that a triple regimen containing ranitidine bismuth❻ plus clarithromycin plus metronidazole versus a triple regimen containing ranitidine bismuth plus clarithromycin plus amoxicillin significantly increases eradication at 5–7 days.

### UNLIKELY TO BE BENEFICIAL

#### *H pylori* eradication in people with gastro-oesophageal reflux disease

One RCT in people with gastro-oesophageal reflux disease found no significant difference between *H pylori* eradication treatment and placebo in symptomatic relapse.

**DEFINITION**  *Helicobacter pylori* is a Gram negative flagellated spiral bacterium found in the stomach. Infection with *H pylori* is predominantly acquired in childhood. The organism is associated with lifelong chronic gastritis and may cause other gastroduodenal disorders.[1]

**INCIDENCE/ PREVALENCE**  *H pylori* prevalence rates vary with birth cohort and social class in the developed world. Prevalence rates in many developed countries tend to be much higher (50–80%) in those born before 1950 in comparison to rates (< 20%) in individuals born more recently.[2] In many developing countries the infection has a high prevalence (80–95%) irrespective of the period of birth.[3] Adult prevalence is believed to represent the persistence of a historically higher rate of infection acquired in childhood, rather than increasing acquisition of infection during life.

**AETIOLOGY/ RISK FACTORS**  Overcrowded conditions associated with childhood poverty lead to increased transmission and higher prevalence rates. Adult reinfection rates are low — less than 1% a year.[3]

▶

# *Helicobacter pylori* infection

◀ **PROGNOSIS**   *H pylori* infection is believed to be causally related to the development of duodenal and gastric ulceration, gastric B cell lymphoma, and distal gastric cancer. About 15% of people infected with *H pylori* will develop a peptic ulcer, and 1% of people will develop gastric cancer during their lifetime.[4] *H pylori* infection is not associated with a specific type of dyspeptic symptom.

Please refer to CD-ROM for full text and references.

Digestive system disorders

## What are the effects of surgical treatments in people with pancreatic cancer that is considered suitable for complete tumour resection?

### UNKNOWN EFFECTIVENESS

**Pylorus-preserving pancreaticoduodenectomy**
Four small RCTs found no evidence that pylorus-preserving surgery improved overall quality of life or 5 year survival compared with classical Whipple's procedure🄖. The studies may have lacked power to detect clinically important differences for these outcomes.

**Surgery\***
We found no RCTs comparing surgery versus non-surgical treatment in people with resectable pancreatic cancer. Observational data provide limited evidence that surgery may reduce mortality compared with non-surgical treatment, although results may be confounded by differences in disease stage.

\*RCTs comparing surgery versus no surgery may be considered unethical in people with pancreatic cancer that is considered suitable for complete tumour resection.

## What are the effects of adjuvant treatments in people with resected pancreatic cancer?

### LIKELY TO BE BENEFICIAL

**Systemic fluorouracil-based chemotherapy after resection**
One RCT has found that adjuvant fluorouracil-based chemotherapy improves median survival compared with no adjuvant chemotherapy in people with resected pancreatic cancer. However, it found no evidence that fluorouracil improved 5 year survival directly, although the study may have lacked power to detect a difference. A second RCT did not directly compare chemotherapy alone versus no chemotherapy.

### UNKNOWN EFFECTIVENESS

**Systemic gemcitabine-based chemotherapy after resection**
One systematic review found insufficient evidence about effects of adjuvant gemcitabine compared with no adjuvant chemotherapy in people with resected pancreatic cancer.

**DEFINITION**     Primary adenocarcinoma of the pancreas. Other pancreatic malignancies, such as carcinoid tumour, are not considered in the present review. Pancreatic cancer is staged according to disease spread. Stage I disease is limited to the pancreas, duodenum, bile duct, or peri-pancreatic tissues, with no distant metastases or regional lymph node involvement. Stages II–IV describe disease that has spread more extensively or become metastatic. A pancreatic tumour is considered resectable if surgery aims to completely remove all cancerous tissue. Early stage tumours in the tail or body of the pancreas are more likely to be resectable than the more common, later stage cancers in the head of the pancreas. Other factors that influence resectability include proximity of the tumour to major blood vessels and perceived peri-operative risk. Symptoms include pain, jaundice, nausea, weight loss, loss of appetite, and symptoms of gastrointestinal obstruction and diabetes. ▶

# Pancreatic cancer

**INCIDENCE/ PREVALENCE**
Pancreatic cancer is the eighth most frequent cancer in the UK.[1] Annual incidence in England and Wales is about 12/100 000. Prevalence is similar in males and females, with 5–10% presenting with resectable disease.[2] Pancreatic cancer is the fourth most common cause of cancer death in higher income countries, responsible for about 30 000 deaths each year in the US.[3]

**AETIOLOGY/ RISK FACTORS**
Pancreatic cancer is more likely in people who smoke and have high alcohol intake. Dietary factors, such as lack of fruit and vegetables, are also reported risk factors.[4] One meta-analysis of observational studies found that people with diabetes mellitus of more than 5 years' duration are more likely to develop pancreatic cancer compared with the general population.[5] However, estimates of the magnitude of increased risk vary. Additional risk factors include pancreatitis and, in some cases, a family history.[1]

**PROGNOSIS**
Prognosis is poor. One year survival is about 12%, with 5 year survival ranging from less than 1% in those with advanced cancer at presentation to 5% in those with early stage cancer at presentation.[1,6]

---

Please refer to CD-ROM for full text and references.

## *What are the effects of treatments?*

### LIKELY TO BE BENEFICIAL

#### Complete surgical resection*

RCTs of complete surgical resection are unlikely to be conducted. Observational studies and multivariate analysis of RCTs have found a strong association between survival and complete resection of the primary tumour.

#### Subtotal gastrectomy (as effective as total gastrectomy) for resectable distal tumours

RCTs in people with primary tumours in the distal stomach have found no significant difference with total⊙ versus subtotal⊙ gastrectomy in 5 year survival or postoperative mortality.

*Observational evidence only; RCTs unlikely to be conducted.

### UNKNOWN EFFECTIVENESS

#### Adjuvant chemotherapy

Systematic reviews and subsequent RCTs have found conflicting evidence that adjuvant chemotherapy⊙ increases survival compared with surgery alone. Two RCTs found that adjuvant chemotherapy increased postoperative complications. The size of any benefit remains uncertain, and many recent adjuvant chemo-therapy regimens have not been evaluated fully in RCTs.

#### Radical versus conservative lymphadenectomy

Two large RCTs found no significant difference in 5 year survival rates between radical and conservative lymphadenectomy. However, confounding factors may have affected reliability of results, and we found conflicting data from subgroup analyses of prospective cohort studies.

### LIKELY TO BE INEFFECTIVE OR HARMFUL

#### Removal of adjacent organs

One RCT found no significant difference between radical gastrectomy plus splenectomy and radical gastrectomy alone in 5 year survival rates or postopera-tive mortality. The RCT found that radical gastrectomy plus splenectomy signifi-cantly increased the number of postoperative infections compared with radical gastrectomy alone. Retrospective analyses of observational studies and RCTs in people with stomach cancer found that removal of additional organs (spleen and distal pancreas) increased morbidity and mortality compared with no organ removal.

**DEFINITION**    Stomach cancer is usually an adenocarcinoma arising in the stomach and includes tumours arising at or just below the gastro-oesophageal junction (type II and III junctional tumours). Tumours are staged according to degree of invasion and spread❶. Only non-metastatic stomach cancers are considered in this topic.

**INCIDENCE/**    The incidence of stomach cancer varies among countries and by sex (inci-
**PREVALENCE** dence per 100 000 population a year in Japanese men is about 80, Japanese women 30, British men 18, British women 10, white American men 11, white American women 7).[1] Incidence has declined dramatically in North America, Australia, and New Zealand since 1930, but the decline in Europe has been ▶

# Stomach cancer

slower.[2] In the USA, stomach cancer remains relatively common among particular ethnic groups, especially Japanese–Americans and some Hispanic groups. The incidence of cancer of the proximal stomach and gastro-oesophageal junction is rising rapidly in many European populations and in North America.[3,4] The reasons for this are poorly understood.

**AETIOLOGY/ RISK FACTORS**  Distal stomach cancer is strongly associated with lifelong infection with *Helicobacter pylori* and poor dietary intake of antioxidant vitamins (A, C, and E).[5,6] In Western Europe and North America, distal stomach cancer is associated with relative socioeconomic deprivation. Proximal stomach cancer is strongly associated with smoking (OR about 4),[7] and is probably associated with gastro-oesophageal reflux, obesity, high fat intake, and medium to high socioeconomic status.

**PROGNOSIS**  Invasive stomach cancer (stages T2–T4) is fatal without surgery. Mean survival without treatment is less than 6 months from diagnosis.[8,9] Intramucosal or submucosal cancer (stage T1) may progress slowly to invasive cancer over several years.[10] In the USA, over 50% of people recently diagnosed with stomach cancer have regional lymph node metastasis or involvement of adjacent organs. The prognosis after macroscopically and microscopically complete resection (R0) is related strongly to disease stage⊙, particularly penetration of the serosa (stage T3) and lymph node involvement. Five year survival rates range from over 90% in intramucosal cancer to about 20% in people with stage T3N2 disease⊙. In Japan, the 5 year survival rate for people with advanced disease is reported to be about 50%, but the explanation for the difference remains unclear. Comparisons between Japanese and Western practice are confounded by factors such as age, fitness, and disease stage, as well as by tumour location, because many Western series include gastro-oesophageal junction adenocarcinoma with a much lower survival after surgery.

Please refer to CD-ROM for full text and references.

## What are the effects of treatments in people with clinically diagnosed acute sinusitis? New

### UNKNOWN EFFECTIVENESS

**Antibiotics**

One RCT found no evidence that amoxicillin reduced or cured symptoms compared with placebo in people with clinically diagnosed acute sinusitis. It found that diarrhoea was more common with amoxicillin than with placebo.

**Antihistamines; decongestants; steroids**

We found no RCTs examining the effects of antihistamines, decongestants, or steroids in people with clinically diagnosed acute sinusitis.

## What are the effects of treatments in people with radiologically or bacteriologically confirmed acute sinusitis? New

### LIKELY TO BE BENEFICIAL

**Cefalosporins and macrolides**

One systematic review in people with radiologically or bacteriologically confirmed acute sinusitis found no significant difference in clinical resolution between amoxicillin or amoxicillin–clavulanate and cefalosporins or macrolides. However, cefalosporins and macrolides caused fewer adverse effects than amoxicillin and amoxicillin–clavulanate. One RCT found no significant difference in clinical improvement or clinical cure between cefalosporins and azithromycin (a macrolide).

### TRADE OFF BETWEEN BENEFITS AND HARMS

**Amoxicillin and amoxicillin-clavulanate**

One systematic review identified two RCTs in people with radiologically or bacteriologically confirmed acute maxillary sinusitis, which found that amoxicillin improved early clinical cure rate compared with placebo, but was associated with more frequent adverse effects, mainly gastrointestinal. One systematic review in people with radiologically or bacterological confirmed acute sinusitis found no significant difference in clinical resolution between amoxicillin or amoxicillin–clavulanate and cefalosporins or macrolides. However, amoxicillin and amoxicillin–clavulanate caused more adverse effects.

### UNKNOWN EFFECTIVENESS

**Different dosages of antibiotics**

One RCT in people with radiologically or bacteriologically confirmed acute sinusitis found no significant difference in clinical resolution rates or adverse events between two and three daily doses of cefaclor.

**Antihistamines; decongestants; steroids**

We found no RCTs examining effects of antihistamines, decongestants, or steroids in people with radiologically or bacteriologically confirmed acute sinusitis.

# Acute sinusitis

**UNLIKELY TO BE BENEFICIAL**

## Long course antibiotic regimens

RCTs in people with confirmed acute sinusitis found no significant difference in clinical resolution rates between a 10 day course and 3–5 day courses of either co-trimoxazole or cefuroxime up to 3 weeks after treatment. One RCT found that adverse effects, which were mainly gastrointestinal, were more frequent with longer course cefuroxime than with shorter course cefuroxime.

**DEFINITION**  Acute sinusitis is defined pathologically, by transient inflammation of the mucosal lining of the paranasal sinuses lasting less than 4 weeks. Clinically, it is characterised by nasal congestion, rhinorrhoea**G**, facial pain, hyposmia**G**, sneezing, and, if more severe, additional malaise and fever. The diagnosis is usually made clinically (on the basis of history and examination, but without radiological or bacteriological investigation). Clinically diagnosed acute sinusitis is less likely to be due to bacterial infection than is acute sinusitis confirmed by radiological or bacteriological investigation.[1] In this chapter, we have excluded studies in children, in people with symptoms for more than 4 weeks (chronic sinusitis), and in people with symptoms following facial trauma. We have made it clear in each section whether we are dealing with clinically diagnosed acute sinusitis or acute sinusitis that has been confirmed by bacteriological or radiological investigation, because the effects of treatment may be different in these groups.

**INCIDENCE/ PREVALENCE**  Each year in Europe, between 1% and 5% of adults are diagnosed with acute sinusitis by their general practitioner.[2] Extrapolated to the British population, this is estimated to cause 6 million restricted working days per year.[3,4] Most people with acute sinusitis are assessed and treated in a primary care setting. The prevalence varies according to whether diagnosis is made on clinical grounds or on the basis of radiological or bacteriological investigation.

**AETIOLOGY/ RISK FACTORS**  One systematic review reported that about 50% of people with a clinical diagnosis of acute sinusitis have bacterial sinus infection.[1] The usual pathogens in acute bacterial sinusitis are *Streptococcus pneumoniae* and *Haemophilus influenza*, with occasional infection with *Moraxella catarrhalis*. Preceding viral upper respiratory tract infection is often the trigger for acute bacterial sinusitis,[5] with about 0.5% of common colds becoming complicated by the development of acute sinusitis.[6]

**PROGNOSIS**  One meta-analysis of RCTs found that up to two thirds of people with acute sinusitis had spontaneous resolution of symptoms without active treatment.[7] One non-systematic review reported that people with acute sinusitis are at risk of chronic sinusitis and irreversible damage to the normal mucociliary mucosal surface.[8] One further non-systematic review reported rare life-threatening complications, such as orbital cellulitis**G** and meningitis following acute sinusitis.[9] However, we found no reliable data to quantify these risks.

Please refer to CD-ROM for full text and references.

# Chronic suppurative otitis media

**Search date March 2003**

*Jose Acuin*

## What are the effects of treatments in adults?

We found no RCTs with long term follow up.

### Topical antibiotics

We found no RCTs with long term follow up. Two RCTs found limited evidence that topical quinolone antibiotics improved otoscopic appearances compared with placebo in adults with chronic suppurative otitis media. Six RCTs found no clear evidence of clinically important differences among topical antibiotics in adults. One systematic review found that topical antibiotics were more effective than systemic antibiotics for reducing otoscopic features of chronic suppurative otitis media. One RCT found no significant effect of adding topical ceftizoxime to systemic ceftizoxime compared with systemic ceftizoxime alone. One RCT found no significant effect of preoperative topical antibiotics compared with no preoperative treatment in people undergoing tympanoplasty. Short term topical antibiotics have been associated with few adverse events in RCTs. Uncontrolled case studies have reported vestibular ototoxicity after topical non-quinolone antibiotics.

### Ear cleansing (aural toilet)

We found no RCTs comparing ear cleansing❸ versus no treatment.

### Systemic antibiotics

We found insufficient evidence about the effects of systemic antibiotics compared with placebo, no treatment, or topical antiseptics. One systematic review found that systemic antibiotics were less effective than topical antibiotics in reducing otoscopic features of chronic suppurative otitis media. We found no evidence about long term treatment.

### Topical antibiotics plus topical steroids

One systematic review found insufficient evidence from three RCTs about effects on symptoms of topical antibiotics plus topical steroids versus placebo or topical steroids alone.

### Topical antiseptics

We found no RCTs comparing topical antiseptics versus placebo or no treatment. One RCT compared topical antiseptics plus ear cleansing under microscopic control versus topical antibiotics alone or versus oral antibiotics. It found no significant difference in the rate of persistent activity on otoscopy. However, the RCT was too small to exclude a clinically important difference.

### Topical steroids

We found no RCTs comparing topical steroids versus placebo or no treatment.

### Tympanoplasty with or without mastoidectomy

We found no RCTs comparing tympanoplasty❸ with or without mastoidectomy❸ versus no surgery for chronic suppurative otitis media without cholesteatoma❸. ▶

# Chronic suppurative otitis media

◄ *What are the effects of treatments in children?*

**UNKNOWN EFFECTIVENESS**

### Ear cleansing

One systematic review found no significant difference in persistent otorrhoea or tympanic perforations with a simple form of ear cleansing versus no ear cleansing. However, a clinically important effect cannot be excluded.

### Systemic antibiotics

RCTs found insufficient evidence about the effects of systemic antibiotics in children with chronic suppurative otitis media.

### Topical antibiotics

We found no RCTs comparing topical antibiotics versus placebo.

### Topical antibiotics plus topical steroids

We found insufficient evidence from small RCTs to compare topical antibiotics plus topical steroids versus cleansing only or topical antiseptics. We found no RCTs comparing topical antibiotics plus topical steroids versus either topical treatment alone.

### Topical antiseptics

Two RCTs found no significant reduction in otorrhoea with topical antiseptics versus placebo after 2 weeks. One RCT found no significant difference in otorrhoea with topical antiseptics versus topical antibiotic plus steroid. However, the RCTs were too small to exclude a clinically important effect.

### Topical steroids

We found no RCTs comparing topical steroids versus placebo.

### Tympanoplasty with or without mastoidectomy

We found no RCTs comparing tympanoplasty with or without mastoidectomy versus no surgery for chronic suppurative otitis media without cholesteatoma.

**DEFINITION**
Chronic suppurative otitis media is persistent inflammation of the middle ear or mastoid cavity. Synonyms include "chronic otitis media (without effusion)", chronic mastoiditis, and chronic tympanomastoiditis. Chronic suppurative otitis media is characterised by recurrent or persistent ear discharge (otorrhoea) over 2–6 weeks through a perforation of the tympanic membrane. Typical findings also include thickened granular middle ear mucosa, mucosal polyps, and cholesteatoma🅖 within the middle ear. Chronic suppurative otitis media is differentiated from chronic otitis media with effusion, in which there is an intact tympanic membrane with fluid in the middle ear but no active infection. Chronic suppurative otitis media does not include chronic perforations of the eardrum that are dry, or only occasionally discharge, and have no signs of active infection.

**INCIDENCE/**
**PREVALENCE**
The worldwide prevalence of chronic suppurative otitis media is 65–330 million people. Between 39–200 million (60%) suffer from clinically significant hearing impairment. Otitis media was estimated to have caused 28 000 deaths and loss of over 2 million Disability Adjusted Life Years🅖 in 2000,[1] 94% of which were in developing countries. Most of these deaths were probably due to chronic suppurative otitis media because acute otitis media is a self limiting infection. Estimates of prevalence are shown in table A on web extra.[2–32]

**AETIOLOGY/**
**RISK FACTORS**
Chronic suppurative otitis media is assumed to be a complication of acute otitis media, but the risk factors for chronic suppurative otitis media are not clear. Frequent upper respiratory tract infections and poor socioeconomic conditions ▶

(overcrowded housing,[33] hygiene, and nutrition) may be related to the development of chronic suppurative otitis media.[34,35] Improvement of housing, hygiene, and nutrition in Maori children was associated with a halving of the prevalence of chronic suppurative otitis media between 1978 and 1987.[36] See also acute otitis media, p 47.

**PROGNOSIS** Most children with chronic suppurative otitis media have mild to moderate hearing impairment (about 26–60 dB increase in hearing thresholds) based on surveys among children in Africa, Brazil,[37] India,[38] and Sierra Leone,[39] and among the general population in Thailand.[40] In many developing countries, chronic suppurative otitis media represents the most frequent cause of moderate hearing loss (40–60 dB).[41] Persistent hearing loss during the first 2 years of life may increase learning disabilities and poor scholastic performance.[42] Spread of infection may lead to life threatening complications such as intracranial infections and acute mastoiditis.[43] The frequency of serious complications fell from 20% in 1938 to 2.5% in 1948 and is currently estimated to be about 0.24% in Thailand and 1.8% in Africa. This is believed to be associated with increased use of antibiotic treatment, tympanoplasty, and mastoidectomy.[44-46] Cholesteatoma is another serious complication that has been found in a variable proportion of people with chronic suppurative otitis media (range 0–60%).[47-50] In the West, the incidence of cholesteatoma is low (in 1993 in Finland the age standardised incidence of cholesteatoma was eight new cases per 100 000 population/year).[51]

Please refer to CD-ROM for full text and references.

# Menière's disease

**Search date October 2002**

*Adrian James and Marc Thorp*

---

## What are the effects of treatments for acute attacks?

**UNKNOWN EFFECTIVENESS**

### Anticholinergics; benzodiazepines; betahistine

We found no RCTs on the effects of these interventions.

---

## What are the effects of prophylactic interventions?

**UNKNOWN EFFECTIVENESS**

### Betahistine (for vertigo or tinnitus)

Six RCTs found insufficient evidence about the effects of betahistine versus placebo on the frequency and severity of attacks of vertigo, tinnitus, and aural fullness. Two small RCTs in people with definite or possible Menière's disease found no significant difference with betahistine versus trimetazidine in hearing or tinnitus. One of these RCTs found that betahistine versus trimetazidine significantly decreased the proportion of people reporting that the intensity of vertigo was "substantially better or cured". The other RCT found no significant difference with betahistine versus trimetazidine in vertigo intensity.

### Diuretics

One small crossover RCT in people with possible Menière's disease found no significant difference with triamterene plus hydrochlorothiazide versus placebo in change in hearing over 17 weeks, and found insufficient evidence on vertigo and tinnitus

### Trimetazidine

We found no RCTs comparing trimetazidine versus placebo to prevent attacks of Menière's disease. Two small RCTs in people with definite or possible Menière's disease found no significant difference with trimetazidine versus betahistine in hearing or tinnitus. One of these RCTs found that trimetazidine versus betahistine significantly increased the number of people reporting that the intensity of vertigo was "substantially better or cured". The other RCT found no significant difference with trimetazidine versus betahistine in vertigo intensity.

### Dietary modification; psychological support; systemic aminoglycosides; vestibular rehabilitation

We found no RCTs on the effects of these interventions.

**UNLIKELY TO BE BENEFICIAL**

### Betahistine (for hearing loss)

Four RCTs found no change in hearing as assessed by changes in pure tone audiograms with betahistine versus placebo. Two small RCTs in people with definite or possible Menière's disease found no significant difference with betahistine versus trimetazidine in hearing or tinnitus.

## Lithium

Two small crossover RCTs in people with possible Menière's disease found no difference with lithium versus placebo in vertigo, tinnitus, aural fullness, or hearing, and found that lithium was associated with tremor, thirst, and polyuria in some people.

**DEFINITION** Menière's disease is characterised by recurrent episodes of spontaneous rotational vertigo and sensorineural hearing loss with tinnitus and a feeling of fullness or pressure in the ear. It may be unilateral or bilateral. Acute episodes may occur in clusters of about 6–11 a year, although remission may last several months.[1] The diagnosis is made clinically.[2] It is important to distinguish Menière's disease from other types of vertigo that might occur independently with hearing loss and tinnitus, and respond differently to treatment (e.g. benign positional vertigo, acute labyrinthitis). Strict diagnostic criteria help. In this review we applied the classification of the American Academy of Otolaryngology–Head and Neck Surgery to indicate the diagnostic rigour used in RCTs❶.

**INCIDENCE/ PREVALENCE** Menière's disease is most common between 40–60 years of age, although younger people can be affected.[6,7] In Europe, the incidence is about 50–200/ 100 000 a year. A survey of general practitioner records of 27 365 people in the UK found an incidence of 43 affected people in a 1 year period (157/100 000).[8] Diagnostic criteria were not defined in this survey. A survey of over 8 million people in Sweden found an incidence of 46/100 000 a year with diagnosis strictly based on the triad of vertigo, hearing loss, and tinnitus.[9] From smaller studies, the incidence appears lower in Uganda[10] and higher in Japan (350/100 000 based on a national survey of hospital attendances during a single wk).[7]

**AETIOLOGY/ RISK FACTORS** Menière's disease is associated with endolymphatic hydrops (raised endolymph pressure in the membranous labyrinth of the inner ear),[11] but a causal relationship between Menière's disease and endolymphatic hydrops remains unproven.[12] Specific disorders associated with hydrops (such as temporal bone fracture, syphilis, hypothyroidism, Cogan's syndrome❸, and Mondini dysplasia❸, can produce similar symptoms to Menière's disease.

**PROGNOSIS** Menière's disease is progressive, but fluctuates unpredictably. It is difficult to distinguish natural resolution from the effects of treatment. Significant improvement of vertigo is usually seen in the placebo arm of RCTs.[13,14] Acute attacks of vertigo often increase in frequency during the first few years after presentation then decrease in frequency in association with sustained deterioration in hearing.[6] In most people, vertiginous episodes eventually cease completely.[15] In one 20 year cohort study in 34 people, 28 (82%) people had at least moderate hearing loss (mean pure tone hearing loss > 50 dB)[1] and 16 (47%) developed bilateral disease. Symptoms other than hearing loss improve in 60–80% of people irrespective of treatment.[16]

Please refer to CD-ROM for full text and references.

# Middle ear pain and trauma during air travel

**Search date November 2002**

*Simon Janvrin*

Ear, nose, and throat disorders

## What are the effects of preventive interventions?

### LIKELY TO BE BENEFICIAL

**Oral decongestants in adults**

One RCT in adult passengers with a history of ear pain during air travel found limited evidence that oral pseudoephedrine versus placebo significantly decreased symptoms of barotrauma during air travel. One other RCT in adult passengers with a history of ear pain during air travel found limited evidence that oral pseudoephedrine versus placebo significantly decreased ear pain and hearing loss during air travel.

### UNKNOWN EFFECTIVENESS

**Oral decongestants in children**

One small RCT in children up to the age of 6 years found no significant difference with oral pseudoephedrine versus placebo in ear pain at take off or landing.

**Topical nasal decongestants**

One small RCT in adults with a history of ear pain during air travel found no significant difference with oxymetazoline nasal spray versus placebo in symptoms of barotrauma.

**DEFINITION** The effects of air travel on the middle ear can include ear drum pain, vertigo, hearing loss, and ear drum perforation.

**INCIDENCE/ PREVALENCE** The prevalence of symptoms depends on the altitude, type of aircraft, and characteristics of the passengers. One point prevalence study found that 20% of adult and 40% of child passengers had negative pressure in the middle ear after flight, and that 10% of adults and 22% of children had auroscopic evidence of damage to the ear drum.[1] We found no data on the incidence of perforation, which seems to be extremely rare in commercial passengers.

**AETIOLOGY/ RISK FACTORS** During aircraft descent, the pressure in the middle ear drops relative to that in the ear canal. A narrow, inflamed, or poorly functioning Eustachian tube impedes the necessary influx of air. As the pressure difference between the middle and outer ear increases, the ear drum is pulled inward.

**PROGNOSIS** In most people, symptoms resolve spontaneously. Experience in military aviation shows that most ear drum perforations will heal spontaneously.[2]

Please refer to CD-ROM for full text and references.

## What are the effects of empirical treatment? *New*

### LIKELY TO BE BENEFICIAL

### Topical aluminium acetate drops (as effective as topical anti-infective agents)

We found no RCTs that compared topical aluminium acetate versus placebo. One RCT found no significant difference in clinical cure between aluminium acetate drops and topical polymyxin–neomycin–hydrocortisone drops at 4 weeks.

### Topical anti-infective agents (antibiotics or antifungals with or without steroids)

One RCT found that methylprednisolone–neomycin drops improved symptoms and signs compared with placebo at 28 days. Two RCTs found no significant difference in cure rate between topical quinolones and other topical anti-infective agents. One RCT found that triamcinolone–neomycin drops improved resolution rates compared with hydrocortisone–neomycin–polymyxin B drops. We found limited evidence from two RCTs that neomycin–dexamethasone–acetic acid spray improved clinical cure compared with topical anti-infective drops that did not contain acetic acid.

### Topical steroids alone

One RCT found that topical budesonide improved symptoms and signs compared with placebo in people with mild to moderately severe otitis externa. One RCT found no significant difference in symptom scores between topical hydrocortisone and topical hydrocortisone butyrate after 1 week.

### UNKNOWN EFFECTIVENESS

### Oral antibiotics

We found no RCTs of oral antibiotics versus placebo or topical anti-infective agents.

### Specialist aural toilet

We found no RCTs comparing specialist aural toilet❻ versus no aural toilet. One RCT found no significant difference in clinical cure between an ear wick with anti-infective drops versus ribbon gauze impregnated with anti-infective ointment.

### UNLIKELY TO BE BENEFICIAL

### Oral antibiotics plus topical anti-infective agents (compared with topical anti-infective agents alone)

We found limited evidence from one RCT of no clinical effect of oral antibiotics plus topical anti-infective agents compared with topical anti-infective agents alone.

**DEFINITION**  Otitis externa is inflammation, often with infection, of the external ear canal. This inflammation is usually generalised throughout the ear canal so it is often referred to as "diffuse otitis externa". The present topic excludes localised inflammations such as furuncles. Otitis externa has acute (< 6 weeks), chronic (> 3 months), and necrotising forms. Acute otitis externa may present as a single episode, or recur. It causes severe pain with aural ▶

# Otitis externa

discharge and associated hearing loss.[1] If the ear canal is visible, it appears red and inflamed. Chronic otitis externa may result in canal stenosis with associated hearing loss, for which it may be difficult to fit hearing aids. Necrotising otitis externa is defined by destruction of the temporal bone, usually in people with diabetes or in people who are immunocompromised. Necrotising otitis externa can be life-threatening.[2]

**INCIDENCE/ PREVALENCE**  Otitis externa is common in all parts of the world. The incidence is not known precisely, but 10% of people are thought to have been affected at some time.[3] The condition affects children, but is more common in adults. It accounts for a large proportion of the workload of otolaryngology departments, but milder cases are often managed in primary care.[3]

**AETIOLOGY/ RISK FACTORS**  Otitis externa may be associated with local or generalised eczema of the ear canal. It is more common in swimmers, in humid environments, in people with an absence of ear wax or narrow external ear canals, in hearing aid users, and after mechanical trauma.[4]

**PROGNOSIS**  We found few reliable data. Many cases of otitis externa resolve spontaneously over several weeks or months. Acute episodes have a tendency to recur, although the risk of recurrence is unknown. Experience suggests that chronic inflammation affects a small proportion of people after a single episode of acute otitis externa, and may rarely lead to canal stenosis.[1] We found no reliable data about risks of necrotising otitis externa, although it is thought to be a complication that only affects people with diabetes or who are immunosuppressed.

Please refer to CD-ROM for full text and references.

**Search date November 2002**

*Ian Williamson*

## What are the effects of preventive interventions?

### UNKNOWN EFFECTIVENESS

**Change in modifiable risk factors**

We found no RCTs on the effects of avoiding risk factors such as passive smoking and bottle feeding in preventing otitis media with effusion (OME).

## What are the effects of treatments?

### LIKELY TO BE BENEFICIAL

**Autoinflation with nasal balloon (short term benefit)**

One systematic review has found that autoinflation with a nasal balloon significantly improves effusion compared with no treatment. Some children may find autoinflation difficult.

### TRADE OFF BETWEEN BENEFITS AND HARMS

**Antimicrobial drugs (possible short term benefit)**

One systematic review found limited evidence that antimicrobial drugs significantly increased resolution of effusion at up to 1 month compared with placebo or no treatment. However, a a subsequent systematic review found no significant difference between antimicrobial drugs and placebo. Timing to outcome of included RCTs was unclear. Adverse effects of antibiotics (mainly nausea, vomiting, and diarrhoea) have been reported in 2–32% of children.

### UNKNOWN EFFECTIVENESS

**Topical steroids**

One small RCT found no significant difference between topical steroids alone and placebo for resolution of effusion. A second small RCT found limited evidence that topical steroids plus antibiotics improved short term symptoms as compared with antibiotics alone. It did not report on adverse events.

**Grommets with or without adenoidectomy; other autoinflation devices; tonsillectomy**

We found insufficient evidence on the effects of these interventions.

### UNLIKELY TO BE BENEFICIAL

**Mucolytics**

One systematic review found no significant difference between 1–3 month courses of carbocisteine and placebo or no treatment in resolution of effusion. Three small RCTs of bromhexine versus placebo found conflicting results.

### LIKELY TO BE INEFFECTIVE OR HARMFUL

**Antihistamines plus oral decongestants**

One systematic review found no significant difference between antihistamines plus oral decongestants and placebo in clearance of effusion after 4 weeks.

# Otitis media with effusion

## Oral steroids

One systematic review found no significant difference between oral steroids and placebo in clearance of effusion after 2 weeks. It found limited evidence that oral steroids plus antibiotics improved resolution rates compared with antibiotic alone. Oral steroids may cause behavioural changes, increased appetite, and weight gain.

**DEFINITION**    OME, or "glue ear", is serous or mucoid but not mucopurulent fluid in the middle ear. Children usually present with hearing loss and speech problems. In contrast to those with acute otitis media (see topic, p 47), children with OME do not suffer from acute ear pain, fever, or malaise. Hearing loss is usually mild and often identified when parents express concern regarding their child's behaviour, school performance, or language development.

**INCIDENCE/**    One study in the UK found that, at any time, 5% of children aged 2–4 years
**PREVALENCE**    have persistent (at least 3 months) bilateral hearing loss associated with OME. The prevalence declines considerably beyond age 6 years.[1] About 80% of children aged 10 years have been affected by OME at some time in the past. OME is the most common reason for referral for surgery in children in the UK. Middle ear effusions also occur infrequently in adults after upper respiratory tract infection or after air travel, and may persist for weeks or months after an episode of acute otitis media.[2]

**AETIOLOGY/**    Contributory factors include upper respiratory tract infection and narrow upper
**RISK FACTORS** respiratory airways. Case control studies have identified risk factors, including age 6 years or younger at first onset, day care centre attendance, high number of siblings, low socioeconomic group, frequent upper respiratory tract infection, bottle feeding, and household smoking.[3,4] Most factors are associated with about twice the risk of developing OME.[5]

**PROGNOSIS**    In 5% of preschool children, OME (identified by tympanometric screening) persists for at least 1 year.[6,7] One large cohort study (534 children) found that middle ear disease increased reported hearing difficulty at age 5 years (OR 1.44, 95% CI 1.18 to 1.76) and was associated with delayed language development in children up to age 10 years.[8]

Please refer to CD-ROM for full text and references.

### Search date January 2003

*Aziz Sheikh, Sukhmeet Panesar, and Sangeeta Dhami*

## What are the effects of treatments on quality of life?

### BENEFICIAL

**Oral fexofenadine**
Three RCTs found that fexofenadine improved quality of life and rhinitis symptoms compared with placebo.

### LIKELY TO BE BENEFICIAL

**Oral leukotriene receptor antagonists**
Two large RCTs found that oral montelukast improved quality of life compared with placebo.

**Oral leukotriene receptor antagonists plus oral antihistamines**
Two RCTs found that oral montelukast plus oral loratadine improved quality of life compared with loratadine alone or placebo.

### UNKNOWN EFFECTIVENESS

**Intranasal antihistamines; intranasal ipratropium bromide; oral decongestants; oral decongestants plus oral antihistamines; other oral antihistamines**
We found no RCTs evaluating the effects of these interventions on quality of life.

## What are the effects of treatments on rhinitis symptoms?

### BENEFICIAL

**Intranasal levocabastine**
RCTs found that intranasal levocabastine improved symptoms of seasonal allergic rhinitis compared with placebo.

**Oral antihistamines (acrivastine, azatadine, brompheniramine, cetirizine, ebastine, fexofenadine, loratadine, or mizolastine)**
Numerous RCTs have found that oral antihistamines (acrivastine, azatadine, brompheniramine, cetirizine, ebastine, loratadine, or mizolastine) versus placebo significantly improved rhinitis symptoms. Drowsiness, sedation, or somnolence were the most commonly reported adverse events.

**Oral pseudoephedrine plus oral antihistamines**
RCTs have found that pseudoephedrine plus oral antihistamines (fexofenadine, acrivastine, cetirizine, terfenadine, triprolidine, loratadine, or azatadine) improved overall symptoms of seasonal allergic rhinitis compared with pseudoephedrine or oral antihistamine or placebo alone. The most common adverse effects reported with combination treatment were headache and insomnia.

### LIKELY TO BE BENEFICIAL

**Oral leukotriene receptor antagonists**
Two large RCTs found that oral montelukast improved daytime nasal symptom score compared with placebo.

Ear, nose, and throat disorders

◀ **Oral leukotriene receptor antagonists plus oral antihistamines**

Two RCTs found that oral montelukast plus oral loratadine improved nasal symptoms compared with placebo, although they found conflicting effects compared with single treatments.

**TRADE OFF BETWEEN BENEFITS AND HARMS**

**Oral astemizole**

RCTs have found that astemizole versus placebo significantly improves rhinitis symptoms but astemizole has been associated with prolongation of the QTc interval, and may induce ventricular arrhythmias.

**Oral terfenadine**

RCTs have found conflicting results about effectiveness of terfenadine versus placebo on rhinitis symptoms. Terfenadine is associated with risk of fatal cardiac toxicity if used in conjunction with macrolide antibiotics, oral antifungal agents, or grapefruit juice.

**UNKNOWN EFFECTIVENESS**

**Intranasal azelastine**

RCTs have found conflicting results on effectiveness of intranasal azelastine versus placebo on symptoms of seasonal allergic rhinitis. Two small RCTs found no significant difference in nasal symptoms between intranasal antihistamines (azelastine, levocabastine) and oral antihistamines (cetirizine, terfenadine)

**Intranasal ipratropium bromide**

We found no systematic review or published RCTs.

**DEFINITION**    Seasonal allergic rhinitis is a symptom complex that may affect several organ systems. Symptoms will typically consist of seasonal sneezing, nasal itching, nasal blockage, and watery nasal discharge.[1] Eye symptoms (red eyes, itchy eyes, and tearing) are common. Other symptoms may include peak seasonal coughing, wheezing, and shortness of breath, oral allergy syndrome (manifesting as an itchy swollen oropharynx on eating stoned fruits), and systemic symptoms such as tiredness, fever, a pressure sensation in the head, and itchiness. Confirming the presence of pollen hypersensitivity using objective allergy tests such as skin prick tests, detection of serum specific IgE, and nasal provocation challenge testing may improve diagnostic accuracy.

**INCIDENCE/**    Seasonal allergic rhinitis is found throughout the world. Epidemiological
**PREVALENCE**    evidence suggests that there is considerable geographical variation in its prevalence. Prevalence is highest in socioeconomically developed countries, where the condition may affect as much as 25% of the population.[2–4] Prevalence and severity are increasing. It is thought that improved living standards and reduced risk of childhood infections may lead to immune deviation of T helper cells in early life, which may increase susceptibility to seasonal allergic rhinitis (the so called "hygiene hypothesis").[5,6] Although people of all ages may be affected, the peak age of onset is adolescence.[7]

**AETIOLOGY/**    The symptoms of seasonal allergic rhinitis are caused by an IgE mediated type
**RISK FACTORS**  1 hypersensitivity reaction to grass, tree, or weed pollen. Allergy to other seasonal aeroallergens such as fungal spores may also provoke symptoms. Typically, symptoms become worse during the relevant pollen season and in the open, when pollen exposure is increased. Risk factors include a personal or family history of atopy or other allergic disorders, male sex, birth order (increased risk being seen in first born), and small family size.[8,9]

▶

◀ **PROGNOSIS**  Seasonal allergic rhinitis may impair quality of life, interfering with work, sleep, and recreational activities.[10] Other allergic problems such as asthma and eczema frequently coexist, adding to the impact of rhinitis.[11]

Please refer to CD-ROM for full text and references.

*Ear, nose, and throat disorders*

# Tinnitus

Search date October 2002

*Angus Waddell and Richard Canter*

---

## What are the effects of treatments for chronic tinnitus?

### LIKELY TO BE BENEFICIAL

#### Tricyclic antidepressants

One small RCT in people with depression and chronic tinnitus found that tricyclic antidepressants (nortriptyline) versus placebo significantly improved tinnitus related disability, audiometric tinnitus loudness matching, and symptoms of depression, but found no significant difference in tinnitus severity at 6 weeks. One small RCT in people with tinnitus but without depression found that a greater proportion of people rated themselves as improved with tricyclic antidepressants (amitriptyline) versus placebo at 6 weeks

### UNKNOWN EFFECTIVENESS

#### Psychotherapy

One systematic review found insufficient evidence about effects of cognitive behavioural treatment, relaxation therapy, counselling, education, hypnosis, bio-feedback, or stress management compared with other or no treatment in people with chronic tinnitus.

#### Acupuncture; antiepileptics; baclofen; benzodiazepines; cinnarizine; electromagnetic stimulation; hyperbaric oxygen; hypnosis; low power laser; nicotinamide; tinnitus masking devices; zinc

We found insufficient evidence about the effects of these interventions.

### LIKELY TO BE INEFFECTIVE OR HARMFUL

#### Ginkgo biloba

One systematic review and one subsequent RCT found no significant difference with ginkgo biloba versus placebo in tinnitus symptoms.

#### Tocainide

One RCT found no significant difference with tocainide versus placebo in improving symptoms, but found evidence that tocainide caused significantly more adverse effects after 30 days' treatment.

**DEFINITION** Tinnitus is defined as the perception of sound, which does not arise from the external environment, from within the body (e.g. vascular sounds), or from auditory hallucinations related to mental illness. This review concerns the management of chronic tinnitus, where tinnitus is the only, or the predominant, symptom in an affected person.

**INCIDENCE/ PREVALENCE** Up to 18% of the general population in industrialised countries are mildly affected by chronic tinnitus, and 0.5% report tinnitus having a severe effect on their ability to lead a normal life.[1]

**AETIOLOGY/ RISK FACTORS** Tinnitus may occur as an isolated idiopathic symptom or in association with any type of hearing loss. Tinnitus may be a particular feature of presbyacusis, noise induced hearing loss, Ménière's disease ⑥ (see Ménière's disease, p 108), or the presence of an acoustic neuroma. In people with toxicity from aspirin or quinine, tinnitus can occur while hearing thresholds remain normal. Tinnitus is also associated with depression, although it may be unclear whether the tinnitus is a manifestation of the depressive illness or a factor contributing to its development.[2]

Ear, nose, and throat disorders

**PROGNOSIS** Tinnitus may have an insidious onset, with a long delay before clinical presentation. It may persist for many years or decades, particularly when associated with a sensorineural hearing loss. In Menière's disease both the presence and intensity of tinnitus can fluctuate. Tinnitus may cause disruption of sleep patterns, an inability to concentrate, and depression.[3]

Please refer to CD-ROM for full text and references.

# Tonsillitis

## Search date August 2002

*William McKerrow*

---

## What are the effects of tonsillectomy for severe tonsillitis in children and adults?

### TRADE OFF BETWEEN BENEFITS AND HARMS

**Tonsillectomy versus antibiotics in children**

Two systematic reviews found limited evidence that tonsillectomy may benefit some children with severe tonsillitis, but found insufficient evidence to compare surgical versus medical treatment. One subsequent RCT in less severely affected children found that surgery significantly reduced the frequency of tonsillitis compared with medical treatment over 3 years. The modest benefit may be outweighed by morbidity associated with the generation in populations with low incidence of tonsillitis.

### UNKNOWN EFFECTIVENESS

**Tonsillectomy versus antibiotics in adults**

We found no RCTs evaluating tonsillectomy in adults.

| | |
|---|---|
| **DEFINITION** | Tonsillitis is infection of the parenchyma of the palatine tonsils. The definition of severe recurrent tonsillitis is arbitrary, but recent criteria have defined tonsillitis as five or more episodes of true tonsillitis a year, symptoms for at least a year, and episodes that are disabling and prevent normal functioning.[1] |
| **INCIDENCE/ PREVALENCE** | Recurrent sore throat has an incidence in general practice in the UK of 100/1000 population a year.[2] Acute tonsillitis is more common in childhood. |
| **AETIOLOGY/ RISK FACTORS** | Common bacterial pathogens include β haemolytic and other streptococci. Bacteria are cultured successfully only from a minority of people with tonsillitis. The role of viruses is uncertain. |
| **PROGNOSIS** | We found no good data on the natural history of tonsillitis or recurrent sore throat in children or adults. Participants in RCTs who were randomised to medical treatment (courses of antibiotics as required) have shown a tendency towards improvement over time.[3,4] Recurrent severe tonsillits results in significant morbidity, including time lost from school or work. |

---

Please refer to CD-ROM for full text and references.

Search date April 2003

*George Browning*

## What are the effects of methods to remove symptomatic ear wax?

### TRADE OFF BETWEEN BENEFITS AND HARMS

**Ear syringing***

There is consensus that ear syringing is effective but we found no RCTs comparing ear syringing versus no treatment or versus other treatment. Reported complications of ear syringing include otitis externa, perforation of the ear drum, damage to the skin of the external canal, tinnitus, pain, and vertigo.

### UNKNOWN EFFECTIVENESS

**Manual removal (other than ear syringing)***

We found no RCTs about other mechanical methods of removing ear wax.

**Wax softeners**

One small RCT in people with impacted wax found that active treatment (with a proprietary softening agent, sodium bicarbonate, or sterile water) reduced the risk of persisting impaction after 5 days compared with no treatment, but found no significant difference among active treatments. Three RCTs found no consistent evidence that any one type of wax softener was superior to the others. RCTs found insufficient evidence to assess the effects of wax softeners prior to syringing.

*Although many practitioners consider these to be standard treatments, we found no RCTs of these interventions.

| | |
|---|---|
| **DEFINITION** | Ear wax is normal and becomes a problem only if it produces deafness, pain, or other aural symptoms. Ear wax may also need to be removed if it prevents inspection of the ear drum. The term "impacted"⊕ is used in different ways and can merely imply the coexistence of wax obscuring the ear drum with symptoms in that ear.[1,2] |
| **INCIDENCE/ PREVALENCE** | We found four surveys of the prevalence of impacted wax⊕.[3–6] The prevalence was higher in men than in women, in the elderly than in the young, and in people with intellectual impairment.[7] One survey found that 289 Scottish general practitioners each saw an average of nine people a month requesting removal of ear wax.[1] |
| **AETIOLOGY/ RISK FACTORS** | Factors that prevent the normal extrusion of wax from the ear canal (e.g. wearing a hearing aid, using cotton buds) increase the chance of ear wax accumulating. |
| **PROGNOSIS** | Most ear wax emerges from the external canal spontaneously. Without impaction or adherence to the drum, there is likely to be minimal, if any, hearing loss. |

Please refer to CD-ROM for full text and references.

# Foot ulcers and amputations in diabetes

**Search date January 2003**

*Hertzel Gerstein and Dereck Hunt*

---

## What are the effects of preventive interventions?

### LIKELY TO BE BENEFICIAL

**Screening and referral to foot care clinics (for major amputations in those at high risk)**

One RCT found that a diabetes screening and protection programme (involving referral to a foot clinic) reduced the risk of major amputation compared with usual care after 2 years.

### UNKNOWN EFFECTIVENESS

**Education (for foot ulceration, serious foot lesions, amputation)**

One systematic review found insufficient evidence about the effects of patient education for the prevention of foot complications.

**Therapeutic footwear (for ulcer recurrence)**

In people with diabetes and previous diabetic foot ulcer, one RCT found no significant difference in rates of foot ulceration between therapeutic footwear and usual footwear.

---

## What are the effects of treatments?

### BENEFICIAL

**Pressure off-loading with non-removable cast (for non-infected foot ulcer healing)**

We found evidence that pressure off-loading⊕ with total contact casting⊕ or non-removable fibreglass casts improved non-infected diabetic foot ulcer healing compared with other treatments.

### LIKELY TO BE BENEFICIAL

**Human skin equivalent (for chronic neuropathic non-infected foot ulcer healing)**

One RCT found that human skin equivalent⊕ increased ulcer healing rates compared with saline moistened gauze in people with chronic neuropathic non-infected foot ulcers.

**Systemic hyperbaric oxygen (for infected ulcers)**

We found evidence that systemic hyperbaric oxygen⊕ plus usual care reduced the risk of foot amputation compared with usual care alone in people with severely infected foot ulcers.

**Topical growth factors (for non-infected foot ulcer healing)**

One systematic review found that topical growth factors⊕ increased healing rates compared with placebo in people with non-infected diabetic foot ulcers.

### UNKNOWN EFFECTIVENESS

**Cultured human dermis (for non-infected foot ulcer healing)**

We found insufficient evidence of the effects of cultured human dermis⊕ on ulcer healing.

◀ **Pressure off-loading with felted foam versus pressure relief half shoe**
We found insufficient evidence that a pressure off-loading felted foam dressing improved ulcer healing compared with a pressure relief half-shoe.

**DEFINITION** Diabetic foot ulceration is full thickness penetration of the dermis of the foot in a person with diabetes. Ulcer severity is often classified using the Wagner system. Grade 1 ulcers are superficial ulcers involving the full skin thickness but no underlying tissues. Grade 2 ulcers are deeper, penetrating down to ligaments and muscle, but not involving bone or abscess formation. Grade 3 ulcers are deep ulcers with cellulitis or abscess formation, often complicated with osteomyelitis. Ulcers with localised gangrene are classified as grade 4 and those with extensive gangrene involving the entire foot are classified as grade 5.

**INCIDENCE/ PREVALENCE** Studies conducted in Australia, Finland, the UK, and the USA have reported the annual incidence of foot ulcers among people with diabetes as 2.5–10.7%, and the annual incidence of amputation as 0.25–1.8%.[1–10]

**AETIOLOGY/ RISK FACTORS** Long term risk factors for foot ulcers and amputation include duration of diabetes, poor glycaemic control, microvascular complications (retinopathy, nephropathy, and neuropathy) and peripheral vascular disease. The strongest predictors of foot complications are altered foot sensation, foot deformities, and previous foot ulcer or amputation.[1–10]

**PROGNOSIS** People with diabetes are at risk of foot ulcers, infections, and vascular insufficiency. Amputation is indicated if these are severe or do not improve with conservative treatment. As well as affecting quality of life, these complications account for a large proportion of the healthcare costs of diabetes. For people with healed diabetic foot ulcers, the 5 year cumulative rate of ulcer recurrence is 66% and of amputation is 12%.[11]

Please refer to CD-ROM for full text and references.

# Glycaemic control in diabetes

**Search date December 2002**

*Bazian Ltd*

---

## What are the effects of intensive versus conventional glycaemic control?

### BENEFICIAL

**Intensive control of hyperglycaemia in people aged 13–75 years**

Large RCTs have found that diabetic complications increase with HbA1c concentrations above the non-diabetic range.

One systematic review and large subsequent RCTs in people with type 1 or type 2 diabetes have found strong evidence that intensive versus conventional glycaemic control significantly reduces the development and progression of microvascular and neuropathic complications. A second systematic review has found that intensive versus conventional treatment is associated with a small reduction in cardiovascular risk.

RCTs have found that intensive treatment increases the incidence of hypoglycaemia and weight gain, without adverse impact on neuropsychological function or quality of life.

The benefit of intensive treatment is limited by the complications of advanced diabetes (such as blindness, end stage renal disease, or cardiovascular disease), major comorbidity, and reduced life expectancy.

### TRADE OFF BETWEEN BENEFITS AND HARMS

**Intensive control of hyperglycaemia in people with frequent severe hypoglycaemia**

The benefits of intensive treatment of hyperglycaemia are described above.

It is difficult to weigh the benefit of reduced complications against the harm of increased hypoglycaemia. The risk of intensive treatment is increased by a history of severe hypoglycaemia or unawareness of hypoglycaemia, advanced autonomic neuropathy or cardiovascular disease, and impaired ability to detect or treat hypoglycaemia (such as altered mental state, immobility, or lack of social support). For people likely to have limited benefit or increased risk with intensive treatment, it may be more appropriate to negotiate less intensive goals for glycaemic management that reflect the person's self determined goals of care and willingness to make lifestyle modifications.

**DEFINITION**   Diabetes mellitus is a group of disorders characterised by hyperglycaemia (definitions vary slightly, one current US definition is fasting plasma glucose $\geq 7.0$ mmol/L or $\geq 11.1$ mmol/L 2 h after a 75 g oral glucose load, on 2 or more occasions). Intensive treatment is designed to achieve blood glucose values as close to the non-diabetic range as possible. The components of such treatment are education, counselling, monitoring, self management, and pharmacological treatment with insulin or oral antidiabetic agents to achieve specific glycaemic goals.

**INCIDENCE/**   Diabetes is diagnosed in about 5% of adults aged 20 years or older in the
**PREVALENCE**   USA.[1] A further 2.7% have undiagnosed diabetes on the basis of fasting glucose. The prevalence is similar in men and women, but diabetes is more common in some ethnic groups. The prevalence in people aged 40–74 years has increased over the past decade.

**AETIOLOGY/ RISK FACTORS**  Diabetes results from deficient insulin secretion, decreased insulin action, or both. Many processes can be involved, from autoimmune destruction of the β cells of the pancreas to incompletely understood abnormalities that result in resistance to insulin action. Genetic factors are involved in both mechanisms. In type 1 diabetes there is an absolute deficiency of insulin. In type 2 diabetes, insulin resistance and an inability of the pancreas to compensate are involved. Hyperglycaemia without clinical symptoms but sufficient to cause tissue damage can be present for many years before diagnosis.

**PROGNOSIS**  Severe hyperglycaemia causes numerous symptoms, including polyuria, polydipsia, weight loss, and blurred vision. Acute, life threatening consequences of diabetes are hyperglycaemia with ketoacidosis or the non-ketotic hyperosmolar syndrome. There is increased susceptibility to certain infections. Long term complications of diabetes include retinopathy (with potential loss of vision), nephropathy (leading to renal failure), peripheral neuropathy (increased risk of foot ulcers, amputation, and Charcot joints), autonomic neuropathy (cardiovascular, gastrointestinal, and genitourinary dysfunction), and greatly increased risk of atheroma affecting large vessels (macrovascular complications of stroke, myocardial infarction, or peripheral vascular disease). The physical, emotional, and social impact of diabetes and the demands of intensive treatment can also create problems for people with diabetes and their families. One systematic review (search date 1998) of observational studies in people with type 2 diabetes found a positive association between increased blood glucose concentration and mortality.[2] It found no minimum threshold level.

Please refer to CD-ROM for full text and references.

# Obesity

### Search date January 2003

*David E Arterburn*

## What are the effects of drug treatments in adults?

### TRADE OFF BETWEEN BENEFITS AND HARMS

**Diethlyproprion**

One systematic review found that diethylpropion promotes modest weight loss compared with placebo in healthy obese adults. We found two case reports describing pulmonary hypertension and psychosis with diethylpropion. We found insufficient evidence on weight regain and long term safety. A European Commission review concluded that a link between diethylpropion and heart and lung problems could not be excluded.

**Fluoxetine**

One systematic review found that fluoxetine promotes modest weight loss compared with placebo in healthy obese adults. We found insufficient evidence on weight regain and long term safety of fluoxetine in obesity. One systematic review of antidepressant treatment has found an association between selective serotonin reuptake inhibitors and uncommon but serious adverse events, including bradycardia, bleeding, granulocytopenia, seizures, hyponatraemia, hepatotoxicity, serotonin syndrome❻, and extrapyramidal effects❻.

**Mazindol**

One systematic review found that mazindol promotes modest weight loss compared with placebo in healthy obese adults. We found one case report of pulmonary hypertension diagnosed 1 year after stopping treatment with mazindol. We found one case series of mazindol in people with stable cardiac disease that reported cardiac events such as atrial fibrillation and syncope. We found insufficient evidence on weight regain and long term safety.

**Orlistat**

Systematic reviews and subsequent RCTs have found that, in addition to a low energy diet, orlistat modestly increases weight loss compared with placebo in healthy obese adults (body mass index❻ 25–40 kg/m$^2$) and in obese people with diabetes, hyperlipidaemia, and hypertension. Adverse effects such as oily spotting from the rectum, flatulence, and faecal urgency occurred in a high proportion of people taking orlistat. We found insufficient evidence on weight regain and long term safety.

**Phentermine**

One systematic review found that phentermine promotes modest weight loss compared with placebo in healthy obese adults. We found insufficient evidence on weight regain and long term safety. A European Commission review concluded that a link between phentermine and heart and lung problems could not be excluded.

**Sibutramine**

A systematic review and RCTs have found that sibutramine promotes modest weight loss compared with placebo in healthy obese adults (body mass index 25–40 kg/m$^2$) and in obese people with diabetes and hypertension. One RCT has found that sibutramine is more effective than placebo for weight maintenance after weight loss in healthy, obese adults, but weight regain occurs when sibutramine is discontinued. Sibutramine was temporarily suspended from the market in Italy for use in obesity because of concerns about severe adverse reactions, including arrhythmias, hypertension, and two deaths resulting from cardiac arrest. ▶

◀ Two RCTs found no difference in the incidence of valvular heart disease between sibutramine and placebo, although these trials may have been too small to detect clinically important differences.

## UNKNOWN EFFECTIVENESS

### Sibutramine plus orlistat (v sibutramine alone)

We found insufficient evidence about the effects of sibutramine plus orlistat versus sibutramine alone.

## LIKELY TO BE INEFFECTIVE OR HARMFUL

### Dexfenfluramine

One systematic review found that dexfenfluramine promotes weight loss compared with placebo in healthy obese adults. Dexfenfluramine has been associated with valvular heart disease and pulmonary hypertension.

### Fenfluramine

One systematic review found that fenfluramine promotes modest weight loss compared with placebo in healthy obese adults. Fenfluramine has been associated with valvular heart disease and pulmonary hypertension.

### Fenfluramine plus phentermine

One RCT found that fenfluramine plus phentermine promotes weight loss compared with placebo. The combination of fenfluramine plus phentermine has been associated with valvular heart disease and pulmonary hypertension.

### Phenylpropanolamine

One systematic review found that phenylpropanolamine promotes modest weight loss compared with placebo in healthy obese adults. One case control study found that phenylpropanolamine increased risk of haemorrhagic stroke in the first 3 days of use.

**DEFINITION** Obesity is a chronic condition characterised by an excess of body fat. It is most often defined by the body mass index (BMI), a mathematical formula that is highly correlated with body fat. BMI is weight in kilograms divided by height in metres squared ($kg/m^2$). Worldwide, people with BMIs between 25–30 $kg/m^2$ are categorised as overweight, and those with BMIs above 30 $kg/m^2$ are categorised as obese.[1,2] Nearly 5 million US adults used prescription weight loss medication between 1996 and 1998. A quarter of users were not overweight, suggesting that weight loss medication may be inappropriately used. This is thought to be especially the case among women, white people, and Hispanic people.[3] The National Institutes of Health has issued guidelines for obesity treatment, which indicate that all obese adults (BMI ≥ 30 $kg/m^2$) and all adults with a BMI ≥ 27 $kg/m^2$ and concomitant risk factors or diseases are candidates for drug therapy.[1]

**INCIDENCE/ PREVALENCE** Obesity has increased steadily in many countries since 1900. In the UK in 2001, it was estimated that 21% of men and 24% of women were obese.[4] In the past decade alone, the prevalence of obesity in the USA has increased from 22.9% between 1988 and 1994, to 30.5% between 1999 and 2000.[5]

**AETIOLOGY/ RISK FACTORS** Obesity is the result of long term mismatches in energy balance where daily energy intake exceeds daily energy expenditure.[6] Energy balance is modulated by a myriad of factors, including metabolic rate, appetite, diet, and physical activity.[7] Although these factors are influenced by genetic traits, the increase in obesity prevalence in the past few decades cannot be explained by changes in ▶

# Obesity

the human gene pool, and is more often attributed to environmental changes that promote excessive food intake and discourage physical activity.[7,8] Obesity may also be induced by drugs (e.g. high dose glucocorticoids), or be secondary to a variety of neuroendocrine disorders such as Cushing's syndrome and polycystic ovary syndrome.[9]

**PROGNOSIS**  Obesity is a risk factor for several chronic diseases, including hypertension, dyslipidaemia, diabetes, cardiovascular disease, sleep apnoea, osteoarthritis, and some cancers.[1] The relationship between increasing body weight and mortality is curvilinear, where the mortality rate is highest among adults with low body weight (BMI $< 18.5$ kg/m$^2$) and among adults with the highest body weight (BMI $> 35$ kg/m$^2$).[2] Results from five prospective cohort studies and 1991 national statistics suggest that the number of annual deaths attributable to obesity among US adults is about 280 000.[10] Obese adults also have more annual hospitalisations, more outpatient visits, higher prescription drug costs, and worse health related quality of life than normal weight adults.[11,12]

Please refer to CD-ROM for full text and references.

# Prevention of cardiovascular events in diabetes

### Search date December 2002

*Janine Malcolm, Hilary Meggison, and Ronald Sigal*

## What are the effects of promoting smoking cessation in people with diabetes?

### LIKELY TO BE BENEFICIAL

**Smoking cessation**
> We found no RCTs on promotion of smoking cessation. Observational evidence and extrapolation from evidence in people without diabetes suggest that promotion of smoking cessation is likely to reduce cardiovascular events.

## What are the effects of controlling blood pressure in people with diabetes?

### BENEFICIAL

**Antihypertensive treatment versus no antihypertensive treatment**
> One systematic review and RCTs have found that blood pressure lowering with antihypertensive agents in people with diabetes and hypertension reduces cardiovascular morbidity and mortality compared with no antihypertensive treatment.

**Lower target blood pressures**
> Large RCTs including people with diabetes and hypertension have found that control of blood pressure to a target diastolic blood pressure of no more than 80 mm Hg reduces the risk of major cardiovascular events. One RCT in normotensive people with diabetes found that intensive blood pressure lowering reduced cerebral vascular accidents but found no significant difference in cardiovascular death, myocardial infarction, congestive heart failure, or all cause mortality.

### TRADE OFF BETWEEN BENEFITS AND HARMS

**Different antihypertensive drugs**
> Systematic reviews and RCTs have found that angiotensin converting enzyme inhibitors, diuretics, β blockers, and calcium channel blockers all reduce cardiovascular morbidity and mortality in people with diabetes and hypertension. However, there are differences in the types of adverse effects reported with different antihypertensive drugs. RCTs have found that people taking atenolol gained more weight than those taking captopril, an increase in risk of congestive heart failure with lisinopril compared with chlorthalidone, a higher frequency of headache with diltiazem compared with diuretics or β blockers, and a higher rate of withdrawal from treatment because of adverse effects with atenolol compared with losartan.

## What are the effects of treating dyslipidaemia in people with diabetes?

### BENEFICIAL

**Statins versus placebo**
> One systematic review and RCTs have found that statins reduce cardiovascular morbidity and mortality compared with placebo.

▶

Endocrine disorders

# Prevention of cardiovascular events in diabetes

◀ **LIKELY TO BE BENEFICIAL**

### Aggressive versus moderate lipid lowering with statins

One RCT found that, compared with usual care, treatment with atorvastatin to achieve a target low density lipoprotein (LDL) concentration below 2.6 mmol/L (< 100 mg/dL) reduces cardiovascular morbidity and mortality. Another RCT found no significant difference between a lower target LDL (1.55–2.20 mmol/L) using lovastatin, along with cholestyramine if necessary, and a moderate target LDL (3.36–3.62 mmol/L) in 4 year event rate for myocardial infarction and death.

### Fibrates

One RCT found that gemfibrozil reduced cardiovascular events over 5 years compared with placebo whereas another smaller RCT found no significant difference. One RCT found that bezafibrate reduced cardiovascular events compared with placebo, whereas another RCT found no significant difference in myocardial infarction between fenofibrate and placebo.

### Low versus standard statin dose in older people

One RCT found no significant difference in cardiovascular events between low dose pravastatin (5 mg/day) and standard dose pravastatin (10–20 mg/day) over 4 years.

---

## What are the effects of antiplatelet drugs in people with diabetes?

**BENEFICIAL**

### Clopidogrel *New*

We found no RCTs comparing only clopidogrel versus placebo. One RCT in people with diabetes and with recent ischaemic stroke, myocardial infarction, or established peripheral arterial disease found no significant difference between clopidogrel and aspirin at 28 days in cardiovascular events. This RCT also found a lower proportion of people hospitalised for a bleeding event with clopidogrel than with aspirin.

### Prophylactic aspirin

One systematic review and RCTs have found that prophylactic aspirin reduces cardiovascular morbidity and mortality compared with controls. One RCT found that aspirin increased non-fatal major bleeds and minor bleeds but not fatal bleeds compared with placebo. Another RCT found no increase in the risks of vitreous, retinal, gastrointestinal, or cerebral haemorrhage with aspirin compared with placebo.

**LIKELY TO BE BENEFICIAL**

### Adding glycoprotein IIb/IIIa inhibitors to heparin in acute coronary syndromes

One RCT in people presenting with unstable angina or acute myocardial infarction ⊕ without ST segment elevation found that addition of tirofiban (a glycoprotein IIb/IIIa inhibitor) to heparin reduced the composite outcome of death, myocardial infarction, or refractory ischaemia at 180 days compared with heparin alone. This RCT found no significant difference between tirofiban plus heparin and heparin alone in risk of bleeding in people already taking aspirin.

▶

## Adding clopidogrel to aspirin in acute coronary syndromes

One RCT in people presenting with unstable angina or non-Q-wave myocardial infarction and also taking aspirin found no significant reduction in cardiovascular events after 12 months with addition of clopidogrel compared with placebo. This RCT also found a higher proportion of major bleeds with addition of clopidogrel than with placebo.

## What are the effects of blood glucose control for prevention of cardiovascular disease in diabetes?

LIKELY TO BE BENEFICIAL

### Metformin versus diet alone in obese people

One RCT in obese people with type 2 diabetes found that intensive treatment with metformin compared with conventional treatment with diet alone reduced myocardial infarction but not stroke over 5 years. This RCT found no significant increase in major hypoglycaemic episodes in the metformin group compared with the diet only group.

UNLIKELY TO BE BENEFICIAL

### Intensive versus conventional glycaemic control

Three RCTs found no significant difference in cardiovascular morbidity and mortality between intensive and conventional treatment for blood glucose control. These RCTs also found an increase in hypoglycaemic episodes and weight gain with intensive compared with conventional treatment.

## What are the effects of revascularisation procedures in people with diabetes?

BENEFICIAL

### Coronary artery bypass graft (CABG) versus percutaneous transluminal coronary angioplasty (PTCA)

One large RCT in people with diabetes and multivessel coronary artery disease has found that CABG reduces mortality or myocardial infarction within 8 years compared with PTCA. Another smaller RCT found a non-significant reduction in mortality with CABG compared with PTCA at 4 years.

### Stent plus glycoprotein IIb/IIIa inhibitors in people undergoing PTCA

RCTs in people with diabetes undergoing PTCA have found that the combination of stent and a glycoprotein IIb/IIIa inhibitor reduces cardiovascular morbidity and mortality compared with stent plus placebo.

TRADE OFF BETWEEN BENEFITS AND HARMS

### CABG plus stent versus PTCA plus stent

One RCT in people with diabetes and multivessel coronary artery disease found no significant difference between CABG plus stent and PTCA plus stent in cardiovascular morbidity or mortality (to time of discharge). However, it found that CABG plus stent compared with PTCA plus stent in the short term increased cardiovascular risk at 1 year.

**Prevention of cardiovascular events in diabetes**

◀ **UNKNOWN EFFECTIVENESS**

## PTCA versus thrombolysis

We found no systematic review or RCTs comparing PTCA versus thrombolysis for prevention of cardiovascular events in people with diabetes.

**DEFINITION**  **Diabetes mellitus:** See definition under glycaemic control in diabetes, p 124. **Cardiovascular disease:** Atherosclerotic disease of the heart and/or the coronary, cerebral, or peripheral vessels leading to clinical events such as acute myocardial infarction❺, congestive heart failure, sudden cardiac death, stroke, gangrene, and/or need for revascularisation procedures. **Population:** In previous versions of *Clinical Evidence* we attempted to differentiate between primary and secondary prevention in this topic. However, in middle aged and older people with type 2 diabetes this distinction may not be clinically important. We are not aware of any intervention that has been shown to be effective in secondary prevention but ineffective in primary prevention, or vice versa, in people with diabetes. In most cases a large proportion of people with diabetes entered into cardiovascular disease prevention trials are middle aged and older with additional cardiovascular disease risk factors, and a large portion of these actually have undiagnosed cardiovascular disease.

**INCIDENCE/**  Diabetes mellitus is a major risk factor for cardiovascular disease. In the USA,
**PREVALENCE**  60–75% of people with diabetes die from cardiovascular causes.[1] The annual incidence of cardiovascular disease is increased in people with diabetes (men: RR 2–3; women: RR 3–4, adjusted for age and other cardiovascular risk factors).[2] About 45% of middle aged and older white people with diabetes have evidence of coronary artery disease, compared with about 25% of people without diabetes in the same populations.[2] In a Finnish population based cohort study (1059 people with diabetes and 1373 people without diabetes, aged 45–64 years), the 7 year risk of acute myocardial infarction was as high in adults with diabetes without previous cardiac disease (20.2/100 person years) as it was in people without diabetes with previous cardiac disease (18.8/100 person years).[3]

**AETIOLOGY/**  Diabetes mellitus increases the risk of cardiovascular disease. Cardiovascular
**RISK FACTORS**  risk factors in people with diabetes include conventional risk factors (age, prior cardiovascular disease, cigarette smoking, hypertension, dyslipidaemia, sedentary lifestyle, family history of premature cardiovascular disease) and more diabetes specific risk factors (elevated urinary protein excretion, poor glycaemic control). Conventional risk factors for cardiovascular disease contribute to increasing the relative risk of cardiovascular disease in people with diabetes to about the same extent as in those without diabetes (see aetiology under primary prevention, p 28). One prospective cohort study (164 women and 235 men with diabetes [mean age 65 years] and 437 women and 1099 men without diabetes [mean age 61 years] followed for mortality for a mean 3.7 years following acute myocardial infarction) found that more people with diabetes died compared with people without diabetes (116/399 [29%] v 204/1536 [13%]; RR 2.2, 95% CI 1.8 to 2.7).[4] It also found that the mortality risk after myocardial infarction associated with diabetes was higher for women than for men (adjusted HR 2.7, 95% CI 1.8 to 4.2 for women v 1.3, 95% CI 1 to 1.8 for men). Physical inactivity is a significant risk factor for cardiovascular events in both men and women. One cohort study of women with diabetes found that participation in little (< 1 hour/week) or no physical activity compared with physical activity for at least 7 hours a week was associated with doubling of the risk of a cardiovascular event.[5] Another cohort study (1263 men with diabetes, mean follow up 12 years) found that low baseline cardiorespiratory fitness increased overall mortality compared with moderate or high fitness (RR 2.9, 95% CI 2.1 to 3.6), and overall mortality was higher in those reporting no recreational exercise in the previous 3 months compared with those reporting any recreational physical activity in the same period (RR 1.8, ▶

95% CI 1.3 to 2.5).[6] The absolute risk of cardiovascular disease is almost the same in women as in men with diabetes. Diabetes specific cardiovascular risk factors include the duration of diabetes during adulthood (the years of exposure to diabetes before age 20 years add little to risk of cardiovascular disease); raised blood glucose concentrations (reflected in fasting blood glucose or HbA1c**G**); and any degree of microalbuminuria (albuminuria 30–299 mg/24 hours).[7] People with diabetes and microalbuminuria have a higher risk of coronary morbidity and mortality than people with normal levels of urinary albumin and a similar duration of diabetes (RR 2–3).[8,9] Clinical proteinuria increases the risk of major cardiac events in type 2 diabetes (RR 3)[10] and in type 1 diabetes (RR 9)[7,11,12] compared with individuals with the same type of diabetes having normal albumin excretion. An epidemiological analysis of people with diabetes enrolled in the Heart Outcomes Prevention Evaluation (HOPE) clinical trial (3498 people with diabetes and at least 1 other cardiovascular risk factor, age > 55 years, of whom 1140 [32%] had microalbuminuria at baseline, 5 years' follow up) found higher risk for major cardiovascular events in for those with microalbuminuria (albumin : creatinine [ACR] ratio ≥ 2.0 mg/mmol) compared with those without microalbuminuria (adjusted RR 1.97, 95% CI 1.68 to 2.31), and for all cause mortality (RR 2.15, 95% CI 1.78 to 2.60).[13] It also found an association between ACR and the risk of major cardiovascular events (ACR 0.22 to 0.57 mg/mmol: RR 0.85, 95% CI 0.63 to 1.14; ACR 0.58 to 1.62 mg/mmol: RR 1.11, 95% CI 0.86 to 1.43; ACR 1.62 to 1.99 mg/mmol: RR 1.89, 95% CI 1.52 to 2.36).

**PROGNOSIS** Diabetes mellitus increases the risk of mortality or serious morbidity after a coronary event (RR 1.5–3).[2,3,14,15] This excess risk is partly accounted for by increased prevalence of other cardiovascular risk factors in people with diabetes. A systematic review (search date 1998) found that, in people with diabetes admitted to hospital for acute myocardial infarction, "stress hyperglycaemia" versus lower blood glucose levels was associated with increased mortality in hospital (RR 1.7, 95% CI 1.2 to 2.4).[16] One large prospective cohort study (91 285 men aged 40–84, 5 years' follow up) found higher all cause and coronary heart disease (CHD) mortality in men with diabetes versus men without coronary artery disease or diabetes (age adjusted RR 3.3, 95% CI 2.6 to 4.1 in men with diabetes and without coronary artery disease v RR 2.3%, 95% CI 2.0 to 2.6 in healthy people; RR 5.6, 95% CI 4.9 to 6.3 in men with coronary artery disease but without diabetes v RR 2.2%, 95% CI 2.0 to 2.4 in healthy people; RR 12.0, 95% CI 9.9 to 14.6 in men with both risk factors v RR 4.7%, 95% CI 4.0 to 5.4 in healthy people).[17] Multivariate analysis did not materially alter these associations. These findings support previous studies. Diabetes mellitus alone is associated with a two fold increase in risk for all cause death, a three fold increase in risk of death from CHD and, in people with pre-existing CHD, a 12-fold increase in risk of death from CHD compared with people with neither risk factor.

---

Please refer to CD-ROM for full text and references.

# Primary hypothyroidism

Search date April 2003

*Birte Nygaard*

## What are the effects of treatments for clinical (overt) hypothyroidism?

### BENEFICIAL

**Levothyroxine (L-thyroxine)**

We found no RCTs comparing levothyroxine (L-thyroxine) versus placebo, although there is consensus that treatment is beneficial. Treating clinical (overt) hypothyroidism with thyroid hormone (levothyroxine; L-thyroxine) can induce hyperthyroidism and reduce bone mass in postmenopausal women and increase the risk of atrial fibrillation.

### UNKNOWN EFFECTIVENESS

**Levothyroxine (L-thyroxine) plus liothyronine**

We found insufficient evidence about the effects of levothyroxine (L-thyroxine) plus liothyronine versus levothyroxine alone in people with clinical (overt) hypothyroidism. Thyroid hormone treatment can induce hyperthyroidism and reduce bone mass in postmenopausal women and increase the risk of atrial fibrillation.

## What are the effects of treatments for subclinical hypothyroidism?

### UNKNOWN EFFECTIVENESS

**Levothyroxine (L-thyroxine)**

One RCT in women with biochemically defined subclinical hypothyroidism found no significant difference between levothyroxine (L-thyroxine) and placebo for dry skin, cold intolerance, and constipation at 1 year. The RCT may, however, have lacked power to exclude a clinically important difference between treatments. Another RCT found no significant difference in health related quality of life scores between levothyroxine and placebo. One RCT found inconclusive results about the effect of levothyroxine versus placebo on cognitive function in people with subclinical hypothyroidism. One RCT found that levothyroxine improved left ventricular function at 6 months compared with placebo. Treating subclinical hypothyroidism with thyroid hormone can induce hyperthyroidism and reduce bone mass in postmenopausal women and increase the risk of atrial fibrillation.

**DEFINITION** Hypothyroidism is characterised by low levels of blood thyroid hormone. **Clinical (overt) hypothyroidism** is diagnosed on the basis of characteristic clinical features consisting of mental slowing, depression, dementia, weight gain, constipation, dry skin, hair loss, cold intolerance, hoarse voice, irregular menstruation, infertility, muscle stiffness and pain, bradycardia, hypercholesterolaemia, combined with a raised blood level of thyroid stimulating hormone (TSH) (serum TSH levels > 12 mU/L), and a low serum thyroxine ($T_4$ level (serum $T_4$ < 60 nmol/L). **Subclinical hypothyroidism** is diagnosed when serum TSH is raised (serum TSH levels > 4 mU/L) but serum thyroxine is normal and there are no symptoms or signs, or only minor symptoms or signs, of thyroid dysfunction. **Primary hypothyroidism** is seen after destruction of the thyroid gland because of autoimmunity (the most common cause), or medical intervention such as surgery, radioiodine, and radiation. **Secondary** ▶

**hypothyroidism** is seen after pituitary or hypothalamic damage, and results in insufficient production of TSH. Secondary hypothyroidism is not covered in this review. **Euthyroid sick syndrome** is diagnosed when levels of tri-iodothyronine ($T_3$❸) are low, serum thyroxine is low, and TSH levels are normal or low. Euthyroid sick syndrome is not covered in this review.

**INCIDENCE/ PREVALENCE**

Hypothyroidism is more common in women than in men (the female : male ratio in the UK is 6 : 1). One study (2779 people in the UK with a median age of 58 years) found the incidence of clinical (overt) hypothyroidism was 40/10 000 women per year and 6/10 000 men per year. The prevalence was 9.3% in women and 1.3% in men.[1] In areas with high iodine intake, the incidence of hypothyroidism can be higher than in areas with normal or low iodine intake. In Denmark, where there is moderate iodine insufficiency, the overall incidence of hypothyroidism is 1.4/10 000 per year increasing to 8/10 000 per year in people older than 70 years.[2] The incidence of subclinical hypothyroidism increases with age. Up to 10% of women over the age of 60 years have subclinical hypothyroidism (evaluated from data from the Netherlands and USA).[3,4]

**AETIOLOGY/ RISK FACTORS**

Primary thyroid gland failure can occur as a result of chronic autoimmune thyroiditis, postradioactive iodine treatment, or thyroidectomy. Other causes include drug adverse effects (e.g. amiodarone and lithium), transient hypothyroidism due to silent thyroiditis, subacute thyroiditis, or postpartum thyroiditis.

**PROGNOSIS**

Hypothyroidism results in mental slowing, depression, dementia, weight gain, constipation, dry skin, hair loss, cold intolerance, hoarse voice, irregular menstruation, infertility, muscle stiffness and pain, bradycardia, and hypercholesterolaemia. In people with subclinical hypothyroidism, the risk of developing overt hypothyroidism is described in the UK Whickham Survey (25 years' follow up; for women: OR 8, 95% CI 3 to 20; for men: OR 44, 95% CI 19 to 104; if both a raised TSH and positive antithyroid antibodies were present; for women: OR 38, 95% CI 22 to 65; for men: OR 173, 95% CI 81 to 370). For women, the survey found an annual risk of 4.3%/year (if both raised serum TSH and antithyroid antibodies were present), 2.6%/year (if raised serum TSH was present alone); the minimum number of people with raised TSH and antithyroid antibodies who would need treating to prevent this progression to clinical (overt) hypothyroidism in one person over 5 years is 5–8.[1] **Cardiovascular disease:** A large cross-sectional study (25 862 people with serum TSH between 5.1–10 mU/L) found significantly higher mean total cholesterol concentrations in hypothyroid people compared with euthyroid people (5.8 v 5.6 mmol/L).[3] Another study (124 elderly women with subclinical hypothyroidism, 931 euthyroid women) found a significantly increased risk of myocardial infarction in women with subclinical hypothyroidism (OR 2.3, 95% CI 1.3 to 4.0) and for aortic atherosclerosis (OR 1.7, 95% CI 1.1 to 2.6).[4] **Mental health:** Subclinical hypothyroidism is associated with depression.[5] People with subclinical hypothyroidism may have depression that is refractory to both antidepressant drugs and thyroid hormone alone. Memory impairment, hysteria, anxiety, somatic complaints, and depressive features without depression have been described in people with subclinical hypothyroidism.[6]

Please refer to CD-ROM for full text and references.

# Acute anterior uveitis

**Search date June 2003**

*André Curi, Kimble Matos, and Carlos Pavesio*

## What are the effects of topical anti-inflammatory eye drops?

**UNKNOWN EFFECTIVENESS**

### Topical non-steroidal anti-inflammatory drug eye drops

One RCT found no significant difference between non-steroidal anti-inflammatory drug and placebo eye drops in clinical cure rate after 21 days. Three RCTs found no significant difference between non-steroidal anti-inflammatory drug and steroid eye drops in clinical cure rate.

### Topical steroid eye drops

One small RCT found no significant difference with steroid (betamethasone phosphate/clobetasone butyrate) eye drops compared with placebo eye drops in symptom severity after 14 or 21 days. Two RCTs found no significant difference between prednisolone and rimexolone, in the anterior chamber cell count (a marker of disease severity). One RCT found that prednisolone increased the proportion of people with fewer than five anterior chamber cells per examination field compared with loteprednol after 28 days. The results of a second RCT comparing prednisolone with loteprednol were difficult to interpret. RCTs found that rimexolone and loteprednol were less likely than prednisolone to be associated with increased intraocular pressure, although differences were not statistically significant. Three RCTs found no significant difference between steroid and non-steroidal anti-inflammatory drug eye drops in clinical cure rate after 14 or 21 days.

**DEFINITION**
Anterior uveitis is inflammation of the uveal tract, and includes iritis⊙ and iridocyclitis⊙. It can be classified according to its clinical course into acute or chronic anterior uveitis, or according to its clinical appearance into granulomatous or non-granulomatous anterior uveitis. Acute anterior uveitis is characterised by an extremely painful red eye, often associated with photophobia and occasionally with decreased visual acuity. Chronic anterior uveitis is defined as inflammation lasting over 6 weeks. It is usually asymptomatic, but many people have mild symptoms during exacerbations.

**INCIDENCE/ PREVALENCE**
Acute anterior uveitis is rare, with an annual incidence of 12/100 000 population.[1] It is particularly common in Finland (annual incidence 22.6/100 000 population, prevalence 68.7/100 000 population), probably because of genetic factors such as the high frequency of HLA-B27 in the Finnish population.[2] It is equally common in men and women and more that 90% of cases occur in people older than 20 years of age.[2,3]

**AETIOLOGY/ RISK FACTORS**
No cause is identified in 60–80% of people with acute anterior uveitis. Systemic disorders that may be associated with acute anterior uveitis include ankylosing spondylitis; Reiter's syndrome; juvenile chronic arthritis; Kawasaki syndrome; infectious uveitis; Behçet's syndrome; inflammatory bowel disease; interstitial nephritis; sarcoidosis; multiple sclerosis; Wegener's granulomatosis; Vogt-Koyanagi-Harada syndrome; and masquerade syndromes⊙. Acute anterior uveitis also occurs in association with HLA-B27 expression not linked to any systemic disease, and it may also be the manifestation of an isolated eye disorder such as Fuchs' iridocyclitis, Posner-Schlossman syndrome, or Schwartz syndrome. Acute anterior uveitis may also occur following surgery or as an adverse drug or hypersensitivity reaction.[2,3]

**PROGNOSIS** Acute anterior uveitis is often self limiting, but we found no evidence about how often it resolves spontaneously, in which people, or over what time period. Complications include posterior synechiae⊙, cataract, glaucoma, and chronic uveitis. In a study of 154 people (232 eyes) with acute anterior uveitis (119 people HLA-B27 positive), visual acuity was better than 20/60 in 209/232 (90%) eyes, 20/60 or worse in 23/232 (10%) eyes, and worse than 20/200 (classified as legally blind) in 11/232 (5%) eyes.[4]

Please refer to CD-ROM for full text and references.

# Age related macular degeneration

**Search date November 2002**

*Jennifer Arnold and Shirley Sarks*

## What are the effects of interventions to prevent progression?

### LIKELY TO BE BENEFICIAL

**Antioxidant vitamin and zinc supplementation** *New*

One systematic review found modest evidence from one large RCT that, compared with placebo, antioxidant vitamins plus zinc supplements reduce the risk of progression to late age related macular degeneration⊙ over 6 years in people who already have moderate amounts of drusen⊙ in both eyes; or choroidal neovascularisation⊙, or geographic atrophy⊙ in one eye.

### UNKNOWN EFFECTIVENESS

**Laser to drusen**

We found insufficient evidence that drusen reduction by laser⊙ prevents late age related macular degeneration — choroidal neovascularisation or geographic atrophy. One RCT found that, compared with no laser treatment, laser treatment to eyes with high risk drusen significantly improved visual acuity after 2 years. A second RCT found that, compared with no laser treatment, visual acuity with laser treatment only improved in a subgroup of eyes with a reduction in the number of drusen of greater than 50%. It also found that, compared with no treatment, laser treatment increased the short term incidence of choroidal neovascularisation in eyes with unilateral (but not bilateral) drusen.

## What are the effects of treatments for exudative age related macular degeneration?

### BENEFICIAL

**Photodynamic treatment with verteporfin**

Two RCTs in selected people with exudative age related macular degeneration found that, compared with placebo, photodynamic treatment⊙ with verteporfin⊙ reduced the risk of moderate and severe visual loss after 1–2 years. In the first RCT, subgroup analysis suggests the benefit is greatest in people with predominantly classic lesions⊙ on fluorescein angiography. In the second RCT, a more modest benefit was seen in the second year of treatment in people with only occult (no classic) lesions on fluorescein angiography. Both RCTs found that photodynamic treatment with verteporfin was associated with an initial loss of vision and photosensitive reactions in a small proportion of people.

### TRADE OFF BETWEEN BENEFITS AND HARMS

**Thermal laser photocoagulation**

Four large RCTs in people with exudative age related macular degeneration and well demarcated lesions have found that, compared with no treatment, thermal laser photocoagulation decreases the rate of severe visual loss after 2–3 years and preserves contrast sensitivity. Choroidal neovascularisation recurs within 2 years in about half of those treated. Photocoagulation may reduce visual acuity initially.

### UNKNOWN EFFECTIVENESS

**Proton beam and scleral plaque radiotherapy**

We found no RCTs.

▶

◀ **Submacular surgery**

We found insufficient evidence on the effects of submacular surgery◯. Case series have found that rates of recurrent choroidal neovascularisation are high, and there is a clinically important risk of ocular complications resulting in visual loss and a need for further surgical intervention

## UNLIKELY TO BE BENEFICIAL

### External beam radiation

One large RCT found no significant difference between low dose external beam radiation and placebo in the proportion of people with exudative age related macular degeneration and moderate visual loss after 1 year. Smaller RCTs comparing both low and high dose external beam radiation versus placebo or no treatment found conflicting evidence. We found insufficient evidence on long term safety, although RCTs found no evidence of toxicity to the optic nerve or retina after 12–24 months.

## LIKELY TO BE INEFFECTIVE OR HARMFUL

### Subcutaneous interferon alfa-2a

One large RCT found that subcutaneous interferon alfa-2a increased visual loss after 1 year compared with placebo, although the difference was not significant, and found evidence of serious ocular and systemic adverse effects.

**DEFINITION**   Age related macular degeneration (AMD) has two forms in the late (sight threatening) stage: atrophic (or dry) AMD, characterised by geographic atrophy; and exudative (or wet) AMD, characterised by choroidal neovascularisation, which eventually causes a disciform scar.

**INCIDENCE/**   AMD is a common cause of blind registration in industrialised countries.
**PREVALENCE**   Atrophic AMD is more common than the more sight threatening exudative AMD, affecting about 85% of people with AMD.[1] End stage (blinding) AMD is found in about 2% of all people aged over 50 years, and incidence rises with age (0.7–1.4% of people aged 65–75 years; 11–19% of people aged > 85 years).[2–4]

**AETIOLOGY/**   Proposed hypotheses for the cause of AMD involve vascular factors and
**RISK FACTORS**   oxidative damage coupled with genetic predisposition.[5] Age is the strongest risk factor. Ocular risk factors for the development of exudative AMD include the presence of soft drusen, macular pigmentary change, and choroidal neovascularisation in the other eye. Systemic risk factors include hypertension, smoking, and a family history of AMD.[5–7] Hypertension, diet (especially intake of antioxidant micronutrients), and oestrogen use are suspected as aetiological agents, but this remains unproved.[5]

**PROGNOSIS**   AMD impairs central vision, which is required for reading, driving, face recognition, and all fine visual tasks. **Atrophic AMD** progresses slowly over many years, and time to legal blindness◯ is highly variable (usually about 5–10 years).[8,9] **Exudative AMD** is more often threatening to vision; 90% of people with severe visual loss owing to AMD have the exudative type. This condition usually manifests with a sudden worsening and distortion of central vision. A modelling exercise (derived primarily from cohort studies) found the risk of developing exudative AMD in people with bilateral soft drusen was 1–5% at 1 year and 13–18% at 3 years.[10] The observed 5 year rate in a population survey was 7%.[11] Most eyes (estimates vary from 60–90%) with exudative AMD progress to legal blindness and develop a central defect (scotoma) in the visual ▶

# Age related macular degeneration

field.[12–15] Peripheral vision is preserved, allowing the person to be mobile and independent. The ability to read with visual aids depends on the size and density of the central scotoma and the degree to which the person retains sensitivity to contrast. Once exudative AMD has developed in one eye, the other eye is at high risk (cumulative estimated incidence: 10% at 1 year, 28% at 3 years, and 42% at 5 years).[5]

Please refer to CD-ROM for full text and references.

### Search date June 2003
*Justine Smith*

## What are the effects of antibiotic treatment?

### BENEFICIAL

**Antibiotic treatment in culture positive bacterial conjunctivitis**

One systematic review has found that antibiotics (polymyxin–bacitracin, cipro-floxacin, or ofloxacin) increase rates of clinical and microbiological cure compared with placebo. Four RCTs found no significant difference among antibiotics in clinical or microbiological cure. One RCT found that fusidic acid increased clinical cure rate compared with chloramphenicol. One RCT found that topical netilmicin increased clinical cure rate compared with topical gentamicin. One RCT found that topical levofloxacin increased microbiological cure rate, but not clinical cure rate, compared with topical ofloxacin.

### LIKELY TO BE BENEFICIAL

**Empirical antibiotic treatment of suspected bacterial conjunctivitis**

One systematic review found limited evidence from one RCT that topical nor-floxacin increased rates of clinical and microbiological improvement or cure after 5 days compared with placebo. RCTs comparing different topical antibiotics versus each other found no significant difference in rates of clinical or microbiological cure. One RCT found no significant difference between topical polymyxin–bacitracin ointment and oral cefixime for clinical or microbiological improvement or cure.

**DEFINITION**
Conjunctivitis is any inflammation of the conjunctiva, generally characterised by irritation, itching, foreign body sensation, and watering or discharge. Bacterial conjunctivitis may often be distinguished from other types of conjunctivitis by the presence of a yellow–white mucopurulent discharge. There is also usually a papillary reaction (small bumps with fibrovascular cores on the palpebral conjunctiva, appearing grossly as a fine velvety surface). Bacterial conjunctivitis is usually bilateral. This review covers non-gonococcal bacterial conjunctivitis.

**INCIDENCE/ PREVALENCE**
We found no good evidence on the incidence or prevalence of bacterial conjunctivitis.

**AETIOLOGY/ RISK FACTORS**
Conjunctivitis may be infectious (caused by bacteria or viruses) or allergic. In adults, bacterial conjunctivitis is less common than viral conjunctivitis, although estimates vary widely (viral conjunctivitis has been reported to account for 8–75% of acute conjunctivitis).[1-3] *Staphylococcus* species are the most common pathogens for bacterial conjunctivitis in adults, followed by *Strepto-coccus pneumoniae* and *Haemophilus influenzae*.[4,5] In children, bacterial conjunctivitis is more common than viral, and is mainly caused by *H influenzae*, *S pneumoniae*, and *Moraxella catarrhalis*.[6,7]

**PROGNOSIS**
Most bacterial conjunctivitis is self limiting. One systematic review (search date 2001) found clinical cure or significant improvement with placebo within 2–5 days in 64% of people (99% CI 54% to 73%).[8] Some organisms cause corneal or systemic complications, or both. Otitis media may develop in 25% of children with *H influenzae* conjunctivitis,[9] and systemic meningitis may complicate primary meningococcal conjunctivitis in 18% of people.[10]

Please refer to CD-ROM for full text and references.

# Diabetic retinopathy

**Search date September 2002**

*Simon Harding*

---

## What are the effects of treatments for diabetic retinopathy?

### BENEFICIAL

**Control of diabetes (see glycaemic control in diabetes, p 124)**

**Control of hypertension (see primary prevention, p 25)**

**Macular photocoagulation in people with clinically significant macular oedema**

One large RCT has found that laser photocoagulation to the macula versus no treatment significantly reduces visual loss at 3 years in eyes with macular oedema and mild to moderate diabetic retinopathy, with some evidence of greater benefit in eyes with better vision. Subgroup analysis found that focal laser treatment☉ was significantly more effective in reducing visual loss in eyes with clinically significant macular oedema☉, particularly in people in whom the centre of the macula was involved or imminently threatened.

**Peripheral retinal laser photocoagulation in people with preproliferative (*moderate/severe non-proliferative\**) retinopathy and maculopathy**

RCTs in eyes with preproliferative retinopathy and maculopathy have found that peripheral retinal photocoagulation versus no treatment significantly reduces the risk of severe visual loss at 5 years.

**Peripheral retinal laser photocoagulation in people with proliferative retinopathy**

RCTs have found that peripheral retinal photocoagulation versus no treatment significantly reduces the risk of severe visual loss at 2–3 years. One RCT in eyes with high risk proliferative diabetic retinopathy found that low intensity versus standard intensity argon laser significantly reduced vitreous haemorrhage☉ and macular oedema. It found no significant difference between treatments for visual acuity, although it may have lacked power to detect clinically important effects.

**Smoking cessation (see primary prevention, p 25)**

### LIKELY TO BE BENEFICIAL

**Grid photocoagulation to zones of retinal thickening in people with diabetic maculopathy**

One RCT found a significant improvement in visual acuity in eyes treated with grid photocoagulation versus untreated eyes at 12 months and at 24 months. Photocoagulation versus no photocoagulation reduced the risk of moderate visual loss by 50–70%.

### UNKNOWN EFFECTIVENESS

**Macular photocoagulation in people with maculopathy but without clinically significant macular oedema**

We found no RCTs of macular photocoagulation in this population.

**Peripheral retinal laser photocoagulation in people with background or preproliferative (*non-proliferative\**) retinopathy without maculopathy**

We found no RCTs in people with background or preproliferative☉ retinopathy without maculopathy.

## What are the effects of treatments for vitreous haemorrhage?

### LIKELY TO BE BENEFICIAL

**Vitrectomy in people with severe vitreous haemorrhage and proliferative retinopathy (if performed early)**

One RCT found that early versus deferred (for 1 year) vitrectomy🛈 significantly reduced visual loss at 1, 2, and 3 years in eyes with severe vitreous haemorrhage and proliferative retinopathy. Subgroup analysis showed significant benefit in people with type 1 diabetes but not those with type 2.

### UNKNOWN EFFECTIVENESS

**Vitrectomy in people with maculopathy**

The role of vitrectomy in this population remains unclear.

| | |
|---|---|
| **DEFINITION** | Diabetic retinopathy is characterised by varying degrees of microaneurysms, haemorrhages, exudates *(hard exudates)*, venous changes, new vessel formation, and retinal thickening. It can involve the peripheral retina or the macula, or both. The range of severity of retinopathy includes background🛈 *(mild non-proliferative)*, preproliferative *(moderate/severe non-proliferative)*, proliferative🛈, and advanced retinopathy🛈. Involvement of the macula can be focal🛈, diffuse🛈, ischaemic🛈, or mixed. |
| **INCIDENCE/ PREVALENCE** | Diabetic eye disease is the most common cause of blindness in the UK, responsible for 12% of registrable blindness in people aged 16–64 years.[1] |
| **AETIOLOGY/ RISK FACTORS** | Risk factors include age, duration and control of diabetes, raised blood pressure, and raised serum lipids.[2] |
| **PROGNOSIS** | Natural history studies from the 1960s found that at least half of people with proliferative diabetic retinopathy progressed to Snellen visual acuity🛈 of less than 6/60 (20/200) within 3-5 years.[3–5] After 4 years' follow up the rate of progression to less than 6/60 (20/200) visual acuity in the better eye was 1.5% in people with type 1 diabetes, 2.7% in people with non-insulin requiring type 2 diabetes, and 3.2% in people with insulin requiring type 2 diabetes.[6] |

\* Terms in italics indicate US definitions🛈.

Please refer to CD-ROM for full text and references.

# Glaucoma

Search date August 2002

*Rajiv Shah and Richard Wormald*

---

## What are the effects of treatments for established primary open angle glaucoma?

### LIKELY TO BE BENEFICIAL

**Laser trabeculoplasty (v medical treatment)**

One RCT found that combined treatment with initial laser trabeculoplasty⊙ followed by medical treatment versus medical treatment alone significantly reduced intraocular pressure and deterioration in optic disc appearance, and significantly improved visual fields after a mean of 7 years.

**Topical medical treatment**

One systematic review found limited evidence that topical medical treatments versus placebo significantly reduced intraocular pressure after a minimum of 3 months, but found no significant difference between treatments in visual field loss on long term follow up. The systematic review did not clearly define the medical treatments involved.

### TRADE OFF BETWEEN BENEFITS AND HARMS

**Surgical trabeculectomy**

RCTs found that surgical trabeculectomy⊙ versus medical treatment significantly reduced both visual field loss and intraocular pressures, but found no significant difference between treatments in visual acuity after about 5 years. RCTs found that surgical trabeculectomy versus laser trabeculoplasty significantly reduced intraocular pressure, but found conflicting results for changes in visual acuity after 5–7 years. Observational studies have found limited evidence that surgical trabeculectomy may reduce central vision.

### UNKNOWN EFFECTIVENESS

**Laser trabeculoplasty (v surgical treatment)**

RCTs found that laser trabeculoplasty reduced intraocular pressures significantly less than surgical trabeculectomy, but found conflicting results for changes in visual acuity after 5–7 years.

---

## What are the effects of lowering intraocular pressure in normal tension glaucoma?

### LIKELY TO BE BENEFICIAL

**Medical treatments for lowering intraocular pressure in normal pressure glaucoma**

One RCT found that surgical or medical treatment significantly reduced progression of visual field loss after 8 years.

### TRADE OFF BETWEEN BENEFITS AND HARMS

**Surgical treatments for lowering intraocular pressure in normal pressure glaucoma**

One RCT found that surgical or medical treatment significantly reduced progression of visual field loss after 8 years. However, it found that surgery significantly increased cataract formation.

▶

◄ *What are the effects of treatments for acute angle closure glaucoma?*

UNKNOWN EFFECTIVENESS

### Medical treatments of acute angle closure glaucoma

We found no placebo controlled RCTs, but strong consensus suggests that medical treatments are effective. One RCT found no significant difference in intraocular pressure after 2 hours with low dose pilocarpine versus an intensive pilocarpine regimen versus pilocarpine ocular inserts. We found no RCTs of other medical treatments.

### Surgical treatments of acute angle closure glaucoma

We found no placebo controlled RCTs, but strong consensus suggests that surgical treatments are effective. One RCT found no significant difference with surgical iridectomy⊕ versus laser iridotomy⊕ in visual acuity or intraocular pressure after 3 years.

**DEFINITION**     Glaucoma is a group of diseases that are characterised by progressive optic neuropathy. It is usually bilateral but asymmetric and may occur at any point within a wide range of intraocular pressures. All forms of glaucoma show optic nerve cupping with pallor associated with peripheral visual field loss. **Primary open angle glaucoma** occurs in people with an open drainage angle and no secondary identifiable cause. **Normal tension glaucoma** occurs in people with intraocular pressures that are consistently below 21 mm Hg (a point two standard deviations above the population mean). **Acute angle closure glaucoma** is a rapid and severe rise in intraocular pressure caused by physical obstruction of the anterior chamber drainage angle.

**INCIDENCE/**     Glaucoma occurs in 1–2% of white people aged over 40 years, rising to 5% at
**PREVALENCE**     70 years. Primary open angle glaucoma accounts for two thirds of those affected, and normal tension glaucoma for about a quarter.[1,2] In black people glaucoma is more prevalent, presents at a younger age with higher intraocular pressures, is more difficult to control, and is the main irreversible cause of blindness.[1,3] Glaucoma related blindness is responsible for 8% of new blind registrations in the UK.[4]

**AETIOLOGY/**     The major risk factor for developing primary open angle glaucoma is raised
**RISK FACTORS** intraocular pressure. Lesser risk factors include family history and ethnic origin. The relationship between systemic blood pressure and intraocular pressure may be an important determinant of blood flow to the optic nerve head and, as a consequence, may represent a risk factor for glaucoma.[5] Systemic hypotension, vasospasm (including Raynaud's disease and migraine), and a history of major blood loss have been reported as risk factors for normal tension glaucoma in hospital based studies. Risk factors for acute angle closure glaucoma include family history, female sex, being long sighted, and cataract. A recent systematic review failed to find any evidence supporting the theory that routine pupillary dilatation with short acting mydriatics was a risk factor for acute angle closure glaucoma.[6]

**PROGNOSIS**     Advanced visual field loss is found in about 20% of people with primary open angle glaucoma at diagnosis,[7] and is an important risk factor for glaucoma related blindness.[8] Blindness results from gross loss of visual field or loss of central vision. Once early field defects have appeared, and where the intraocular pressure is greater than 30 mm Hg, untreated people may lose the ▶

# Glaucoma

remainder of the visual field in 3 years or less.[9] As the disease progresses, people with glaucoma have difficulty moving from a bright room to a darker room, and judging steps and kerbs. Progression of visual field loss is often slower in normal tension glaucoma. Acute angle glaucoma leads to rapid loss of vision, initially from corneal oedema and subsequently from ischaemic optic neuropathy.

Please refer to CD-ROM for full text and references.

## What are the effects of treatments for epithelial ocular herpes simplex?

### BENEFICIAL

**Interferons**

One systematic review has found that topical interferons (alpha or beta) significantly increase healing after 7 and 14 days compared with placebo. The review found no significant difference between a topical interferon and a topical antiviral agent in healing after 7 days, but found that a topical interferon significantly increased healing after 14 days. "Healing" was not clearly defined.

**Topical antiviral agents**

One systematic review has found that idoxuridine or vidarabine significantly increases healing after 14 days compared with placebo, and that trifluridine or aciclovir (acyclovir) significantly increases healing compared with idoxuridine after 7 and 14 days. "Healing" was not clearly defined.

### UNKNOWN EFFECTIVENESS

**Debridement**

One systematic review has found no significant difference between debridement and placebo in the proportion of people healed, but has found that debridement plus antiviral treatment versus dibridement alone significantly increases the proportion of people healed after 7 and 14 days. "Healing" was not clearly defined.

## What are the effects of treatments for stromal ocular herpes simplex?

### BENEFICIAL

**Topical corticosteroids**

One RCT in people receiving topical antiviral treatment found that topical corticosteroids significantly reduced the progression and shortened the duration of stromal keratitis⊙ compared with placebo.

### UNLIKELY TO BE BENEFICIAL

**Oral aciclovir**

One RCT in people receiving topical corticosteroids plus antiviral treatment found no significant difference between oral aciclovir and placebo in rates of treatment failure at 16 weeks.

## What are the effects of treatments to prevent recurence of epithelial or stromal ocular herpes simplex?

### BENEFICIAL

**Long term (1 year) oral aciclovir**

One large RCT in people with at least one previous episode of epithelial⊙ or stromal keratitis found that long term (1 year) oral aciclovir significantly reduced recurrence after 1 year compared with placebo.

▶

# Ocular herpes simplex

## UNLIKELY TO BE BENEFICIAL

### Short term (3 wks) oral aciclovir

One RCT in people with epithelial keratitis receiving topical trifluridine found no significant difference between short term prophylaxis with oral aciclovir and placebo in the rate of stromal keratitis or iritis at 1 year.

---

## *What are the effects of treatments to prevent recurrence of ocular herpes simplex in people with corneal grafts?*

## LIKELY TO BE BENEFICIAL

### Oral aciclovir

One small RCT found limited evidence that prophylactic use of oral aciclovir significantly reduced recurrence and improved graft survival compared with placebo.

**DEFINITION**
Ocular herpes simplex is usually caused by herpes simplex virus type 1 (HSV-1), but also occasionally by type 2 virus (HSV-2). Ocular manifestations of HSV are varied and include blepharitis (inflammation of the eyelids), canalicular obstruction, conjunctivitis, epithelial keratitis, stromal keratitis, iritis, and retinitis. HSV infections are classified as neonatal, primary (HSV in a person with no previous viral exposure), and recurrent (previous viral exposure with humoral and cellular immunity present).

**INCIDENCE/ PREVALENCE**
Infections with HSV are usually acquired in early life. A US study found antibodies against HSV-1 in about 50% of people with high socioeconomic status and 80% of people with low socioeconomic status by the age of 30 years.[1] However, only about 20–25% of people with HSV antibodies had any history of clinical manifestations of ocular or cutaneous herpetic disease.[2] Ocular HSV is the most common cause of corneal blindness in high income countries and the most common cause of unilateral corneal blindness in the world.[3] A 33 year study of the population of Rochester, Minnesota, found the annual incidence of new cases of ocular herpes simplex was 8.4/100 000 (95% CI 6.9 to 9.9) and the annual incidence of all episodes (new and recurrent) was 20.7/100 000 (95% CI 18.3 to 23.1).[4] The prevalence of ocular herpes was 149 cases/100 000 population (95% CI 115 to 183). Twelve per cent of people had bilateral disease.

**AETIOLOGY/ RISK FACTORS**
Epithelial keratitis results from productive, lytic viral infection of the corneal epithelial cells. Stromal keratitis and iritis are thought to result from a combination of viral infection and compromised immune mechanisms. Observational evidence (346 people with ocular HSV in the placebo arm of an RCT) has found that the risk of developing stromal keratitis was 4% in people with no previous history of stromal keratitis (RR 1.0) as compared with 32% (RR 10, 95% CI 4.32 to 23.38) with previous stromal keratitis, but that a history of epithelial keratitis was not a risk factor for recurrent epithelial keratitis.[5] Age, sex, ethnicity, and previous experience of non-ocular HSV disease were not associated with an increased risk of recurrence.[5]

**PROGNOSIS**
HSV epithelial keratitis tends to resolve within 1–2 weeks. In a trial of 271 people treated with topical trifluorothymidine and randomly assigned to receive either oral aciclovir or placebo, the epithelial lesion had resolved completely or was at least less than 1 mm after 1 week of treatment with placebo in 89% of people and after 2 weeks in 99% of people.[6] Stromal keratitis or iritis occurs in about 25% of people following epithelial keratitis.[7] The effects of HSV stromal keratitis include scarring, tissue destruction, neovascularisation, glaucoma, and persistent epithelial defects. Rate of recurrence of ocular herpes for people with one episode is 10% at 1 year, 23% at 2 years, and 50% at 10 years.[8] The ►

risk of recurrent ocular HSV infection (epithelial or stromal) has also been found to increase with the number of previous episodes reported (2 or 3 previous episodes: RR 1.41, 95% CI 0.82 to 2.42; 4 or more previous episodes: RR 2.09, 95% CI 1.24 to 3.50).[5] Of corneal grafts performed in Australia over a 10 year period, 5% were in people with visual disability or with actual or impending corneal perforation following stromal ocular herpes simplex. The recurrence of HSV in a corneal graft has a major effect on graft survival. The Australian Corneal Graft Registry has found that, in corneal grafts performed for HSV keratitis, there was at least one HSV recurrence in 58% of corneal grafts that failed over a follow up period of 9 years.[9]

Please refer to CD-ROM for full text and references.

# Trachoma

**Search date February 2003**

*Denise Mabey and Nicole Fraser-Hurt*

---

## What are the effects of interventions to prevent scarring trachoma by reducing active trachoma?

### LIKELY TO BE BENEFICIAL

**Promotion of face washing plus topical tetracycline**

One RCT found that promotion of face washing plus topical tetracycline reduced the rate of severe trachoma after 1 year compared with topical tetracycline alone, but found no significant difference in the overall rate of trachoma. However, the RCT may lack power to rule out a clinically important effect. One RCT found that face washing plus topical tetracycline reduced the proportion of children with trachoma after 3 months compared with no intervention.

### UNKNOWN EFFECTIVENESS

**Antibiotics (v placebo or no treatment)**

One systematic review found insufficient evidence on the effects of antibiotics versus placebo or no treatment in active trachoma. However, RCTs were heterogeneous and the review may not exclude clinically important effects.

**Face washing alone**

One RCT found no significant difference between face washing alone and no intervention rate of trachoma in children after 3 months.

**Oral azithromycin (v topical tetracycline)**

One systematic review found insufficient evidence on the effects of oral azithromycin versus topical tetracycline in active trachoma. However, RCTs were heterogeneous and the review may not exclude clinically important effects.

---

## What are the effects of surgical treatments for scarring trachoma (entropion and trichiasis)?

### LIKELY TO BE BENEFICIAL

**Bilamellar tarsal rotation or tarsal advance and rotation (v other eyelid surgery)**

In people with major trichiasis, one RCT found limited evidence that bilamellar tarsal rotation increased operative success after 2 weeks compared with eversion splinting, tarsal advance, or tarsal grooving, but found no significant difference between bilamellar tarsal rotation and tarsal advance and rotation in operative success after 2 weeks. A second RCT found that bilamellar tarsal rotation increased operative success after 25 months compared with tarsal advance and rotation. In both RCTs, one experienced surgeon performed most of the operations. In people with minor trichiasis, one of the RCTs found that tarsal rotation increased operative success after 25 months compared with cryoablation or electrolysis. One further RCT reporting combined results for major and minor trichiasis found no significant difference in recurrence between bilamellar tarsal rotation and tarsal advance and lid margin rotation after 3 months, although there were more minor complications (lid notching and pyogenic granuloma) with the bilamellar procedure. In this RCT, the procedures were undertaken by less experienced surgeons under supervision.

**DEFINITION** **Active trachoma** is chronic inflammation of the conjunctiva caused by infection with *Chlamydia trachomatis*. The World Health Organization classification for active trachoma defines mild trachoma (grade TF) as the presence of five or more follicles in the upper tarsal conjunctiva of at least 0.5 mm in diameter. Severe trachoma (grade TI) is defined as pronounced inflammatory thickening of the upper tarsal conjunctiva that obscures more than half of the normal deep vessels. **Scarring trachoma** is caused by repeated active infection by *C trachomatis* in which the upper eyelid is shortened and distorted (entropion) and the lashes abrade the eye (trichiasis). Scarring can exist without entropion/trichiasis but if entropion/trichiasis is present, there will be scarring. Blindness results from corneal opacification, which is related to the degree of entropion/trichiasis.

**INCIDENCE/ PREVALENCE** Trachoma is the world's leading cause of preventable blindness and is second only to cataract as an overall cause of blindness.[1] Globally, active trachoma affects an estimated 150 million people, most of them children. About 5.5 million people are blind or at risk of blindness as a consequence. Trachoma is a disease of poverty regardless of geographical region. Scarring trachoma is prevalent in large regions of Africa, the Middle East, south west Asia, the Indian subcontinent, and Aboriginal communities in Australia, and there are also small foci in Central and South America.[1] In areas where trachoma is constantly present at high prevalence, active disease is found in more than 50% of preschool children and may have a prevalence as high as 60–90%.[2] The prevalence of active trachoma decreases with increasing age, with fewer than 5% of adults showing signs of active disease.[2] Although similar rates of active disease are observed in boys and girls, the later sequelae of trichiasis, entropion, and corneal opacification are more common in women than men.[2] As many as 75% of women and 50% of men over the age of 45 years may show signs of scarring disease.[3]

**AETIOLOGY/ RISK FACTORS** Active trachoma is associated with youth and close contact between people. Discharge from the eyes and nose may be a source of further reinfection.[4] Sharing a bedroom with someone who has active trachoma is a risk factor for infection.[5] Facial contact with flies is held to be associated with active trachoma, but studies reporting this relationship used weak methods.[6]

**PROGNOSIS** Corneal damage from trachoma is caused by multiple processes. Scarring may cause an inadequate tear film, and a dry eye may be more susceptible to damage from inturned lashes, leading to corneal opacification. The prevalence of scarring and consequent blindness increases with age, and therefore is most commonly seen in older adults.[7]

Please refer to CD-ROM for full text and references.

# HIV infection

**Search date November 2002**

*David Wilkinson and Martin Talbot*

---

## What are the effects of preventive interventions?

### BENEFICIAL

**Early diagnosis and treatment of sexually transmitted diseases (STDs)**

One RCT has found that early diagnosis and treatment of STDs reduces the risk of acquiring HIV infection over 2 years.

### LIKELY TO BE BENEFICIAL

**Postexposure prophylaxis in healthcare workers***

One case control study found limited evidence suggesting that postexposure prophylaxis with zidovudine may reduce the risk of HIV infection over 6 months. Evidence from other settings suggests that combining several antiretroviral drugs is likely to be more effective than zidovudine alone.

*Based on observational studies and indirectly from RCTs in other settings.

### UNKNOWN EFFECTIVENESS

**Presumptive mass treatment of STDs**

One RCT found no significant difference with presumptive, mass treatment for STDs versus no treatment in the incidence of HIV over 20 months.

---

## What are the effects of treatments?

### BENEFICIAL

**Three drug antiretroviral regimens**

One systematic review has found that three drug regimens are beneficial compared with two drug regimens. Some of the reviewed trials included a non-nucleoside reverse-transcriptase inhibitor as a third drug, and some a protease inhibitor.

### TRADE OFF BETWEEN BENEFITS AND HARMS

**Two drug versus single drug antiretroviral regimens**

Large RCTs, with follow up of 1–3 years, have found that two drug regimens (zidovudine plus another nucleoside analogue or protease inhibitor drug) reduce the risk of new AIDS defining illnesses and death compared with zidovudine alone. Adverse events were common in all treatment groups.

### UNKNOWN EFFECTIVENESS

**Early versus delayed antiretroviral treatment**

We found no RCTs evaluating delayed versus early treatment with two or three drug regimens. RCTs conducted when zidovudine was the only drug available found no difference between early versus delayed treatment in survival at 1 year.

**DEFINITION** HIV infection refers to infection with the human immunodeficiency virus type 1 or type 2. Clinically, this is characterised by a variable period (average around 8–10 years) of asymptomatic infection, followed by repeated episodes of illness of varying and increasing severity as immune function deteriorates. The type of illness varies greatly by country, availability of specific treatment for HIV, and prophylaxis for opportunistic infections.

**INCIDENCE/ PREVALENCE**  Worldwide estimates suggest that, by December 1999, about 50 million people had been infected with HIV, about 16 million people had died as a result, and about 16 000 new HIV infections were occurring each day.[1] About 90% of HIV infections occur in the developing world.[1] Occupationally acquired HIV infection in healthcare workers has been documented in 95 definite and 191 possible cases, although this is likely to be an underestimate.[2]

**AETIOLOGY/ RISK FACTORS**  The major risk factor for transmission of HIV is unprotected heterosexual or homosexual intercourse. Other risk factors include needlestick injury, sharing drug injecting equipment, and blood transfusion. An HIV infected woman may also transmit the virus to her baby. This has been reported in 15–30% of pregnant women with HIV infection. Not everyone who is exposed to HIV will become infected, although risk increases if exposure is repeated, at high dose, or through blood. There is at least a two to five times greater risk of HIV infection among people with sexually transmitted diseases.[3]

**PROGNOSIS**  Without treatment, about half of people infected with HIV will become ill and die from AIDS over about 10 years. A meta-analysis of 13 cohort studies from Europe and the USA looked at 12 574 treatment naive people starting highly active antiretroviral therapy with a combination of at least three drugs.[4] During 24 310 person years of follow up, 1094 people developed AIDS or died. Baseline CD4 cell count and baseline HIV-1 viral load were associated with the probability of progression to AIDS or death. Other independent predictors of poorer outcome were advanced age, infection through injection drug use, and a previous diagnosis of AIDS. The CD4 cell count at initiation was the dominant prognostic factor in people starting highly active antiretroviral therapy. Genetic factors have been shown to affect response to antiretroviral treatment, but were not considered in the meta-analysis.[4]

Please refer to CD-ROM for full text and references.

# HIV: mother to child transmission

Search date September 2002

*Jimmy Volmink*

---

## *What are the effects of measures to reduce mother to child transmission of HIV?*

**BENEFICIAL**

### Antiretroviral drugs

One systematic review has found that zidovudine versus placebo significantly reduces the incidence of HIV in infants. One RCT has found that the longer versus shorter courses of zidovudine (long–long versus short–short courses) given to mother and infant significantly reduces the incidence of HIV in infants. One RCT has found that nevirapine versus zidovudine given to the mother and to her newborn significantly reduces the risk of HIV transmission. One RCT found no additional advantage in giving nevirapine to the mother and baby when transmission rates are already reduced by mothers receiving standard antiretroviral treatment. One RCT has found that zidovudine plus lamivudine versus placebo given in the antenatal and intrapartum period, or in the intrapartum and postpartum period, significantly reduces the risk of transmission of HIV.

**LIKELY TO BE BENEFICIAL**

### Elective caesarean section

One RCT found limited evidence that elective caesarean section versus vaginal delivery in women with HIV reduced the incidence of HIV in infants at 18 months.

**TRADE OFF BETWEEN BENEFITS AND HARMS**

### Avoiding breast feeding

One RCT in women with HIV who had access to clean water and health education has found that versus formula feeding breast feeding significantly reduces the incidence of HIV in infants after 24 months without increasing infant mortality.

**UNKNOWN EFFECTIVENESS**

### Immunotherapy

One RCT found no significant difference in the incidence of HIV in infants of mothers taking hyperimmune globulin versus immunoglobulin without HIV antibody in addition to a standard zidovudine regimen, but it may have been too small to exclude a clinically important difference.

### Vaginal microbicides

We found insufficient evidence about the effects of vaginal microbicides on the transmission of HIV to infants.

**LIKELY TO BE INEFFECTIVE OR HARMFUL**

### Vitamin supplements

RCTs found no significant difference in the incidence of HIV at birth, 6 weeks, or 3 months in the infants of pregnant women given vitamin A or multivitamins versus placebo.

**DEFINITION**      Mother to child transmission of HIV-1🛇 infection can occur during pregnancy, in the intrapartum period, or postnatally through breast feeding.[1] By contrast, HIV-2🛇 is rarely transmitted from mother to child.[2] Infected children usually have no symptoms and signs of HIV at birth, but develop them over subsequent months or years.[3] ▶

**INCIDENCE/ PREVALENCE**  A review of 13 cohorts found that the risk of mother to child transmission of HIV without antiviral treatment is on average about 15–20% in Europe, 15–30% in the USA, and 25–35% in Africa.[4] The risk of transmission is estimated to be between 15 and 30% during pregnancy, with an additional risk of about 10–20% postpartum through breast feeding.[5] It has been estimated that 800 000 children below the age of 15 years were newly infected with HIV during 2001, bringing the total number of children with HIV/AIDS to 3 million worldwide.[6] Most of these children were infected from their mother and 90% live in sub-Saharan Africa.

**AETIOLOGY/ RISK FACTORS**  Transmission of HIV to children is more likely if the mother has a high viral load.[1,7,8] Women with detectable viraemia (by p24 antigen or culture) have double the risk of transmitting HIV-1 to their infants than those who do not.[1] Breast feeding has also been shown in prospective studies to be a risk factor.[6,10] Other risk factors include sexually transmitted diseases, chorioamnionitis, prolonged rupture of membranes, and vaginal mode of delivery.[11–15]

**PROGNOSIS**  About 25% of infants infected with HIV progress rapidly to AIDS or death in the first year. Some survive beyond 12 years of age.[3] One European study found a mortality of 15% in the first year of life and a mortality of 28% by the age of 5 years.[16] A recent report estimated the mortality attributable to HIV/AIDS in children under 5 years of age in sub-Saharan Africa after correcting for competing causes of mortality.[17] HIV accounted for 2% of deaths in 1990 rising significantly to almost 8% in 1999. Five countries (Botswana, Namibia, Swaziland, Zambia, and Zimbabwe) had rates of HIV attributable mortality in excess of 30/1000 in children under the age of 5 years.

---

Please refer to CD-ROM for full text and references.

# HIV: prevention of opportunistic infections

**Search date April 2003**

*John Ioannidis and David Wilkinson*

## What are the effects of prophylaxis for Pneumocystis carinii pneumonia (PCP) and toxoplasmosis?

**BENEFICIAL**

### Trimethoprim/sulfamethoxazole (TMP/SMX — co-trimoxazole) for PCP

Systematic reviews have found that TMP/SMX reduces the incidence of PCP compared with placebo or pentamidine. Two systematic reviews have found that TMP/SMX reduced incidence of PCP compared with dapsone (with or without pyrimethamine), although only one of these reviews found that the reduction was significant. One systematic review and one subsequent RCT found no significant difference between high and low dose TMP/SMX for PCP prophylaxis, although adverse effects were more common with the higher dose.

**LIKELY TO BE BENEFICIAL**

### Atovaquone (no difference compared with dapsone or aerosolised pentamidine for PCP in people intolerant of TMP/SMX)

We found no RCTs of atovaquone versus placebo. RCTs found no significant difference in the incidence of PCP with atovaquone versus dapsone or versus aerosolised pentamidine, both of which are regarded as effective in people intolerant of TMP/SMX.

### Azithromycin (for PCP)

One RCT has found that azithromycin, either alone or in combination with rifabutin reduces the risk of PCP in people receiving standard PCP prophylaxis compared with rifabutin alone.

**UNKNOWN EFFECTIVENESS**

### TMP/SMX (for toxoplasmosis)

One RCT found no significant difference between TMP/SMX and placebo for preventing toxoplasmosis. One systematic review has found no significant difference between TMP/SMX and dapsone (with or without pyrimethamine) for preventing toxoplasmosis.

## What are the effects of antituberculosis prophylaxis in people with HIV infection?

**BENEFICIAL**

### Tuberculosis prophylaxis versus placebo (in people with positive tuberculin test)

Systematic reviews have found that in people who are HIV and tuberculin skin test positive, antituberculosis prophylaxis reduces the frequency of tuberculosis compared with placebo over 2–3 years. The reviews found no evidence of benefit in people who are HIV positive but tuberculin skin test negative. One RCT found that the benefit of prophylaxis diminished with time after treatment was stopped.

### TRADE OFF BETWEEN BENEFITS AND HARMS

**Isoniazid for 6–12 months (v combination treatment for 2 months — similar benefits, fewer harms)**

RCTs found no evidence of a difference in effectiveness between regimens using combinations of tuberculosis drugs for 2–3 months and those using isoniazid alone for 6–12 months. One RCT found that multidrug regimens increased the number of people with adverse reactions resulting in cessation of treatment.

---

## What are the effects of prophylaxis for disseminated Mycobacterium avium complex (MAC) disease for people without previous MAC disease?

### LIKELY TO BE BENEFICIAL

**Azithromycin**

One RCT has found that azithromycin reduces the incidence of MAC compared with placebo.

**Clarithromycin**

One RCT has found that clarithromycin reduces the incidence of MAC compared with placebo.

### TRADE OFF BETWEEN BENEFITS AND HARMS

**Combination treatment (rifabutin plus either clarithromycin or azithromycin)**

One RCT has found that rifabutin plus clarithromycin or clarithromycin alone reduces the incidence of MAC compared with rifabutin alone. One RCT has found that rifabutin plus azithromycin reduces the incidence of MAC compared with azithromycin alone or rifabutin alone at 1 year. One systematic review and two subsequent RCTs found that toxicity, including uveitis, was more common with combination therapy that with clarithromycin or rifabutin alone.

---

## What are the effects of prophylaxis for disseminated MAC disease for people with previous MAC disease?

### LIKELY TO BE BENEFICIAL

**Clarithromycin, rifabutin, and ethambutol (v clarithromycin plus clofazimine)**

One RCT found that clarithromycin, rifabutin, and ethambutol reduced MAC relapse compared with clarithromycin plus clofazimine.

**Ethambutol added to clarithromycin plus clofazimine**

One RCT found that adding ethambutol to clarithromycin and clofazimine reduced MAC relapse compared with clarithromycin plus clofazimine.

### UNKNOWN EFFECTIVENESS

**Rifabutin added to clarithromycin plus ethambutol**

One RCT found no significant difference in survival by adding rifabutin to clarithromycin plus ethambutol in people with previous MAC.

# HIV: prevention of opportunistic infections

### Clofazimine added to ethambutol plus clarithromycin (v clofazimine plus ethambutol)

One RCT found that adding clarithromycin to clofazimine and ethambutol was associated with higher mortality compared with clofazimine plus ethambutol.

## What are the effects of prophylaxis for cytomegalovirus (CMV), herpes simplex virus (HSV), and varicella zoster virus (VZV)?

### Aciclovir (for HSV and VZV)

One systematic review has found that aciclovir reduces HSV and VZV infection, and reduces overall mortality in people at different clinical stages of HIV infection compared with placebo. It found no reduction in CMV.

### Oral ganciclovir (in people with severe CD4 depletion)

One RCT has found that oral ganciclovir reduces the incidence of CMV in people with severe CD4 depletion compared with placebo. It found that 25% of people taking ganciclovir developed severe neutropenia. A second RCT found no significant differences between treatments.

### Famciclovir (for recurrent HSV)

One small RCT found that famciclovir reduced the rate of viral shedding compared with placebo, but provided insufficient evidence on the effect of famciclovir on HSV recurrence.

### Valaciclovir (v aciclovir for CMV)

One RCT has found that valaciclovir compared with aciclovir reduces the incidence of CMV, but may be associated with increased mortality.

## What are the effects of prophylaxis for invasive fungal disease in people without previous fungal disease?

### Fluconazole or itraconazole

RCTs in people with advanced HIV disease have found that both fluconazole and itraconazole reduce the incidence of invasive fungal infections compared with placebo. One RCT found that fluconazole reduced the incidence of invasive fungal disease and mucocutaneous candidiasis compared with clotrimazole. One RCT found no difference between high and low dose fluconazole.

◀ *What are the effects of prophylaxis for invasive fungal disease in people with previous fungal disease?*

**LIKELY TO BE BENEFICIAL**

**Itraconazole (for *Penicillium marneffei*)**
Two RCTs have found that itraconazole reduces the incidence of relapse of *P marneffei* infection🅖 and candidiasis compared with placebo.

**UNKNOWN EFFECTIVENESS**

**Itraconazole (for histoplasmosis)**
We found no RCTs.

**LIKELY TO BE INEFFECTIVE OR HARMFUL**

**Itraconazole (v fluconazole for maintenance treatment of cryptococcal meningitis)**
One RCT found that itraconazole increased the risk of relapse of cryptococcal meningitis compared with fluconazole.

---

*What are the effects of discontinuing prophylaxis against opportunistic pathogens in people on highly active antiretroviral treatment (HAART)?*

**LIKELY TO BE BENEFICIAL**

**Discontinuing prophylaxis for MAC in people with CD4 > 100/mm³ on highly active antiretroviral treatment (HAART)**
Two RCTs in people taking HAART found that discontinuation of prophylaxis for MAC disease did not increase the incidence of MAC disease.

**Discontinuing prophylaxis for PCP and toxoplasmosis in people with CD4 > 200/mm³ on HAART**
One systematic review of two unblinded RCTs in people taking HAART found that discontinuation of prophylaxis did not increase the incidence of PCP. Two unblinded RCTs found that discontinuation of prophylaxis did not increase the incidence of toxoplasmosis.

**UNKNOWN EFFECTIVENESS**

**Discontinuing prophylaxis for CMV in people with CD4 > 100/mm³ on HAART**
We found insufficient evidence on the effects of discontinuation of maintenance treatment for CMV retinitis or other end organ disease in people taking HAART.

**DEFINITION**    Opportunistic infections are intercurrent infections that occur in people infected with HIV. Prophylaxis aims to avoid either the first occurrence of these infections (primary prophylaxis) or their recurrence (secondary prophylaxis, maintenance treatment). This review includes PCP, *Toxoplasma gondii* encephalitis, *Mycobacterium tuberculosis*, MAC disease, CMV disease (most often retinitis), infections from other herpesviruses (HSV and VZV), and invasive fungal disease (*Cryptococcus neoformans*, *Histoplasma capsulatum*, and *P marneffei*).

**INCIDENCE/**    The incidence of opportunistic infections is high in people with immune
**PREVALENCE**    impairment. Data available before the introduction of HAART suggest that, with a CD4 < 250/mm³, the 2 year probability of developing an opportunistic ▶

# HIV: prevention of opportunistic infections

infection is 40% for PCP, 22% for CMV, 18% for MAC, 6% for toxoplasmosis, and 5% for cryptococcal meningitis.[1] The introduction of HAART has reduced the rate of opportunistic infections. A recent cohort study found that the introduction of HAART decreased the incidence of PCP by 94%, CMV by 82%, and MAC by 64%, as presenting AIDS events. HAART decreased the incidence of events subsequent to the diagnosis of AIDS by 84% for PCP, 82% for CMV, and 97% for MAC.[2]

**AETIOLOGY/ RISK FACTORS**
Opportunistic infections are caused by a wide array of pathogens and result from immune defects induced by HIV. The risk of developing opportunistic infections increases dramatically with progressive impairment of the immune system. Each opportunistic infection has a different threshold of immune impairment, beyond which the risk increases substantially.[1] Opportunistic pathogens may infect the immunocompromised host *de novo*, but usually they are simply reactivations of latent pathogens in such hosts.

**PROGNOSIS**
Prognosis depends on the type of opportunistic infection. Even with treatment they may cause serious morbidity and mortality. Most deaths owing to HIV infection are caused by opportunistic infections.

Please refer to CD-ROM for full text and references.

## What are the effects of preventive interventions?

### BENEFICIAL

**High dose aciclovir (> 3200 mg/day) in people with HIV infection**

One systematic review has found that high dose aciclovir (at least 3200 mg/day) significantly reduces the risk of clinical chickenpox and reduces all cause mortality over 22 months' treatment compared with placebo.

**Live attenuated vaccine in healthy children**

Two RCTs have found that live attenuated varicella vaccine significantly reduces clinical chickenpox compared with placebo, with no significant increase in adverse effects.

### LIKELY TO BE BENEFICIAL

**Zoster immune globulin (ZIG) versus human serum globulin in healthy children**

One small RCT in children exposed to a sibling with chickenpox found that ZIG🅖 significantly reduced the number of exposed children with clinical chickenpox at 20 days compared with human immune serum globulin (ISG)🅖.

### UNKNOWN EFFECTIVENESS

**Aciclovir in people with immunocompromise other than HIV**

We found no RCTs.

**Live attenuated vaccine in immunocompromised people**

We found no RCTs in immunocompromised people on the effects of live attenuated varicella vaccine.

**ZIG versus varicella zoster immune globulin (VZIG) in immunocompromised children**

One RCT in immunocompromised children exposed to a sibling with chickenpox found no significant difference in clinical chickenpox with ZIG compared with VZIG🅖 at 12 weeks.

## What are the effects of treatments?

### BENEFICIAL

**Oral aciclovir in healthy people (given < 24 h of onset of the rash)**

Two systematic reviews have found that oral aciclovir compared with placebo reduces the symptoms of chickenpox in healthy people.

### LIKELY TO BE BENEFICIAL

**Intravenous aciclovir for treatment of chickenpox in children with malignancy**

Two RCTs compared intravenous aciclovir versus placebo; one large RCT has found that aciclovir significantly reduces clinical deterioration, and the other small RCT found no significant difference in clinical deterioration. ▶

# Chickenpox

**Oral aciclovir in healthy people (given > 24 h after the onset of the rash)**
One systematic review and one additional RCT have found that oral aciclovir given beyond 24 hours after onset of rash does not significantly reduce the symptoms of chickenpox compared with placebo.

**DEFINITION**   Chickenpox is due to primary infection with varicella zoster virus (VZV). In healthy people it is usually a mild self limiting illness, characterised by low grade fever, malaise, and a generalised, itchy vesicular rash.

**INCIDENCE/ PREVALENCE**   Chickenpox is extremely contagious. Over 90% of unvaccinated people become infected, but infection occurs at different ages in different parts of the world: over 80% of people have been infected by the age of 10 years in the USA, UK, and Japan, but by 30 years of age in India, Southeast Asia, and the West Indies.[1,2]

**AETIOLOGY/ RISK FACTORS**   Chickenpox is caused by exposure to VZV.

**PROGNOSIS**   **Infants and children:** In healthy children the illness is usually mild and self limiting. In the USA, death rates in infants and children aged 1–14 years with chickenpox are about 7/100 000 and 1.4/100 000, respectively.[3] In Australia, mortality in children aged between 1 and 11 years with chickenpox is about 0.5–0.6/100 000, and in infants with chickenpox it is about 1.2/100 000.[4] Bacterial skin sepsis is the most common complication in children under 5 years of age, and acute cerebellar ataxia is the most common complication in older children; both cause hospital admission in 2–3/10 000 children.[5] **Adults:** Mortality in adults is higher, at about 31/100 000.[3] Varicella pneumonia is the most common complication, causing 20–30 hospital admissions/10 000 adults.[5] Activation of latent VZV infection can cause herpes zoster, also known as shingles (see postherpetic neuralgia, p 185). **Cancer chemotherapy:** One case series (77 children with cancer and chickenpox) found that more children receiving chemotherapy versus those in remission developed progressive chickenpox with multiple organ involvement (19/60 [32%] v 0/17 [0%]) and more children died (4/60 [7%] v 0/17 [0%]).[6] **HIV infection:** One retrospective case series found that one in four children with HIV who acquired chickenpox in hospital developed pneumonia and 5% died.[7] In a retrospective cohort study (73 children with HIV and chickenpox), infection beyond 2 months occurred in 10 children (14%) and recurrent VZV infections occurred in 38 children (55%).[8] Half of recurrent infections involved generalised rashes and the other half had zoster. **Newborns:** We found no cohort studies of untreated children with perinatal exposure to chickenpox. One cohort study (281 neonates receiving VZIG because their mothers had developed a chickenpox rash during the month before or after delivery) found that 134 (48%) developed a chickenpox rash and 19 (14%) developed severe chickenpox.[9] Severe chickenpox occurred in neonates of mothers whose rash had started during the 7 days before delivery.

Please refer to CD-ROM for full text and references.

### Search date November 2002

*Piero Olliaro*

## What are the effects of treating toxoplasmosis in pregnancy?

### UNKNOWN EFFECTIVENESS

### Spiramycin and other antiparasitic drugs

Two systematic reviews of cohort studies in women who seroconvert during pregnancy found insufficient evidence on the effects of current antiparasitic treatment compared with no treatment on mother or baby.

**DEFINITION**   Toxoplasmosis is caused by the parasite *Toxoplasma gondii*. Infection is asymptomatic or unremarkable in immunocompetent individuals, but leads to a lifelong antibody response. During pregnancy, toxoplasmosis can be transmitted across the placenta and may cause intrauterine death, neonatal growth retardation, mental retardation, ocular defects, and blindness in later life. Congenital toxoplasmosis (confirmed infection of the fetus or newborn) can present at birth, either as subclinical disease, which may evolve with neurological or ophthalmological disease later in life, or as a disease of varying severity, ranging from mild ocular damage to severe mental retardation.

**INCIDENCE/**   Reported rates of toxoplasma seroprevalence vary across and within coun-
**PREVALENCE**   tries, as well as over time. The risk of primary infection is highest in young people, including young women during pregnancy. We found no cohort studies describing annual seroconversion rates in women of childbearing age nor incidence of primary infection. One systematic review (search date 1996) identified 15 studies that reported rates of seroconversion in non-immune pregnant women ranging from 2.4–16/1000 in Europe and from 2–6/1000 in the USA.[1] France began screening for congenital toxoplasmosis in 1978, and during the period 1980–1995 the seroconversion rate during pregnancy in non-immune women was 4–5/1000.[2]

**AETIOLOGY/**   Toxoplasma infection is usually acquired by ingesting either sporocysts (from
**RISK FACTORS** unwashed fruit or vegetables contaminated by cat faeces) or tissue cysts (from raw or undercooked meat). The risk of contracting toxoplasma infection varies with eating habits, contact with cats and other pets, and occupational exposure.

**PROGNOSIS**   One systematic review of studies conducted from 1983–1996 found no population based prospective studies of the natural history of toxoplasma infection during pregnancy.[1] One systematic review (search date 1997) reported nine controlled, non-randomised studies, and found that untreated toxoplasmosis acquired during pregnancy was associated with infection rates in children of between 10–100%.[3] We found two European studies that correlated gestation at time of seroconversion with risk of transmission and severity of disease at birth.[4,5] Risk of transmission increased with gestational age at maternal seroconversion, reaching 70–90% for infections acquired after 30 weeks' gestation. In contrast, the risk of the infected infant developing clinical disease was highest when infection occurred early in pregnancy. The highest risk of early signs of disease (including chorioretinitis and hydrocephaly) was about 10%, and occurred with infection between 24 and 30 weeks' gestation.[5] Infants with untreated congenital toxoplasmosis and generalised neurological abnormalities at birth develop mental retardation, growth retardation, blindness ▶

Infectious diseases

# Congenital toxoplasmosis

or visual defects, seizures, and spasticity. Children with untreated subclinical infection at birth may have cognitive and motor deficits and visual defects or blindness, which may go undiagnosed for many years. One case control study (845 school children in Brazil) found mental retardation and retinochoroiditis to be significantly associated with positive toxoplasma serology (population attributable risk 6–9%).[6]

Please refer to CD-ROM for full text and references.

Infectious diseases

## What are the effects of treatments?

### LIKELY TO BE BENEFICIAL

**Amino acid oral rehydration solution (ORS) (v standard ORS)**

One small RCT has found that amino acid ORS❸ versus standard ORS reduces the total volume and duration of diarrhoea.

**Rice based ORS (v standard ORS)**

One systematic review has found that rice based ORS versus standard ORS significantly reduced the 24 hour stool volume.

### UNKNOWN EFFECTIVENESS

**Bicarbonate ORS (v standard ORS)**

Two RCTs found no significant difference in the duration or volume of diarrhoea with bicarbonate ORS versus standard ORS. One RCT found no significant difference in total stool output or duration of diarrhoea with bicarbonate ORS versus an otherwise identical ORS in which the bicarbonate was replaced with chloride.

**Reduced osmolarity ORS (v standard ORS)**

Three RCTs comparing reduced osmolarity ORS versus standard IRS found a small and inconsistent effect on total stool volume and duration of diarrhoea.

### TRADE OFF BETWEEN BENEFITS AND HARMS

**Antimotility agents**

RCTs have found that loperamide hydrochloride and loperamide oxide versus placebo significantly reduce the time to relief of symptoms, but frequently cause constipation. We found insufficient evidence about the effects of other antimotility agents.

**Empirical antibiotic treatment in community acquired diarrhoea**

RCTs have found that ciprofloxacin versus placebo reduces the duration of community acquired diarrhoea by 1–2 days❶. RCTs found limited evidence that other antibiotics, except for lomefloxacin, reduced duration of diarrhoea compared with placebo. Adverse events varied by agent.

**Empirical antibiotic treatment in travellers' diarrhoea**

One systematic review and one additional RCT have found that empirical use of antibiotics versus placebo significantly increases cure rate at 3 and 6 days. Antibiotic treatment is associated with prolonged presence of bacterial pathogens in the stool and development of resistant strains.

**DEFINITION** Diarrhoea is watery or liquid stools, usually with an increase in stool weight above 200 g daily and an increase in daily stool frequency. This chapter covers empirical treatment of suspected infectious diarrhoea in adults.

**INCIDENCE/ PREVALENCE** An estimated 4000 million cases of diarrhoea occurred worldwide in 1996, resulting in 2.5 million deaths.[1] In the USA, the estimated incidence for infectious intestinal disease is 0.44 episodes per person a year (episode per person every 2.3 years), resulting in about one consultation with a doctor per person every 28 years.[2] A recent community study in the UK reported an incidence of 19 cases per 100 person years, of which 3.3 cases per 100 ▶

Infectious diseases

# Diarrhoea in adults

person years resulted in consultation with a general practitioner.[3] The epidemiology of travellers' diarrhoea (in people who have crossed a national boundary) is not well understood. Incidence is higher in travellers visiting developing countries, but it varies widely by location and season of travel.[4]

**AETIOLOGY/**  The cause of diarrhoea depends on geographic location, standards of food
**RISK FACTORS**  hygiene, sanitation, water supply, and season. Commonly identified causes of sporadic diarrhoea in adults in developed countries include *Campylobacter*, *Salmonella*, *Shigella*, *Escherichia coli*, *Yersinia*, protozoa, and viruses. No pathogens are identified in more than half of people with diarrhoea. In returning travellers, about 50% of episodes are caused by bacteria such as enterotoxigenic *E coli*, *Salmonella*, *Shigella*, *Campylobacter*, *Vibrio*, enteroadherent *E coli*, *Yersinia*, and *Aeromonas*.[5]

**PROGNOSIS**  In developing countries, diarrhoea is reported to cause more deaths in children under 5 years of age than any other condition.[1] Few studies have examined which factors predict poor outcome in adults. In developed countries, death from infectious diarrhoea is rare, although serious complications, including severe dehydration and renal failure, can occur and may necessitate admission to hospital. Elderly people and those in long term care have an increased risk of death.[6]

---

Please refer to CD-ROM for full text and references.

Search date February 2003

*Kamran Siddiqi*

## What are the effects of immunisation in countries with high endemicity? New

**BENEFICIAL**

### Universal immunisation of infants

One non-systematic review and three additional and subsequent RCTs have found that, in countries with high endemicity, universal immunisation of infants, using either recombinent or plasma derived vaccines, reduces acute hepatitis and development of a chronic carrier state compared with placebo. One non-systematic review and four additional and subsequent RCTs have found that universal (both recombinant and plasma derived) hepatitis B immunisation in infants in countries with high endemicity⊙, compared with placebo, reduces acute hepatitis and development of a chronic carrier state⊙. The longest RCT found universal immunisation⊙ protected at 15 years. Two historical cohort studies found reduced secondary mortality from hepatocellular carcinoma in children born after the introduction of a universal plasma derived hepatitis immunisation program. One additional historical cohort study found a lower rate of related chronic liver disease, cirrhosis, and hepatocellular cancer after the introduction of a universal plasma derived immunisation program. Three non-systematic reviews and one RCT found only minor adverse reactions after recombinant hepatitis B immunisation. One cluster RCT found universal immunisation with first plasma and then recombinant vaccine reduced the development of chronic carrier state and acute hepatitis events compared with immunisation of high risk groups.

### Selective immunisation of high risk individuals

The available evidence relates only to children born to HbsAg mothers. One non-systematic review of both plasma derived and recombinant vaccine⊙ in mainly observational studies and three RCTs of plasma hepatitis B immunisation compared with placebo or no treatment, found that immunisation prevents chronic carrier state in children born to HbsAg⊙ positive mothers. One RCT found minor adverse events with immunisation, the other RCTs did not report on adverse events. We found no good evidence in other high risk groups. One cluster RCT found that selective immunisation in high risk individuals was less effective than universal immunisation of infants in reducing the development of chronic carrier state and acute hepatitis events.

## What are the effects of immunisation in countries with low endemicity? New

**LIKELY TO BE BENEFICIAL**

### Selective immunisation of high risk individuals

One systematic review in countries with low endemicity⊙ found that plasma derived hepatitis B immunisation prevented acute hepatitis B and development of chronic carrier state in healthcare workers at high risk of exposure to bodily fluids. Three RCTs found that plasma derived hepatitis B immunisation prevented acute hepatitis B in homosexual men. One small RCT found no significant difference in hepatitis B events in heterosexual partners of infected people. Three RCTs of plasma derived immunisation in people on regular haemodialysis found potentially conflicting results. Two RCTs from France and Belgium found good protective ▶

# Hepatitis B

efficacy⦿ against chronic carrier state. However, one large US based RCT found no good evidence of benefit. The systematic review of plasma derived vaccination found no significant difference between immunisation and placebo in the rate and severity of adverse events. One observational study showed a high prevalence of hepatitis B carrier state and low immunisation uptake in young homosexuals despite a national strategy to immunise high risk groups. We found insufficient evidence to compare the effectiveness of selective immunisation of high risk individuals with other strategies.

## Universal immunisation of infants

One historical cohort study found a reduction in the prevalence of hepatitis B chronic carrier state following universal immunisation. We found insufficient evidence to compare its effectiveness with other strategies. Two cohort studies and surveillance data did not report any links between hepatitis B immunisation and serious adverse reactions.

## UNKNOWN EFFECTIVENESS

### Comparative effectiveness of different strategies

We found no good systematic reviews, RCTs, or observational studies comparing the effectiveness of different immunisation strategies in countries with low endemicity.

### Universal immunisation of adolescents

We found insufficient evidence to assess the effects of universal adolescent immunisation, or to compare its effectiveness with other strategies. One observational study suggests minor adverse effects following hepatitis B immunisation in this group.

**DEFINITION**   Hepatitis B is a viral infectious disease with an incubation period of 40–160 days. Acute hepatitis B infection is characterised by anorexia, vague abdominal discomfort, nausea and vomiting, jaundice, and occasional fever. Illness is associated with deranged liver function tests (especially raised alanine transaminases) and presence of serological markers of acute hepatitis B infection (e.g. HbsAg⦿, antiHBc IgM).[1]

**INCIDENCE/**   The incidence of acute hepatitis B and prevalence of its chronic carrier state⦿
**PREVALENCE**   varies widely across the globe. In areas with high endemicity⦿ (HbsAg prevalence ≥8%, e.g. South East Asia and Africa), more than half of the population becomes infected at some point in their lives.[2] In countries with low endemicity⦿ (HbsAg prevalence <2%, e.g. North America, western Europe, Australia), most of the population do not become infected.[2] Nearly a third of the world population has been infected by hepatitis B at some point, and at least 350 million people (5–6% of world population) are currently chronic carriers of hepatitis B infection.[3]

**AETIOLOGY/**   In countries with high endemicity⦿, most infections occur during childhood
**RISK FACTORS** from an infected mother to her baby (vertical transmission) or from one child to another (horizontal transmission).[4] However, most hepatitis B infection in developed countries occurs later from either sexual activity, injection drug use, or occupational exposure. Less frequent causes of infection include household contact, regular haemodialysis, transmission from a health professional, and receipt of organs or other blood products.[5] The vaccination policy of a country is a large determinant of the risk of developing hepatitis B. Since the development of plasma derived hepatitis B vaccine in the early 1980s, subsequently replaced by recombinant vaccine⦿, many countries have adopted a policy of universal immunisation⦿ of all infants. On the basis of disease burden, the World Health Organization recommended that hepatitis B vaccine be incorporated into routine infant and childhood immunisation programmes in countries ▶

Infectious diseases

with high endemicity by 1995 and in all countries by 1997.[6] Despite this, in many countries with low endemicity**ⓖ**, universal immunisation policy remains controversial and has still not been adopted.[7] Some of these countries have adopted a policy of selective immunisation of high risk individuals, others have adopted a universal adolescent immunisation policy.

**PROGNOSIS**  Hepatitis B infection resolves in most cases after the acute infection. In the remainder, it may result in a number of serious sequelae. Massive hepatic necrosis occurs in 1% of people with acute viral hepatitis, leading to a serious and often fatal condition called acute fulminant hepatitis. Between 2 and 10% of those infected as adults become chronic carriers with hepatitis B surface antigen (HbsAg**ⓖ**), persisting for longer than 6 months. Chronic carriage is more frequent in those infected as children, and reaches up to 90% in those infected during the perinatal period.[1] Between 20 and 25% of chronic carriers develop a progressive chronic liver disease. This progresses to the most important sequelae of hepatitis B infection, cirrhosis and hepatocellular carcinoma. These complications usually arise in older adults and are major causes of mortality in populations with high hepatitis B endemicity**ⓖ**.[4] Observational studies suggest that, in these countries, almost 80% of chronic liver disease and cirrhosis is attributed to hepatitis B, and these complications lead to at least a million deaths every year.[2]

Please refer to CD-ROM for full text and references.

# Influenza

**Search date November 2002**

*Lucy Hansen*

*Infectious diseases*

---

## What are the effects of antiviral treatment of influenza in adults?

### LIKELY TO BE BENEFICIAL

**Oral amantadine for early treatment of influenza A in adults (duration of symptoms reduced)**

One systematic review and three additional RCTs have found that oral amantadine reduces the duration of influenza A symptoms by about 1 day compared with placebo. We found insufficient evidence about adverse effects in this setting. We found no good evidence of benefit if amantadine is started more than 2 days after symptom onset.

**Orally inhaled zanamivir for early treatment of influenza A and B in adults (duration of symptoms reduced)**

One systematic review has found that orally inhaled zanamivir reduces the duration of influenza symptoms by about 1 day compared with placebo. Adverse effects were similar in people taking zanamivir and in people taking placebo. We found no good evidence of benefit if zanamivir is started more than 2 days after symptom onset.

**Oral oseltamivir for early treatment of influenza A and B in adults (duration of symptoms reduced)**

Two RCTs have found that oral oseltamivir reduces the duration of influenza symptoms by about 1 day compared with placebo. Oral oseltamivir increases the incidence of nausea and vomiting compared with placebo. We found no good evidence of benefit if oseltamivir is started more than 1.5 days after symptom onset.

**Oral rimantadine for early treatment of influenza A in adults (duration of symptoms reduced)**

One systematic review has found that oral rimantadine reduces the duration of influenza A symptoms by about 1 day compared with placebo. We found insufficient evidence about adverse effects in this setting. We found no good evidence of benefit if rimantadine is started more than 2 days after symptom onset.

### UNKNOWN EFFECTIVENESS

**All antivirals (reduction of serious influenza complications)**

We found insufficient evidence about the effects of antiviral agents on reducing serious complications of influenza.

**DEFINITION**    Influenza is caused by infection with influenza viruses. Uncomplicated influenza is characterised by the abrupt onset of fever, chills, non-productive cough, myalgias, headache, nasal congestion, sore throat, and fatigue.[1] Influenza is usually diagnosed clinically. Not all people infected with influenza viruses become symptomatic. People infected with other pathogens may have symptoms identical to those of influenza.[2] The percentage of infections resulting in clinical illness can vary from about 40–85%, depending on age ▶

and pre-existing immunity to the virus.[3] Influenza can be confirmed by viral culture, immunofluorescence staining, enzyme immunoassay, or rapid diagnostic testing of nasopharyngeal, nasal or throat swab specimens, or by serological testing of paired sera. Some rapid tests detect influenza A only, some detect and distinguish between influenza A and B, whereas others detect but do not distinguish between influenza A and B.

**INCIDENCE/ PREVALENCE** In temperate areas of the northern hemisphere, influenza activity typically peaks between late December and early March, whereas in temperate areas of the southern hemisphere influenza activity typically peaks between May and September. In tropical areas, influenza can occur throughout the year.[2] The annual incidence of influenza varies yearly, and depends partly on the underlying level of population immunity to circulating influenza viruses.[1] One localised study in the USA found that serological conversion with or without symptoms occurred in 10–20% a year, with the highest infection rates in people aged under 20 years.[4] Attack rates are higher in institutions and in areas of overcrowding.[5]

**AETIOLOGY/ RISK FACTORS** Influenza viruses are transmitted primarily from person to person through respiratory droplets disseminated during sneezing, coughing, and talking.[1,6]

**PROGNOSIS** The incubation period of influenza is 1–4 days and infected adults are usually contagious from the day before symptom onset until 5 days after symptom onset. The signs and symptoms of uncomplicated influenza usually resolve within a week, although cough and fatigue may persist.[1] Complications include otitis media, bacterial sinusitis, secondary bacterial pneumonia, and, less commonly, viral pneumonia and respiratory failure. Complications are also caused by exacerbation of underlying disease.[1,2] In the USA each year, over 110 000 admissions to hospital and about 20 000 deaths are related to influenza.[2] The risk of hospitalisation is highest in people 65 years or older, in very young children, and in those with chronic medical conditions.[1,7,8] Over 90% of influenza related deaths during recent seasonal epidemics in the USA have been in people 65 years or older.[1] During influenza pandemics, morbidity and mortality may be high in younger age groups.[1] Severe illness is more common with influenza A infections than with influenza B infections.[1]

Please refer to CD-ROM for full text and references.

# Leprosy

**Search date March 2003**

*Diana Lockwood*

---

## What are the effects of preventive interventions?

### Bacillus Calmette Guerin (BCG) vaccine

One RCT evaluated four different vaccines and found that the largest effect was with ICRC vaccine and BCG plus killed *M leprae,* followed by BCG alone. The effectiveness of *Mycobacterium w* was only marginal. However, only for the BCG vaccine alone were the findings corroborated by large controlled clinical trials with long term follow up. Only one RCT reported on harms of vaccination; it found these to be minimal.

### BCG plus killed *Mycobacterium leprae*

One RCT evaluated four different vaccines and found that the largest effect was with ICRC vaccine and BCG plus killed *M leprae,* followed by BCG alone. The effectiveness of *Mycobacterium w* was only marginal. However, only for the BCG vaccine alone were the findings corroborated by large controlled clinical trials with long term follow up. Only one RCT reported on harms of vaccination; it found these to be minimal.

### LIKELY TO BE BENEFICIAL

### ICRC vaccine

One RCT evaluated four different vaccines and found that the largest effect was with ICRC vaccine and BCG plus killed *M leprae,* followed by BCG alone. The effectiveness of *Mycobacterium w* was only marginal. However, only for the BCG vaccine alone were the findings corroborated by large controlled clinical trials with long term follow up. Only one RCT reported on harms of vaccination; it found these to be minimal.

### UNKNOWN EFFECTIVENESS

### *Mycobacterium w* vaccine

One RCT evaluated four different vaccines and found that the largest effect was with ICRC vaccine and BCG plus killed *M leprae,* followed by BCG alone. The effectiveness of *Mycobacterium w* was only marginal. Only one RCT reported on harms of vaccination; it found these to be minimal.

---

## What are the effects of treatments?

### BENEFICIAL

### Multidrug treatment for multibacillary leprosy*

We found no reliable comparisons between multidrug treatment with rifampicin plus clofazimine plus dapsone versus dapsone alone, or versus dapsone plus rifampicin, in people with multibacillary leprosy. Observational studies found that multidrug treatment improved skin lesions and was associated with a low relapse rate. The evidence on the incidence of adverse effects is poor. Multidrug treatment was not compared with dapsone alone because rising dapsone resistance rates meant that it would have been unethical to do such a study. The same applies for multidrug treatment for paucibacillary leprosy below. ▶

◀ **Multidrug treatment for paucibacillary leprosy\***

We found no reliable comparison between multidrug treatment with rifampicin plus clofazimine plus dapsone versus dapsone alone, or against dapsone plus rifampicin, in people with multibacillary leprosy Ⓖ. Observational studies found that multidrug treatment improved skin lesions and was associated with a low relapse rate. We found poor evidence on the incidence of adverse effects.

**Multiple dose versus single dose treatment for single lesion leprosy (both increase cure rates but multiple more than single dose)**

One RCT found that multiple dose treatment with rifampicin monthly plus dapsone daily for 6 months achieved higher cure rates at 18 months than single dose treatment with rifampicin plus minocycline plus ofloxacin. Some improvement occurred in 99% of people in both groups. Adverse effects were similar with both regimens.

\*Observational evidence only, RCTs unlikely to be conducted.

**DEFINITION** Leprosy is a chronic granulomatous disease caused by *Mycobacterium leprae*, primarily affecting the peripheral nerves and skin. The clinical outcome of infection is determined by the individual's immune response to *M leprae*. At the tuberculoid end of the Ridley–Jopling scale, individuals have good cell mediated immunity and few skin lesions. At the lepromatous end of the scale, individuals have good cell mediated immunity, causing uncontrolled bacterial spread and skin and mucosal infiltration. Peripheral nerve damage occurs across the spectrum. Nerve damage may occur before, during or, after treatment. Some patients have no nerve damage, others develop anaesthesia of the hands and feet, which puts them at risk of developing neuropathic injury. Weakness and paralysis of the small muscles of the hands, feet, and eyes puts patients at risk of developing deformity and contractures. Loss of the fingers and toes is due to repeated injury in a weak, anaesthetic limb. These visible deformities cause stigmatisation the world over. Classification is based on the clinical appearance and bacterial index of lesions Ⓖ. The World Health Organization field classification Ⓖ is based on the number of skin lesions: single lesion leprosy Ⓖ (1 lesion), paucibacillary leprosy Ⓖ (2–5 skin lesions), and multibacillary leprosy Ⓖ (> 5 skin lesions).[1]

**INCIDENCE/ PREVALENCE** Worldwide, about 720 000 new cases of leprosy are reported each year,[2] and about 2 million people have leprosy related disabilities. Six major endemic countries (India, Brazil, Myanmar, Madagascar, Nepal, and Mozambique) account for 88% of all new cases. Cohort studies show a peak of disease presentation between 10–20 years of age.[3] After puberty there are twice as many male as female cases.

**AETIOLOGY/ RISK FACTORS** *M leprae* is discharged from the nasal mucosa of people with untreated lepromatous leprosy, and transmitted through the nasal mucosa with subsequent spread of mycobacteria to skin and nerves. It is a hardy organism and has been shown to survive in the Indian environment for many months.[4] Risk factors include household contact with a person with leprosy. We found no good evidence of a relationship between HIV infection, nutrition, and socioeconomic status.[5]

**PROGNOSIS** Complications of leprosy include nerve damage, immunological reactions, and bacillary infiltration. Without treatment, tuberculoid infection eventually resolves spontaneously. Most people with borderline tuberculoid and borderline lepromatous leprosy gradually develop lepromatous infection. Many people have peripheral nerve damage at the time of diagnosis, ranging from 15% in Bangladesh to 55% in Ethiopia. Immunological reactions can occur with or without antibiotic treatment. Further nerve damage occurs through immune mediated reactions and neuritis Ⓖ. Erythema nodosum leprosum Ⓖ is an ▶

# Leprosy

immune complex mediated reaction causing fever, malaise, and neuritis, which is reported to occur in 20% of people with lepromatous leprosy and 15% with borderline lepromatous leprosy.[8] Secondary impairments (wounds, contractures, and digit resorption) occur in 33–56% of people with established nerve damage.[9] We found no recent information on mortality.

Please refer to CD-ROM for full text and references.

## What are the effects of preventive interventions and treatments?

### BENEFICIAL

**Lyme disease vaccine in people exposed to North American strains of *Borrelia burgdorferi***

One RCT has found that, compared with placebo, three doses of a vaccine (consisting of recombinant outer surface protein A [Osp–A] of *B burgdorferi* combined with adjuvant**G**) reduces the incidence of Lyme disease in immuno-competent people aged 15–70 years in Lyme disease endemic areas of North America.

**Prophylactic antibiotics after *Ixodes scapularis* tick bites in Lyme disease endemic areas in North America**

One systematic review in people with recognised *I scapularis* tick bites in the preceding 72 hours found that antibiotics reduced the risk of developing clinical Lyme disease compared with placebo, but the difference was not significant. One subsequent large RCT in people who had removed an attached *I scapularis* tick in the preceding 72 hours found that doxycycline reduced the proportion of people with erythema migrans at the site of the tick bite compared with placebo.

### LIKELY TO BE BENEFICIAL

**\*Cefotaxime (more effective than penicillin for late neurological Lyme disease)**

One RCT found weak evidence from a small subgroup analysis of people with late Lyme disease that cefotaxime improved symptoms of neuropathy compared with penicillin.

**\*Cefotaxime (more effective than penicillin for Lyme arthritis)**

One RCT found weak evidence from a small subgroup analysis of people with Lyme arthritis that cefotaxime increased the proportion of people with full recovery compared with penicillin.

**\*Ceftriaxone (more effective than penicillin for Lyme arthritis)**

One RCT found weak evidence from a small subgroup analysis of people with Lyme arthritis that ceftriaxone improved symptoms compared with penicillin.

**Doxycycline (as effective as amoxicillin plus probenecid for Lyme arthritis)**

One RCT in people with Lyme arthritis found no significant difference between doxycycline and amoxicillin plus probenecid in resolution of Lyme arthritis.

**Penicillin (better than placebo for Lyme arthritis)**

One RCT in people with Lyme arthritis has found that penicillin increases resolution of Lyme arthritis compared with placebo.

\*Based on subgroup analysis of RCTs.

### UNKNOWN EFFECTIVENESS

**Ceftriaxone (in late neurological Lyme disease)**

One RCT found insufficient evidence from a small subgroup analysis in people with late neurological Lyme disease about effects of ceftriaxone and cefotaxime. ▶

# Lyme disease

◀ **Lyme disease vaccine in Europe or Asia**

We found no RCTs about the effects of recombinant outer surface protein A (Osp–A) vaccine in European or Asian populations. There is heterogeneity of the species that cause Lyme disease in Europe and Asia. The vaccine may not be as effective in European or Asian populations as it is in North American populations.

## LIKELY TO BE INEFFECTIVE OR HARMFUL

**Ceftriaxone plus doxycycline (in people with late neurological Lyme disease who had been previously treated)**

One RCT comparing ceftriaxone plus doxycycline versus placebo in people with previously treated Lyme disease and persistent neurological symptoms found no significant difference in health related quality of life at interim analysis at 180 days; therefore the RCT was terminated.

**DEFINITION**
Lyme disease is an inflammatory illness resulting from infection with spirochetes of the *B burgdorferi* genospecies transmitted to humans by ticks. Some infected people have no symptoms. The characteristic manifestation of early Lyme disease is erythema migrans: a circular rash at the site of the infectious tick attachment that expands over a period of days to weeks in 80–90% of people with Lyme disease. Early disseminated infection may cause secondary erythema migrans, disease of the nervous system (facial palsy or other cranial neuropathies, meningitis, and radiculoneuritis), musculoskeletal disease (arthralgia), and, rarely, cardiac disease (myocarditis or transient atrioventricular block). Untreated or inadequately treated Lyme disease can cause late disseminated manifestations weeks to months after infection. These late manifestations include arthritis, polyneuropathy, and encephalopathy. Diagnosis of Lyme disease is based primarily on clinical findings and a high likelihood of exposure to infected ticks. Serological testing may be helpful in people with endemic exposure who have clinical findings consistent with later stage disseminated Lyme disease.

**INCIDENCE/ PREVALENCE**
Lyme disease occurs in temperate regions of North America, Europe, and Asia. It is the most commonly reported vector borne disease in the USA, with over 16 000 cases reported a year.[1] Most cases occur in the north-eastern and north-central states, with a reported annual incidence in endemic states as high as 67.9/100 000 people.[1] In highly endemic communities, the incidence of Lyme disease may exceed 1000/100 000 people a year.[2] In some countries of Europe, the incidence of Lyme disease has been estimated to be over 100/100 000 people a year.[3] Foci of Lyme disease have been described in northern forested regions of Russia, in China, and in Japan.[4] Transmission cycles of *B burgdorferi* have not been described in tropical areas or in the southern hemisphere.[4]

**AETIOLOGY/ RISK FACTORS**
Lyme disease is caused by infection with any of the *B burgdorferi* sensu lato genospecies. Virtually all cases of Lyme disease in North America are the result of infection with *B burgdorferi*. In Europe, Lyme disease may be caused by *B burgdorferi*, *B garinii*, or *B afzelii*. The infectious spirochetes are transmitted to humans through the bite of certain *Ixodes* ticks.[4] Humans who have frequent or prolonged exposure to the habitats of infected *Ixodes* ticks are at highest risk of acquiring Lyme disease. Individual risk depends on the likelihood of being bitten by infected tick vectors, which varies with the density of vector ticks in the environment, the prevalence of infection in ticks, and the extent of a person's contact with infected ticks. The risk of Lyme disease is often concentrated in focal areas. In the USA, risk is highest in certain counties within north-eastern and north-central states during the months of April to July.[2] People become infected when they engage in activities in wooded or bushy areas that are favourable habitats for ticks, and deer and rodent hosts.

▶

**PROGNOSIS**  Lyme disease is rarely fatal. Untreated Lyme arthritis resolves at a rate of 10–20% a year; over 90% of facial palsies due to Lyme disease resolve spontaneously, and most cases of Lyme carditis resolve without sequelae.[5] However, untreated Lyme disease can result in arthritis (50% of untreated people), meningitis or neuropathies (15% of untreated people), carditis (5–10% of untreated people with erythema migrans), and, rarely, encephalopathy.

Please refer to CD-ROM for full text and references.

# Malaria in endemic areas

## Search date October 2002

*Aika Omari and Paul Garner*

Infectious diseases

---

## What are the effects of medical treatment for complicated falciparum malaria in non-pregnant people?

### LIKELY TO BE BENEFICIAL

**Artemether (v quinine)**

Two systematic reviews and one subsequent RCT found no significant difference between artemether versus quinine for preventing death in people with severe malaria.

**High first dose quinine**

One systematic review and one additional RCT found no significant difference in mortality between quinine regimens with high initial quinine dose versus no loading dose. The systematic review found that high first dose of quinine reduced parasite and fever clearance times◉ compared with no loading dose.

**Quinine**

We found no RCTs comparing quinine versus placebo or no treatment, but there is consensus that treatment is likely to be beneficial.

**Rectal artemisinin (as effective as quinine)**

One systematic review found no significant difference in mortality with rectal artemisinin versus quinine.

### UNKNOWN EFFECTIVENESS

**Chloroquine versus quinine**

Two RCTs in children found no significant difference in mortality with chloroquine versus quinine. However, these RCTs were conducted in the Gambia between 1988 and 1994, when chloroquine resistance was uncommon.

**Desferrioxamine mesylate**

One systematic review found weak evidence that desferrioxamine mesylate versus placebo reduced the risk of persistent seizures in children with cerebral malaria. However, we were unable to draw reliable conclusions.

**Exchange blood transfusion**

One systematic review has found no suitable RCTs.

**Initial blood transfusion**

One systematic review found no significant difference in deaths in clinically stable children who received an initial blood transfusion for malaria anaemia and found more adverse events.

**Intramuscular versus intravenous quinine**

One RCT in children found no significant difference with intramuscular versus intravenous quinine in recovery times or deaths in Kenya in 1990.

**Sulfadoxine–pyrimethamine versus quinine**

One RCT found that sulfadoxine–pyrimethamine versus quinine cleared parasites faster in children with complicated non-cerebral malaria in 1992–1994 in the Gambia, but found no significant difference in mortality.

## Dexamethasone

One systematic review has found no significant difference in mortality with dexamethasone versus placebo, but gastrointestinal bleeding and seizures were more common with dexamethasone.

| | |
|---|---|
| **DEFINITION** | Severe malaria is caused by the protozoan infection of red blood cells with *Plasmodium falciparum*❻. Clinically complicated malaria presents with life threatening conditions, which include coma, severe anaemia, renal failure, respiratory distress syndrome, hypoglycaemia, shock, spontaneous haemorrhage, and convulsions. The diagnosis of cerebral malaria should be considered where there is encephalopathy in the presence of malaria parasites. A strict definition of cerebral malaria requires the presence of unrousable coma, and no other cause of encephalopathy (e.g. hypoglycaemia, sedative drugs) in the presence of *P falciparum* infection.[1] This review does not currently include the treatment of malaria in pregnancy. |
| **INCIDENCE/ PREVALENCE** | Malaria is a major health problem in the tropics with 300–500 million clinical cases occurring annually, and an estimated 1.1–2.7 million deaths occur each year as a result of severe malaria.[2] Over 90% of deaths occur in children below 5 years of age, mainly from cerebral malaria and anaemia.[2] In areas where malaria transmission is stable (endemic), those most at risk of acquiring severe malaria are children under 5 years old, because adults and older children have partial immunity that offers some protection. In areas where malaria transmission is unstable (non-endemic), severe malaria affects both adults and children. Non-immune travellers and migrants are also at risk from developing severe malaria. |
| **AETIOLOGY/ RISK FACTORS** | Malaria is transmitted by the bite of infected female anopheline mosquitoes. Certain genes are associated with resistance to severe malaria. Human leukocyte antigens (HLA), namely HLA-Bw53 and HLA-DRB1*1302, protect against severe malaria. However, the associations of HLA antigens with severe malaria are limited to specific populations.[3,4] Haemoglobin S[3] and haemoglobin C[5] are also protective against severe malaria. Genes, such as the tumour necrosis factor gene have also been associated with an increased susceptibility to severe malaria (see aetiology under malaria: prevention in travellers, p 182).[6] |
| **PROGNOSIS** | In children under 5 years of age with cerebral malaria, the estimated case fatality of treated malaria is 19%, although reported hospital case fatality may be as high as 10–40%.[1,7] Neurological sequelae persisting for more than 6 months occur in more than 2% of the survivors, and include ataxia, hemiplegia, speech disorders, behavioural disorders, epilepsy, and blindness. Severe malarial anaemia has a case fatality rate higher than 13%.[7] In adults, the mortality of cerebral malaria is 20%; this rises to 50% in pregnancy,[8] and neurological sequelae occur in about 3% of survivors.[9] |

Please refer to CD-ROM for full text and references.

# Malaria: prevention in travellers

Search date November 2002

*Ashley M Croft*

---

## What are the effects of treatments?

### BENEFICIAL

#### Insecticide treated nets in adults

We found no RCTs in travellers. One systematic review in adult and child residents of malaria endemic settings found that insecticide treated nets reduce the number of mild episodes of malaria and reduce child mortality.

### LIKELY TO BE BENEFICIAL

#### Atovaquone plus proguanil in adults

One RCT in migrants with limited immunity found that atovaquone plus proguanil reduced the proportion of people with malaria compared with placebo. One RCT found no significant difference between atovaquone plus proguanil and chloroquine plus proguanil in preventing malaria. One RCT of atovaquone plus proguanil versus mefloquine found no cases of clinical malaria throughout the trial, but found a higher rate of neuropsychiatric harm with mefloquine compared with atovaquone plus proguanil.

#### Doxycycline in adults

One RCT in soldiers and one RCT in migrants with limited immunity found that doxycycline reduces the risk of malaria compared with placebo. One of the RCTs found that doxycycline was associated with nausea and vomiting, diarrhoea, cough, headache, and unspecified dermatological symptoms over 13 weeks.

#### Insecticide treated clothing in adults

Two RCTs in soldiers and refugee householders found that permethrin treated fabric (clothing or sheets) reduces the incidence of malaria.

#### Mefloquine in adults

One systematic review of one RCT in soldiers found that, compared with placebo, mefloquine had 100% protective efficacy. One RCT of mefloquine versus atovaquone plus proguanil found no cases of clinical malaria throughout the trial, but found a higher rate of neuropsychiatric harm with mefloquine compared with atovaquone plus proguanil.

### UNKNOWN EFFECTIVENESS

#### Aerosol insecticides in adults

We found no RCTs on the effects of aerosol insecticides in preventing malaria in travellers. One large questionnaire survey in travellers found insufficient evidence on the effects of aerosol insecticides in preventing malaria. Two community RCTs in residents of malaria endemic areas found that indoor spraying of aerosol insecticides reduced clinical malaria.

#### Air conditioning and electric fans in adults

We found no RCTs on the effects of air conditioning or electric fans in preventing malaria in travellers. One large questionnaire survey found that air conditioning reduced the incidence of malaria. One small observational study found that electric ceiling fans reduced total catches of culicine mosquitos in indoor spaces but did not significantly reduce total catches of anopheline mosquitoes.

### Chloroquine in adults

We found no RCTs on the effects of chloroquine in travellers. One RCT in Austrian workers residing in Nigeria found no significant difference between chloroquine and sulfadoxine plus pyrimethamine in the incidence of malaria after 6–22 months.

### Chloroquine plus proguanil in adults

One RCT found no significant difference between chloroquine plus proguanil and chloroquine plus sulfadoxine plus pyrimethamine in the incidence of *Plasmodium falciparum* malaria. One RCT found no significant difference between chloroquine plus proguanil and proguanil alone in the incidence of *P falciparum* malaria. One RCT found no significant difference between chloroquine plus proguanil and atovaquone plus proguanil in preventing malaria.

### Full length clothing in adults

We found no RCTs on the effects of full length clothing in preventing malaria in travellers. One large questionnaire survey in travellers found that wearing trousers and long sleeved shirts reduced the incidence of malaria.

### Insecticide treated nets in pregnant travellers

We found no RCTs on the effects of insecticide treated nets in preventing malaria in pregnant travellers. One RCT of pregnant residents of a malaria endemic area found insufficient evidence on the effects of permethrin treated nets in preventing malaria.

### Mosquito coils and vaporising mats in adults

We found no RCTs on the effects of coils and vaporising mats in preventing malaria in travellers. One RCT of coils and one observational study of pyrethroid vaporising mats found that these devices reduced numbers of mosquitoes in indoor spaces.

### Pyrimethamine plus dapsone in adults

We found no RCTs in travellers. One RCT in Thai soldiers found insufficient evidence to compare pyrimethamine plus dapsone versus proguanil plus dapsone.

### Smoke in adults

We found no RCTs on the effects of smoke in preventing malaria. One controlled clinical trial found that smoke repelled mosquitoes during the evening.

### Topical (skin applied) insect repellents in adults

We found no RCTs on the effects of topical (skin applied) insect repellents in preventing malaria in travellers. One small crossover RCT found that DEET preparations protected against mosquito bites.

### Vaccines

We found no RCTs in travellers. One systematic review of antimalaria vaccines in residents of malaria endemic areas found that the SPf66 vaccine reduces first attacks of malaria compared with placebo.

### Antimalaria drugs in airline pilots; antimalaria drugs in pregnant travellers; biological control measures⊕ in adults; insect electrocuters and ultrasonic buzzers in adults; insecticide treated clothing in pregnant travellers; mefloquine in children; topical (skin applied) insect repellents in pregnant travellers

We found no RCTs on the effects of these interventions.

# Malaria: prevention in travellers

## LIKELY TO BE INEFFECTIVE OR HARMFUL

### Amodiaquine in adults
We found no RCTs on the effects of amodiaquine in preventing malaria in travellers. We found limited observational evidence that amodiaquine may cause liver damage and hepatitis.

### Doxycycline in children
We found no RCTs in child travellers on the use of doxycycline. Case reports in young children found adverse effects with doxycycline.

### Sulfadoxine plus pyrimethamine in adults
One RCT found no significant difference between chloroquine plus proguanil and chloroquine plus sulfadoxine pyrimethamine in the incidence of *P falciparum* malaria. One retrospective observational study suggested that sulfadoxine plus pyrimethamine was associated with severe cutaneous reactions.

### Topical (skin applied) insect repellents containing DEET in children
We found no RCTs on the effects of DEET in preventing malaria in child travellers. Case reports in young children found serious adverse effects with DEET.

**DEFINITION**  Malaria is caused by a protozoan infection of red blood cells with one of four species of the genus *Plasmodium*: *P falciparum*, *P vivax*, *P ovale*, and *P malariae*.[1] Clinically, malaria may present in different ways but it is usually characterised by fever (which may be swinging), tachycardia, rigors, and sweating. Anaemia, hepatosplenomegaly, cerebral involvement, renal failure, and shock may occur.[2,3] Travellers are defined here as visitors from a malaria free area to a malaria endemic area, and who stay in the endemic area for less than 1 year.

**INCIDENCE/ PREVALENCE**  Each year there are 300–500 million clinical cases of malaria. About 40% of the world's population is at risk of acquiring the disease.[2,3] Each year 25–30 million people from non-tropical countries visit malaria endemic areas, of whom 10 000–30 000 contract malaria.[4,5] Most RCTs of malaria prevention have been conducted in soldiers and travellers. The results of these trials may not be applicable to people such as refugees and migrants, who are likely to differ in their health status and in their susceptibility to disease and adverse drug effects.

**AETIOLOGY/ RISK FACTORS**  Malaria is mainly a rural disease, requiring nearby standing water. It is transmitted by bites of infected female anopheline mosquitoes, mainly at dusk and during the night.[1,6–8] In cities, mosquito bites are usually from female culicine mosquitoes, which are not vectors of malaria.[9] Malaria is resurgent in most tropical countries and risk to travellers is increasing.[10] The sickle cell trait has been shown to convey some protection against malaria in non-immune carriers of that trait. Non-immune adults with the sickle cell trait who develop severe malaria have lower parasite densities, fewer complications (e.g. cerebral malaria), and a reduced mortality compared with adults without the trait.[11] There is little good evidence on the degree of protection afforded by the sickle cell trait.[12]

**PROGNOSIS**  Ninety per cent of tourists and business travellers who contract malaria do not become ill until after they return home.[5] "Imported malaria" is easily treated if diagnosed promptly, and follows a serious course in only about 12% of people.[13,14] The most severe form is cerebral malaria, with a case fatality rate in adult travellers of 2–6% mainly because of delays in diagnosis.[3,15]

Please refer to CD-ROM for full text and references.

Search date March 2003

*J Correia and C A Hart*

## What are the effects of treatments?

**LIKELY TO BE BENEFICIAL**

### Antibiotics for throat carriage (reduce carriage but unknown effect on risk of disease)

RCTs have found that antibiotics reduce throat carriage of meningococci compared with placebo. We found no evidence that eradicating throat carriage reduces the risk of meningococcal disease.

### Pre-admission parenteral penicillin in suspected cases

We found no RCTs on the effects of pre-admission antibiotics in suspected cases🄖. It is unlikely that RCTs will be performed because of the unpredictably rapid course of meningococcal disease in some people, the likely risks involved in delaying treatment, and the low risk of causing harm. Most observational studies suggest benefit with antibiotics, but at least one did not.

### Prophylactic antibiotics in contacts

We found no RCTs on the effects of prophylactic antibiotics on the incidence of meningococcal disease among contacts🄖. RCTs are unlikely to be performed because the intervention has few associated risks whereas meningococcal disease has high associated risks. Observational evidence suggests that antibiotics reduce the risk of meningococcal disease. We found no evidence regarding which contacts should be treated.

**DEFINITION**  Meningococcal disease is any clinical condition caused by *Neisseria meningitidis* (the meningococcus) groups A, B, C, W135, or other serogroups. These conditions include purulent conjunctivitis, septic arthritis, meningitis🄖, and septicaemia🄖 with or without meningitis.

**INCIDENCE/ PREVALENCE**  Meningococcal disease is sporadic in temperate countries, and is most commonly caused by group B or C meningococci. Annual incidence in Europe varies from fewer than 1 case/100 000 people in France, up to 4–5 cases/100 000 people in the UK and Spain, and in the USA it is 0.6–1.5/ 100 000 people.[1,2] Occasional outbreaks occur among close family contacts🄖, secondary school pupils, military recruits, and students living in halls of residence. Sub-Saharan Africa has regular epidemics in countries lying in the expanded "meningitis belt", reaching 500/100 000 people during epidemics, which are usually due to serogroup A, although recent outbreaks of serogroup W135 cause concern.[3–5]

**AETIOLOGY/ RISK FACTORS**  The meningococcus colonises and infects healthy people and is transmitted by close contact, probably by exchange of upper respiratory tract secretions🄣.[6–14] Risk of transmission is greatest during the first week of contact.[9] Risk factors include crowding and exposure to cigarette smoke.[15] In the UK, children younger than 2 years have the highest incidence, with a second peak between ages 15–24 years. There is currently an increased incidence of meningococcal disease among university students, especially among those in their first term and living in catered accommodation,[16] although we found no accurate numerical estimate of risk from close contact in, for example, halls of residence. Close contacts of an index case have a much higher risk of infection than do people in the general population.[9,12,13] The risk of epidemic spread is higher with groups A and C meningococci than with group B meningococci.[6–8,10] It is not known what makes a meningococcus virulent. Certain clones tend to predominate at different times and in different groups. ▶

# Meningococcal disease

Carriage of meningococcus in the throat has been reported in 10–15% of people; recent acquisition of a virulent meningococcus is more likely to be associated with invasive disease.

**PROGNOSIS**  Mortality is highest in infants and adolescents, and is related to disease presentation and availability of therapeutic resources. In developed countries case fatality rates have been around 19–25% for septicaemia, 10–12% for meningitis plus septicaemia, and less than 1% in meningitis alone, but an overall reduction in mortality was observed in recent years in people admitted to paediatric intensive care units.[17–21]

Please refer to CD-ROM for full text and references.

*Infectious diseases*

## What are the effects of interventions to prevent postherpetic neuralgia?

### LIKELY TO BE BENEFICIAL

#### Aciclovir, famciclovir, valaciclovir, netivudine

One systematic review has found limited evidence from RCTs that aciclovir given for 7–10 days reduced pain at 1–3 months. One systematic review has found that famciclovir reduces mean pain duration after acute herpes zoster compared with placebo. One RCT found that valaciclovir reduced the prevalence of postherpetic neuralgia at 6 months compared with aciclovir. One RCT found no significant difference in effectiveness between netivudine and aciclovir. One RCT found no significant difference between valaciclovir and famciclovir in the resolution of postherpetic neuralgia or in adverse effects over 7 days.

### UNKNOWN EFFECTIVENESS

#### Amitriptyline

One small RCT found no significant difference between amitriptyline and placebo started within 48 hours of rash onset in the prevalence of postherpetic neuralgia at 6 months. The RCT may have lacked power to detect a clinically important difference.

#### Adenosine phosphate; amantadine; cimetidine; inosine pranobex; levodopa

RCTs found insufficient evidence on the effects of these interventions.

### UNLIKELY TO BE BENEFICIAL

#### Topical antiviral agents (idoxuridine) for pain at 6 months

One systematic review has found that idoxuridine increases short term pain relief in acute herpes zoster compared with placebo or oral aciclovir, but found no significant difference at 6 months.

### LIKELY TO BE INEFFECTIVE OR HARMFUL

#### Corticosteroids

Systematic reviews found conflicting evidence from RCTs about the effects of corticosteroids alone on postherpetic neuralgia. We found insufficient evidence from two RCTs about effects of high dose steroids plus antiviral agents. There is concern that corticosteroids may cause dissemination of herpes zoster.

## What are the effects of treatments in established postherpetic neuralgia?

### BENEFICIAL

#### Gabapentin

One systematic review has found that gabapentin reduces pain at 8 weeks compared with placebo.

#### Tricyclic antidepressants

One systematic review has found that tricyclic antidepressants increase pain relief in postherpetic neuralgia after 2–6 weeks compared with placebo.

# Postherpetic neuralgia

## TRADE OFF BETWEEN BENEFITS AND HARMS

### Oral opioids (oxycodone, morphine, methodone)

We found no RCTs examining effects of morphine or methadone in people with postherpetic neuralgia. One small RCT found that oral oxycodone reduced pain after 4 weeks compared with placebo, but was associated with more adverse effects.

### Topical counterirritants

Two systematic reviews and one small subsequent RCT found limited evidence that the topical counterirritant, capsaicin, improved pain relief in postherpetic neuralgia compared with placebo, but found that capsaicin may cause painful skin reactions.

## UNKNOWN EFFECTIVENESS

### Topical anaesthesia

We found insufficient evidence from three RCTs about the effects of lidocaine (lignocaine).

### Tramadol

One small RCT found that tramadol reduced pain more than clomipramine after 6 weeks. However, we were unable to draw reliable conclusions from this small study.

## LIKELY TO BE INEFFECTIVE OR HARMFUL

### Dextromethorphan

One systematic review and one subsequent RCT found no evidence that dextromethorphan was more effective than placebo or lorazepam after 3–6 weeks, but found that dextromethorphan was associated with sedation and ataxia at high doses.

### Epidural morphine

One small RCT found that epidural morphine reduced pain by more than 50% compared with placebo but the reduction was not maintained beyond 36 hours. Epidural morphine caused intolerable opioid effects in 75% of people.

**DEFINITION**  Postherpetic neuralgia is pain that sometimes follows resolution of acute herpes zoster and healing of the zoster rash. It can be severe, accompanied by itching, and follows the distribution of the original infection. Herpes zoster is an acute infection caused by activation of latent varicella zoster virus (human herpes virus 3) in people who have been rendered partially immune by a previous attack of chickenpox. Herpes zoster infects the sensory ganglia and their areas of innervation. It is characterised by pain along the distribution of the affected nerve, and crops of clustered vesicles over the area.

**INCIDENCE/**  In a UK general practice survey of 3600–3800 people, the annual incidence
**PREVALENCE**  of herpes zoster was 3.4/1000.[1] Incidence varied with age. Herpes zoster was relatively uncommon in people under the age of 50 years (< 2/1000 a year), but rose to 5–7/1000 a year in people aged 50–79 years, and 11/1000 in people aged 80 years or older. In a population based study of 590 cases in Rochester, Minnesota, USA, the overall incidence was lower (1.5/1000) but there were similar increases in incidence with age.[2] Prevalence of postherpetic neuralgia depends on when it is measured after acute infection. There is no agreed time point for diagnosis.

**AETIOLOGY/**  The main risk factor for postherpetic neuralgia is increasing age. In a UK general
**RISK FACTORS**  practice study (involving 3600–3800 people, 321 cases of acute herpes zoster) there was little risk in those under the age of 50 years, but postherpetic

neuralgia developed in over 20% of people who had had acute herpes zoster aged 60–65 years and in 34% aged over 80 years.[1] No other risk factor has been found to predict consistently which people with herpes zoster will experience continued pain. In a general practice study in Iceland (421 people followed for up to 7 years after an initial episode of herpes zoster), the risk of postherpetic neuralgia was 1.8% (95% CI 0.6% to 4.2%) for people under 60 years of age and the pain was mild in all cases.[2] The risk of severe pain after 3 months in people aged over 60 years was 1.7% (95% CI 0% to 6.2%).

**PROGNOSIS** About 2% of people with acute herpes zoster in the UK general practice survey had pain for more than 5 years.[1] Prevalence of pain falls as time elapses after the initial episode. Among 183 people aged over 60 years in the placebo arm of a UK trial, the prevalence of pain was 61% at 1 month, 24% at 3 months, and 13% at 6 months after acute infection.[3] In a more recent RCT, the prevalence of postherpetic pain in the placebo arm at 6 months was 35% in 72 people over 60 years of age.[4]

Please refer to CD-ROM for full text and references.

# Acute renal failure

**Search date December 2002**

*John A Kellum, Martine Leblanc, and Ramesh Venkataraman*

---

## What are the effects of interventions to prevent acute renal failure in people at high risk?

### BENEFICIAL

**Low osmolality contrast media (better than standard)**

One systematic review comparing low osmolality contrast media🅖 with standard contrast media has found that the development of acute renal failure or need for dialysis is rare in people undertaking diagnostic tests with contrast media. However, nephrotoxicity (evaluated by serum creatinine) was less likely with low osmolality contrast media, especially in people with underlying renal impairment.

### LIKELY TO BE BENEFICIAL

**Fluids**

We found no RCTs of fluids compared with no intervention to prevent acute renal failure. However, dehydration is an important risk factor for acute renal failure, and recommended volumes of fluid have little potential for harm. One RCT found that hydration with 0.9% sodium chloride intravenous infusion compared with 0.45% sodium chloride intravenous infusion reduced the incidence of contrast media associated nephropathy. One RCT found inconclusive evidence on the effects of inpatient compared with outpatient hydration regimens.

**Single dose aminoglycosides (better than multiple doses of aminoglycosides)**

One systematic review in people with fever and neutropenia and receiving antibiotics including aminoglycosides found no significant difference in cure rates or nephrotoxicity between one single daily dose and multiple doses of aminoglycosides. One additional RCT found that in people with fever and requiring antibiotic treatment including aminogylcosides, a single daily dose of aminoglycoside reduced nephrotoxicity compared with multiple doses.

### UNKNOWN EFFECTIVENESS

**Acetylcysteine**

Four RCTs found inconclusive evidence on the effects of *N*-acetylcysteine in preventing radiocontrast induced nephropathy.

**Lipid formulations of amphotericin B (better than standard formulations)**

We found no RCTs. Lipid formulations of amphotericin B seem to cause less nephrotoxicity compared with standard formulations, but direct comparisions of long term safety are lacking.

### UNLIKELY TO BE BENEFICIAL

**Fenoldopam**

Three RCTs found insufficient evidence that fenoldopam is of benefit in the prevention of acute renal failure.

**Mannitol**

Small RCTs in people with traumatic rhabdomyolysis, or in people who had undergone coronary artery bypass, vascular, or biliary tract surgery, found that mannitol did not reduce acute renal failure compared with hydration alone. One ▶

◀ RCT found that mannitol increased the risk of acute renal failure compared with 0.9% sodium chloride infusion, but the difference was not significant.

## Theophylline for preventing acute renal failure induced by contrast media

RCTs found that theophylline does not prevent acute renal failure induced by contrast media compared with placebo when people are adequately hydrated. One RCT also found that theophylline did not prevent acute renal failure after coronary artery bypass surgery compared with placebo.

### LIKELY TO BE INEFFECTIVE OR HARMFUL

## Calcium channel blockers for early allograft dysfunction

One large RCT found no significant difference between isradipine and placebo in reducing graft dysfunction in renal transplantation. We found no RCTs on the effects of calcium channel blockers in other forms of acute renal failure.

## Dopamine

One systematic review and one subsequent RCT found that dopamine does not prevent the onset of acute renal failure, the need for dialysis, or death compared with placebo. One systematic review in people with sepsis found no evidence of harms. One RCT found insufficient evidence on the effects of combined dopamine and diltiazem in people undergoing cardiac surgery. Dopamine is associated with serious adverse effects, such as extravasation necrosis, gangrene, and conduction abnormalities.

## Loop diuretics

One systematic review found that loop diuretics compared with fluids alone do not prevent acute renal failure. One RCT in people with acute tubular necrosis induced by contrast media found that diuretics compared with 0.9% sodium chloride infusion increased acute renal failure. Another RCT found that diuretics compared with 0.9% sodium chloride infusion increased acute renal failure after cardiac surgery.

## Natriuretic peptides

One large RCT found no significant difference in the prevention of acute renal failure induced by contrast media between natriuretic peptides and placebo. Subgroup analysis in another RCT found that atrial natriuretic peptide reduced dialysis free survival in non-oliguric people compared with placebo.

## What are the effects of treatments in critically ill people with acute renal failure?

### LIKELY TO BE BENEFICIAL

## High dose continuous replacement renal therapy (better than low dose)

One RCT has found that high dose continuous renal replacement therapy (haemofiltration) significantly reduces mortality compared with standard dose therapy. A small prospective study found that intensive (daily) intermittent haemodialysis reduced mortality in people with acute renal failure compared with conventional alternate day haemodialysis. A subsequent small three arm RCT found no significant difference in survival at 28 days between early, low volume haemofiltration, early, high volume haemofiltration and late, low volume haemofiltration.

### UNKNOWN EFFECTIVENESS

## Combined diuretics and albumin; continuous versus bolus diuretics

We found insufficient evidence on the effects of these interventions.

# Acute renal failure

### Continuous versus intermittent renal replacement therapy

One systematic review of previously published randomised and observational studies compared intermittent versus continuous renal replacement therapies⊙ and found no overall difference between therapies. However, it found a survival benefit with continuous renal replacement therapy when the analysis was restricted to the subgroup of studies comparing people with similar baseline severity of illness. Weaknesses in included studies preclude a definitive conclusion.

### Synthetic dialysis membranes (better than cellulose-based membranes)

Two systematic reviews found inconclusive evidence on the effects of synthetic based membranes on mortality in critically ill people with acute renal failure compared with cellulose based membranes.

## UNLIKELY TO BE BENEFICIAL

### Loop diuretics

RCTs in people with oliguric acute renal failure found no significant difference in renal recovery, number of days spent on dialysis, or mortality between loop diuretics and placebo. Loop diuretics have been associated with toxicity and low renal perfusion.

## LIKELY TO BE INEFFECTIVE OR HARMFUL

### Dopamine

One systematic review found no significant difference in mortality, or need for dialysis between dopamine and control. One additional RCT found that low dose dopamine did not reduce renal dysfunction compared with placebo. Dopamine has been associated with important adverse effects, including extravasation necrosis, gangrene, tachycardia, and conduction abnormalities.

### Natriuretic peptides

RCTs found no significant difference between atrial natriuretic peptide, ularitide (urodilantin) and placebo in dialysis free survival in oliguric and non-oliguric people. One of the RCTs found that atrial natriuretic peptide may reduce survival in non-oliguric people.

DEFINITION    Acute renal failure is characterised by abrupt and sustained decline in glomerular filtration rate⊙,[1] which leads to accumulation of urea and other chemicals in the blood. There is no clear consensus on a biochemical definition,[2] but most studies define it as a serum creatinine of 2–3 mg/dL (200–250 µmol/L), an elevation of more than 0.5 mg/dL (45 µmol/L) over a baseline creatinine below 2 mg/dL (170 µmol/L), or a twofold increase of baseline creatinine. "Severe" acute renal failure has been defined as a serum concentration of creatinine above 5.5 mg/dL (500 µmol/L) or as requiring renal replacement therapy. Acute renal failure is usually classified according to the location of the predominant primary pathology (prerenal, intrarenal, and postrenal failure). Critically ill people are unstable and at imminent risk of death, which usually implies that they need to be in, or have been admitted to, the intensive care unit.

INCIDENCE/    Two prospective observational studies (2576 people) have found that estab-
PREVALENCE    lished acute renal failure affects nearly 5% of people in hospital and as many as 15% of critically ill people depending on the definitions used.[3,4]

AETIOLOGY/    **For acute renal failure prevention:** Risk factors for acute renal failure that are
RISK FACTORS  consistent across multiple causes include hypovolaemia; hypotension; sepsis; pre-existing renal, hepatic, or cardiac dysfunction; diabetes mellitus; and ▶

exposure to nephrotoxins (e.g. aminoglycosides, amphotericin, immunosuppressive agents, non-steroidal anti-inflammatory drugs, angiotensin converting enzyme inhibitors, iv contrast media) ❶. Isolated episodes of acute renal failure are rarely seen in critically ill people, but are usually part of multiple organ dysfunction syndromes❻. Acute renal failure requiring dialysis is rarely seen in isolation (< 5% of people). The kidneys are often the first organs to fail.[10] In the perioperative setting, acute renal failure risk factors include prolonged aortic clamping, emergency rather than elective surgery, and use of higher volumes (> 100 mL) of intravenous contrast media. One study (3695 people) using multiple logistic regression identified the following independent risk factors: baseline creatinine clearance below 47 mL/minute (OR 1.20, 95% CI 1.12 to 1.30); diabetes (OR 5.5, 95% CI 1.4 to 21.0), and a marginal effect for doses of contrast media above 100 mL (OR 1.01, 95% CI 1.00 to 1.01). Mortality of people with acute renal failure requiring dialysis was 36% during hospitalisation.[11] **For acute renal failure in critically ill people:** Prerenal acute renal failure is caused by reduced blood flow to the kidney from renal artery disease, systematic hypotension, or maldistribution of blood flow. Intrarenal acute renal failure is caused by parenchymal injury (acute tubular necrosis, interstitial nephritis, embolic disease, glomerulonephritis, vasculitis, or small vessel disease). Postrenal acute renal failure is caused by urinary tract obstruction. Observational studies (in several hundred people from Europe, North America, and West Africa with acute renal failure) found a prerenal cause in 40–80%, an intrarenal cause in 10–50%, and a postrenal cause in the remaining 10%.[12–17] Prerenal acute renal failure is the most common type of acute renal failure in people who are critically ill,[12,18] but acute renal failure in this context is usually part of multisystem failure, and most frequently because of acute tubular necrosis resulting from ischaemic or nephrotoxic injury, or both.[19,20]

**PROGNOSIS** One retrospective study (1347 people with acute renal failure) found that mortality was less than 15% in people with isolated acute renal failure.[21] One recent prospective study (> 700 people) found that, in people with acute renal failure, overall mortality and the need for dialysis was higher in an than in a non-intensive care unit (ICU) setting, despite no significant difference between the groups in mean maximal serum creatinine (need for dialysis 71% in ICU v 18% in non-ICU; P < 0.001; mortality 72% in the ICU v 32% in non-ICU settings; P = 0.001).[22]

Please refer to CD-ROM for full text and references.

# Benign prostatic hyperplasia

**Search date November 2002**

*Robyn Webber*

## What are the effects of treatments?

### BENEFICIAL

#### α Blockers

We found evidence that α blockers improve lower urinary tract symptoms compared with placebo. We found limited evidence that different α blockers have similar effects. We found limited evidence that α blockers improve symptoms more than 5α reductase inhibitors. We found no evidence comparing α blockers versus surgical treatment. We found limited evidence that α blockers and saw palmetto are equally effective in improving symptoms.

#### 5α Reductase inhibitors

We found evidence that 5α reductase inhibitors improve symptoms and reduce complications compared with placebo. We found limited evidence that 5α reductase inhibitors were less effective at improving symptoms than α blockers. We found no evidence comparing 5α reductase inhibitors versus surgical treatment.

#### Saw palmetto plant extracts

One systematic review has found that saw palmetto improves symptoms compared with placebo. It found no significant difference in symptom scores between saw palmetto and finasteride. We found evidence of a similar improvement in symptom scores with saw palmetto or tamsulosin. We found evidence of no treatment advantage in combining saw palmetto with tamsulosin.

#### Transurethral microwave thermotherapy

We found evidence that transurethral microwave thermotherapy reduced symptoms compared with sham treatment. We found limited evidence that transurethral resection relieved short term symptoms better than thermotherapy. We found limited evidence that thermotherapy improved symptoms more than α blockers over 18 months.

#### Transurethral resection versus no surgery

We found evidence that transurethral resection reduced symptoms more than watchful waiting, and did not increase the risk of erectile dysfunction or incontinence.

### LIKELY TO BE BENEFICIAL

#### β-Sitosterol plant extract

One systematic review found that β-sitosterol plant extract improved lower urinary tract symptoms compared with placebo in the short term.

### UNKNOWN EFFECTIVENESS

#### Rye grass pollen extract

One systematic review found limited evidence that rye grass pollen extract increased self rated improvement and reduced nocturia in the short term compared with placebo. However, the review identified only two small RCTs, from which we were unable to draw reliable conclusions.

#### Transurethral resection versus less invasive surgical techniques

We found no evidence of a significant difference in symptoms between transurethral resection and transurethral incision or between transurethral resection and ▶

◀ electrical vaporisation. We found limited evidence that transurethral resection improved symptoms more than visual laser ablation but that transurethral resection may be associated with a higher risk of blood transfusion.

### Transurethral resection versus transurethral needle ablation

We found limited evidence from one RCT that transurethral resection reduced symptoms compared with transurethral needle ablation, although transurethral needle ablation caused fewer adverse effects.

**DEFINITION** Benign prostatic hyperplasia is defined histologically. Clinically, it is characterised by lower urinary tract symptoms (urinary frequency, urgency, a weak and intermittent stream, needing to strain, a sense of incomplete emptying, and nocturia), and can lead to complications, including acute urinary retention.

**INCIDENCE/ PREVALENCE** Estimates of the prevalence of symptomatic benign prostatic hyperplasia range from 10–30% for men in their early 70s, depending on how benign prostatic hyperplasia is defined.[1]

**AETIOLOGY/ RISK FACTORS** The mechanisms by which benign prostatic hyperplasia causes symptoms and complications are unclear, although bladder outlet obstruction is an important factor.[2] The best documented risk factors are increasing age and functioning testes.[3]

**PROGNOSIS** Community and practice based studies suggest that men with lower urinary tract symptoms can expect slow progression of the symptoms.[4,5] However, symptoms can wax and wane without treatment. In men with symptoms of benign prostatic hyperplasia, rates of acute urinary retention range from 1–2% a year.[5–7]

---

Please refer to CD-ROM for full text and references.

# Chronic prostatitis

**Search date February 2003**

*Jeffrey Stern and Anthony Schaeffer*

## What are the effects of treatments for chronic bacterial prostatitis?

### LIKELY TO BE BENEFICIAL

#### α Blockers (when added to antimicrobials)

We found no RCTs comparing α blockers versus placebo or no treatment. We found limited evidence from one RCT suggesting that adding α blockers to antimicrobials may improve symptoms and reduce recurrence compared with antimicrobials alone.

### UNKNOWN EFFECTIVENESS

#### Local injection of antimicrobials

We found no RCTs comparing local injection of antimicrobials with placebo or no treatment. One small RCT found that anal submucosal injection of amikacin improved symptom scores and bacterial eradication rates at 3 months compared with intramuscular amikacin.

#### Oral antimicrobial drugs

We found no placebo controlled RCTs. One RCT found no significant difference between lomefloxacin and ciprofloxacin in rates of clinical success or bacteriological cure at 6 months. We found no other RCTs of the effects of oral antimicrobial drugs. Retrospective observational studies reported cure rates of 0–88% depending on the drug used and the duration of treatment.

#### Radical prostatectomy; transurethral resection

We found no RCTs on the effects of these interventions.

## What are the effects of treatments for chronic abacterial prostatitis?

### UNKNOWN EFFECTIVENESS

#### α Blockers

One systematic review found limited evidence from two small RCTs that α blockers may improve maximal flow time and pain compared with placebo. However, we were unable to draw reliable conclusions from these small studies.

#### 5α Reductase inhibitors

One systematic review of one small RCT found insufficient evidence about the effects of 5α reductase inhibitors compared with placebo in men with chronic abacterial prostatitis.

#### Allopurinol

We found insufficient evidence from one small RCT about the effects of allopurinol compared with placebo in men with chronic abacterial prostatitis.

#### Anti-inflammatory medications

We found insufficient evidence about the effects of anti-inflammatory medications compared with placebo or no treatment in men with chronic abacterial prostatitis. ▶

◀ **Transurethral microwave thermotherapy**

One systematic review found limited evidence from one small RCT suggesting that transurethral microwave thermotherapy may significantly improve quality of life at 3 months, and symptoms over 21 months, compared with sham treatment. However, we were unable to draw reliable conclusions from this one small study.

## Biofeedback; prostatic massage; Sitz bath

We found no good evidence on these interventions.

| | |
|---|---|
| **DEFINITION** | **Chronic bacterial prostatitis** is characterised by a positive culture of expressed prostatic secretions. It can be symptomatic (recurrent urinary tract infection, or suprapubic, lower back, or perineal pain), asymptomatic, or associated with minimal urgency, frequency, and dysuria. **Chronic abacterial prostatitis** is characterised by pelvic or perineal pain, often associated with urinary urgency, nocturia, weak urinary stream, frequency, dysuria, hesitancy, dribbling after micturition, interrupted flow, and inflammation (white cells) in prostatic secretions. Symptoms can also include suprapubic, scrotal, testicular, penile, or lower back pain or discomfort, known as prostodynia, in the absence of bacteria in prostatic secretions. |
| **INCIDENCE/ PREVALENCE** | One US community based study (58 955 visits by men ≥ 18 years to office based physicians) estimated that 9% of men have a diagnosis of chronic prostatitis at any one time.[1] Another study found that, of men with genitourinary symptoms, 8% presenting to urologists and 1% presenting to primary care physicians are diagnosed with chronic prostatitis.[2] Most cases of chronic prostatitis are abacterial. Acute bacterial prostatitis, although easy to diagnose, is rare. |
| **AETIOLOGY/ RISK FACTORS** | Organisms commonly implicated in bacterial prostatitis include *Escherichia coli*, other Gram negative Enterobacteriaceae, occasionally *Pseudomonas* species, and rarely Gram positive enterococci. The cause of abacterial prostatitis is unclear, but autoimmunity could be involved.[3] |
| **PROGNOSIS** | One recent study found that chronic abacterial prostatitis had an impact on quality of life similar to that from angina, Crohn's disease, or a previous myocardial infarction.[4] |

Please refer to CD-ROM for full text and references.

# Erectile dysfunction

### Search date December 2002

*Robyn Webber*

## What are the effects of treatments?

### BENEFICIAL

**Intracavernosal alprostadil**

One large RCT found that intracavernosal alprostadil increased the chances of a satisfactory erection compared with placebo.

**Intraurethral alprostadil (in men who had responded to a single test dose)**

One large RCT (in men who had previously responded to alprostadil) found limited evidence that intraurethral alprostadil (prostaglandin E1) increased the chances of successful sexual intercourse and at least one orgasm over 3 months compared with placebo. About a third of men suffered penile ache. We found no direct comparisons of intraurethral alprostadil versus either intracavernosal alprostadil or oral drug treatments.

**Sildenafil**

One systematic review and six subsequent RCTs found that sildenafil improved erections and increased rates of successful intercourse compared with placebo. Adverse effects, including headaches, flushing, and dyspepsia, are reported in up to a quarter of men. Deaths have been reported in men on concomitant treatment with oral nitrates.

**Yohimbine**

One systematic review has found that yohimbine improves self reported sexual function and penile rigidity at 2–10 weeks compared with placebo. Transient adverse effects are reported in up to a third of men.

### TRADE OFF BETWEEN BENEFITS AND HARMS

**Topical alprostadil**

Two quasi randomised trials found limited evidence that topical alprostadil increased the number of men with erections sufficient for intercourse compared with placebo but was commonly associated with akin irritation.

### UNKNOWN EFFECTIVENESS

**L-arginine**

One small RCT found no significant difference in sexual function between L-arginine and placebo, but it may have been too small to exclude a clinically important difference.

**Penile prostheses**

We found no RCTs of penile prostheses in men with erectile dysfunction.

**Trazodone**

One small RCT found no significant difference in erections or libido between trazodone and placebo, but it may have been too small to exclude a clinically important difference.

**Vacuum devices**

Vacuum devices have not been adequately assessed in RCTs. One small RCT found limited evidence that they were as effective as intracavernosal alprostadil (prostaglandin E1) injections for rigidity but not for orgasm.

**DEFINITION** Erectile dysfunction has largely replaced the term "impotence". It is defined as the persistent inability to obtain or maintain sufficient rigidity of the penis to allow satisfactory sexual performance.

**INCIDENCE/ PREVALENCE** We found little good epidemiological information, but one cross sectional study found that age is the variable most strongly associated with erectile dysfunction, and that up to 30 million men in the USA may be affected.[1] Even among men in their 40s, nearly 40% report at least occasional difficulty obtaining or maintaining erection, whereas this approaches 70% in 70 year olds.

**AETIOLOGY/ RISK FACTORS** It is now believed that about 80% of cases of erectile dysfunction have an organic cause, the rest being psychogenic in origin. Risk factors include increasing age, smoking, and obesity. Erectile problems fall into three categories: failure to initiate; failure to fill, caused by insufficient arterial inflow into the penis to allow engorgement and tumescence because of vascular insufficiency; and failure to store because of veno-occlusive dysfunction. Erectile dysfunction is a recognised side effect of a wide variety of pharmaceutical agents.

**PROGNOSIS** We found no good evidence on prognosis in untreated organic erectile dysfunction.

Please refer to CD-ROM for full text and references.

# Prostate cancer (metastatic)

**Search date September 2002**

*M Dror Michaelson, Matthew R Smith, and James A Talcott*

## What are the effects of treatments in men with metastatic prostate cancer?

### LIKELY TO BE BENEFICIAL

**Androgen deprivation**

We found limited evidence from RCTs suggesting that androgen deprivation⦿ reduced mortality compared with no initial treatment. One non-systematic review of RCTs found that orchidectomy⦿, diethylstilbestrol, and gonadorelin analogues initially improved symptoms and objective signs of disease in most men, but found no evidence of a difference between different types of androgen deprivation.

**Combined androgen blockade (androgen deprivation and antiandrogen) versus androgen deprivation alone**

Systematic reviews found limited evidence of a 2–5% improvement in 5 year survival associated with combined androgen blockade⦿ (androgen deprivation plus a non-steroidal antiandrogen) compared with androgen deprivation alone.

### UNKNOWN EFFECTIVENESS

**Intermittent androgen deprivation**

We found no RCTs comparing long term effects of intermittent androgen deprivation versus those of continuous androgen deprivation on mortality, morbidity, or quality of life.

### LIKELY TO BE INEFFECTIVE OR HARMFUL

**Deferred androgen deprivation without surveillance**

One systematic review found limited evidence of a small survival advantage at 10 years for immediate androgen deprivation therapy with gonadorelin analogues or orchidectomy in men with advanced, asymptomatic prostate cancer. There was no significant change in overall survival at 1, 2, or 5 years. The risk of major complications is increased in men whose treatment is deferred until disease progression.

## What are the effects of treatments in men with symptomatic androgen independent metastatic disease?

### LIKELY TO BE BENEFICIAL

**Chemotherapy (palliation but no evidence of an effect on survival)**

RCTs found limited evidence that chemotherapy with some new agents plus corticosteroids reduced pain, lengthened palliation, and improved quality of life, but found no improvement in overall survival compared with corticosteroids alone. Earlier RCTs failed to demonstrate any benefit of chemotherapy in men with metastatic prostate cancer.

**External beam radiation (palliation but no evidence of an effect on survival)\***

We found no RCTs comparing external beam radiation with palliative treatments other than radionuclides. Observational evidence suggests that complete pain relief is achieved in about a quarter of people, and placebo controlled RCTs would probably be considered unethical.

▶

◀ **Radionuclides (palliation but no clear evidence of an effect on survival)**

One systematic review found one small RCT in men with symptomatic bone metastases, which found no significant difference in survival between external beam radiation plus placebo and external beam radiation plus strontium-89. However, strontium-89 significantly reduced the number of new sites of pain. One small subsequent RCT in men with painful bone metastases found that samarium-153 significantly reduced pain scores compared with placebo. A second small subsequent RCT, in a selected population, found an improvement in survival with strontium-89 compared with placebo, but the results are difficult to generalise.

## UNKNOWN EFFECTIVENESS

### Bisphosphonates

One systematic review of two RCTs found insufficient evidence about the effects of bisphosphonates.

*Categorisation based on observational evidence; RCTs unlikely to be conducted.

| | |
|---|---|
| **DEFINITION** | See prostate cancer (non-metastatic), p 201. Androgen independent metastatic disease is defined as disease that progresses despite androgen deprivation. |
| **INCIDENCE/ PREVALENCE** | See prostate cancer (non-metastatic), p 201. |
| **AETIOLOGY/ RISK FACTORS** | See prostate cancer (non-metastatic), p 202. |
| **PROGNOSIS** | Prostate cancer metastasises predominantly to bone. Metastatic prostate cancer can result in pain, weakness, paralysis, and death. |

Please refer to CD-ROM for full text and references.

# Prostate cancer (non-metastatic)

**Search date February 2003**

*Timothy Wilt*

---

## What are the effects of treatments for clinically localised prostate cancer?

### TRADE OFF BETWEEN BENEFITS AND HARMS

#### Radical prostatectomy

Two RCTs found no significant difference in death from any cause between radical prostatectomy❻ and watchful waiting in men with clinically detected disease after median follow up of 6.2 and 23 years. The larger of the RCTs found that radical prostatectomy reduced death due to prostate cancer and metastases at 6 years compared with watchful waiting. Two small RCTs found that radical prostatectomy reduced the risk of treatment failure compared with external beam radiation. Radical prostatectomy carries the risks of major surgery and of sexual and urinary dysfunction.

#### Watchful waiting

Two RCTs found no significant difference in overall survival between watchful waiting and radical prostatectomy in men with clinically detected disease after median follow up of 6 and 23 years. The larger RCT found that radical prostatectomy reduced death rates due to prostate cancer and metastases at 6 years compared with watchful waiting. One RCT found that radical prostatectomy increased erectile dysfunction compared with watchful waiting but found no significant difference in quality of life after 12 months.

### UNKNOWN EFFECTIVENESS

#### Androgen suppression

We found no RCTs of early androgen suppression❻ on length or quality of life in men with asymptomatic, clinically localised prostate cancer. One RCT identified by a systematic review found limited evidence that oestrogen decreased prostate cancer related deaths compared with watchful waiting. It found no significant difference in overall survival. One preliminary report of three large ongoing RCTs in men with localised or locally advanced prostate cancer found that bicalutamide plus standard care reduced rates of radiological progression and bone metastases at 2–3 years compared with standard care alone. There was no significant difference between treatments in overall survival.

#### External beam radiation

We found no RCTs comparing external beam radiation versus watchful waiting. Two RCTs found that external beam radiation increased the risk of treatment failure compared with radical prostatectomy. Two small RCTs found no significant difference between conformal radiotherapy❻ and conventional radiotherapy in overall survival or tumour control at 3–5 years. One systematic review found limited evidence that conformal radiotherapy with dose escalation reduced acute and late treatment related morbidity compared with conventional radiotherapy for men with T1 or T2 low or intermediate risk prostate cancer.

#### Androgen suppression in asymptomatic men with raised prostate specific antigen concentrations after early treatment; brachytherapy❻; cryosurgery

We found no RCTs on the effects of these interventions. ▶

◀ *What are the effects of treatments for locally advanced prostate cancer?*

**BENEFICIAL**

**Immediate androgen suppression after radical prostatectomy and pelvic lymphadenectomy in men with node positive prostate cancer (compared with radical prostatectomy and deferred androgen suppression)**

One small RCT in men with node positive prostate cancer found that immediate androgen suppression compared with deferred androgen suppression after radical prostatectomy☉ and pelvic lymphadenectomy reduced mortality over a median of 7 years' follow up.

**LIKELY TO BE BENEFICIAL**

**Androgen suppression initiated at diagnosis**

RCTs found no significant difference in overall survival between androgen suppression with bicalutamide and no androgen suppression in men with localised or locally advanced prostate cancer at 2–10 years. The RCTs found that bicalutamide reduced objective progression compared with no bicalutamide. One systematic review found that early androgen suppression increased survival at 10 years compared with deferred treatment in men with locally advanced prostate cancer but found no significant difference in survival at 5 years. One RCT found limited evidence that immediate androgen suppression reduced complications compared with deferred androgen suppression.

**Early androgen suppression in addition to external beam radiation (improves survival compared with radiation and deferred androgen suppression)**

RCTs found limited evidence that androgen suppression initiated at diagnosis plus external beam radiation improved long term survival compared with radiation alone or radiation plus deferred androgen suppression. One RCT found limited evidence that immediate androgen suppression reduced complications compared with deferred androgen suppression.

**DEFINITION**  Prostatic cancer is staged according to two systems: the tumour, node, metastasis (TNM) classification system and the American urologic staging system☉. Non-metastatic prostate cancer can be divided into clinically localised disease and locally advanced disease. Clinically localised disease is prostate cancer thought, after clinical examination, to be confined to the prostate gland. Locally advanced disease is prostate cancer that has spread outside the capsule of the prostate gland but has not yet spread to other organs. Metastatic disease is prostate cancer that has spread outside the prostate gland to either local, regional, or systemic lymph nodes, seminal vesicles, or to other body organs (e.g. bone, liver, brain) and is not connected to the prostate gland. We consider clinically localised and locally advanced disease here. Metastatic disease is covered in a separate chapter (see prostate cancer [metastatic], p 198).

**INCIDENCE/**  Prostate cancer is the sixth most common cancer in the world and the third
**PREVALENCE**  most common cancer in men. In 2000, an estimated 513 000 new cases of prostate caner were diagnosed and about 250 000 deaths were attributed to prostate cancers worldwide. Prostate cancer is uncommon under the age of 50 years. About 85% of men with prostate cancer are diagnosed after the age of 65 years. Autopsy studies suggest that the prevalence of subclinical prostate cancer is high at all ages: 30% for men aged 30–39 years, 50% for men aged 50–59 years, and more than 75% for men older than 85 years. ▶

# Prostate cancer (non-metastatic)

Incidence varies widely by ethnic group and around the world. The highest rates occur in men of black ethnic group living in the USA and the lowest among men living in China.[1]

**AETIOLOGY/ RISK FACTORS**  Risk factors for prostate cancer include increasing age, family history of prostate cancer, black race, and possibly higher dietary consumption of fat and meat, low intake of lycopene (from tomato products), low intake of fruit, and high dietary calcium. In the USA, black men have about a 60% higher incidence than white men.[2] The prostate cancer incidence for black men living in the USA is about 90/100 000 in men aged less than 65 years and about 1300/100 000 in men aged 65–74 years. For white men, incidence is about 44/100 000 in men aged less than 65 years and 900/100 000 in men aged 65–74 years.[2]

**PROGNOSIS**  The chance that men with well to moderately differentiated, palpable, clinically localised prostate cancer will remain free of symptomatic progression is 70% at 5 years and 40% at 10 years.[3] The risk of symptomatic disease progression is higher in men with poorly differentiated prostate cancer.[4] One retrospective analysis of a large surgical series in men with clinically localised prostate cancer found that the median time from the increase in prostate specific antigen (PSA) concentration to the development of metastatic disease was 8 years.[5] Time to PSA progression, PSA doubling time, and Gleason score❺ were predictive of the probability and time to development of metastatic disease. Once men developed metastatic disease, the median actuarial time to death was less than 5 years.[5] Morbidity from local or regional disease progression includes haematuria, bladder obstruction, and lower extremity oedema. The age adjusted prostate cancer specific mortality in the USA for all men aged 65 years and older has decreased by about 15% (244 deaths/100 000 to 207 deaths/100 000) from 1991–1997. The reasons for this are unclear, although inaccurate death certification, PSA screening, and earlier, more intensive treatment, including radical prostatectomy❺, radiotherapy, and androgen suppression❺, have been suggested. However, regions of the USA and Canada where PSA testing and early treatment are more common have similar prostate cancer mortality to regions with lower testing and early treatment rates.[6] Similarly, countries with low rates of PSA testing and treatment, such as the UK, have similar age adjusted prostate cancer mortality to countries with high rates of testing and treatment, such as the USA.[7]

Please refer to CD-ROM for full text and references.

Search date August 2002

*Janet Treasure and Ulrike Schmidt*

## What are the effects of treatments?

### UNKNOWN EFFECTIVENESS

**Inpatient versus outpatient treatment setting (in people not so severely ill as to warrant emergency intervention)**

Limited evidence from one small RCT found that outpatient treatment was as effective as inpatient treatment🅖 in increasing weight and improving Morgan Russell scale🅖 global scores at 1, 2, and 5 years in people who did not need emergency intervention.

**Oestrogen treatment (for prevention of fractures)**

We found no good evidence about the effects of hormonal treatment on fracture rates in people with anorexia. One small RCT found no significant effect of oestrogen versus no treatment on bone mineral density in people with anorexia.

**Psychotherapies**

We found insufficient evidence from small RCTs to compare psychotherapies🅖 versus dietary counselling🅖 or versus each other. One small RCT found limited evidence that focal analytical therapy or family therapy🅖 versus usual treatment significantly increased the number of people recovered or improved as assessed by the Morgan Russell scale at 1 year.

**Selective serotonin reuptake inhibitors (fluoxetine)**

We found insufficient evidence from two small RCTs to compare fluoxetine versus placebo in people with anorexia.

**Zinc**

One small RCT found limited evidence that zinc may improve daily body mass index🅖 gain compared with placebo in people managed in an inpatient setting. However, we were unable to draw firm conclusions.

### LIKELY TO BE INEFFECTIVE OR HARMFUL

**Cisapride**

One small RCT found no significant difference with cisapride versus placebo in weight gain at 8 weeks. Cisapride has now been restricted in many countries because of concerns about cardiac irregularities, including ventricular tachycardia, torsades de pointes, and sudden death.

**Cyproheptadine**

Three small RCTs found no significant difference with cyproheptadine versus placebo in weight gain.

**Neuroleptic drugs that increase the QT interval**

We found no RCTs. The QT interval may be prolonged in people with anorexia nervosa, and many neuroleptic drugs (haloperidol, pimozide, sertindole, thioridazine, chlorpromazine, and others) also increase the QT interval. Prolongation of the QT interval may be associated with increased risk of ventricular tachycardia, torsades de pointes, and sudden death.

**Tricyclic antidepressants**

Two small RCTs found no evidence of benefit with amitriptyline compared with placebo. They found that amitriptyline was associated with more adverse effects, such as palpitations, dry mouth, and blurred vision.

# Anorexia nervosa

**DEFINITION**
Anorexia nervosa is characterised by a refusal to maintain weight at or above a minimally normal weight (< 85% of expected weight for age and height, or body mass index◐ < 17.5 kg/m$^2$), or a failure to show the expected weight gain during growth. In association with this, there is often an intense fear of gaining weight, preoccupation with weight, denial of the current low weight and its adverse impact on health, and amenorrhoea. Two subtypes of anorexia nervosa, binge–purge and restricting, have been defined.[1]

**INCIDENCE/ PREVALENCE**
A mean incidence in the general population of 19/100 000 a year in females and 2/100 000 a year in males has been estimated from 12 cumulative studies.[2] The highest rate was in female teenagers (age 13–19 years), where there were 50.8 cases/100 000 a year. A large cohort study of Swedish school children (4291 people, aged 16 years) were screened by weighing and subsequent interview, and the prevalence of anorexia nervosa cases (defined using DSM-III and DSM-III-R criteria) was found to be 7/1000 for girls and 1/1000 for boys.[3] Little is known of the incidence or prevalence in Asia, South America, or Africa.

**AETIOLOGY/ RISK FACTORS**
Anorexia nervosa has been related to family, biological, social, and cultural factors.[4] Studies have found that anorexia nervosa is associated with a family history of anorexia nervosa (HR 11.4, 95% CI 1.1 to 89.0), of bulimia nervosa (adjusted HR 3.5, 95% CI 1.1 to 14.0),[5] depression, generalised anxiety disorder, obsessive compulsive disorder, or obsessive compulsive personality disorder (adjusted RR 3.6, 95% CI 1.6 to 8.0).[6] A twin study suggested that anorexia nervosa may be related to genetic factors but it was unable to estimate reliably the contribution of non-shared environmental factors. Specific aspects of childhood temperament thought to be related include perfectionism, negative self evaluation, and extreme compliance.[7] Perinatal factors include prematurity (OR 3.2, 95% CI 1.6 to 6.2), particularly if the baby was small for gestational age (OR 5.7, 95% CI 1.4 to 4.1).

**PROGNOSIS**
One prospective study followed up 51 people with teenage-onset anorexia nervosa, about half of whom received no or minimal treatment (< 8 sessions). After 10 years, 14/51 people (27%) had a persistent eating disorder, three (6%) had ongoing anorexia nervosa, and six (12%) had experienced a period of bulimia nervosa. People with anorexia nervosa were significantly more likely to have an affective disorder than controls matched for sex, age, and school (lifetime risk of affective disorder 96% in people with anorexia v 23% with controls, ARI 73%, 95% CI 60% to 85%). Obsessive compulsive disorder was, similarly, significantly more likely in people with anorexia nervosa compared with controls (ARI 10%, 95% CI 10% to 41%). However, in 35% of people with obsessive compulsive disorder and anorexia nervosa, obsessive compulsive disorder preceded the anorexia. About half of all participants continued to have poor psychosocial functioning at 10 years (assessed using the Morgan Russell scale and Global Assessment of Functioning Scale).[8] A summary of treatment studies (68 studies published between 1953 and 1989, 3104 people, length of follow up 1–33 years) found that 43% of people recover completely (range 7–86%), 36% improve (range 1–69%), 20% develop a chronic eating disorder (range 0–43%), and 5% die from anorexia nervosa (range 0–21%).[9] Favourable prognostic factors include an early age at onset and a short interval between onset of symptoms and the beginning of treatment. Unfavourable prognostic factors include vomiting, bulimia, profound weight loss, chronicity, and a history of premorbid developmental or clinical abnormalities. The all cause standardised mortality ratio of eating disorders (anorexia nervosa and bulimia nervosa) ▶

has been estimated at 538, about three times higher than other psychiatric illnesses.[10] The average annual risk of mortality was 0.59% a year in females in 10 eating disorder populations (1322 people) with a minimum follow up of 6 years.[11] The mortality risk was higher for people with lower weight and with older age at presentation. Young women with anorexia nervosa are at an increased risk of fractures later in life.[12]

Please refer to CD-ROM for full text and references.

# Bipolar disorder

**Search date April 2002**

*John Geddes*

## What are the effects of treatments in mania? New

### BENEFICIAL

#### Lithium

One RCT in people with bipolar type I disorder experiencing a manic episode found that lithium increased the proportion of people who responded after 3–4 weeks compared with placebo. One systematic review found that lithium increased the proportion of people who had remission of manic symptoms at 3 weeks compared with chlorpromazine, and found no significant difference in symptoms at 3–6 weeks between lithium and haloperidol, olanzapine, valproate, lamotrigine, or clonazepam. One RCT found that lithium was less effective than risperidone in reducing manic symptoms at 4 weeks. Lithium can cause a range of adverse effects. The RCTs provided insufficient evidence about how the adverse effects of lithium compared with those of other antipsychotic drugs.

#### Olanzapine

One systematic review in people with bipolar type I disorder found that olanzapine increased the proportion of people who responded at 3–6 weeks compared with placebo, both as monotherapy and as add on therapy to lithium or valproate, and found no significant difference in symptoms at 28 days between olanzapine and lithium. RCTs found that olanzapine was more effective in reducing symptoms than valproate, but was also more likely to cause adverse effects such as sedation and weight gain. The acceptability of olanzapine may be limited by weight gain.

#### Valproate

One systematic review in people with bipolar type I disorder experiencing a manic episode found that valproate increased the proportion of people who responded over 3 weeks compared with placebo. It found no significant difference in response at 1–6 weeks between valproate and lithium, haloperidol, or carbamazepine. It found that valproate was less effective in reducing manic symptoms than olanzapine, but was also less likely to cause adverse effects such as sedation and weight gain.

### LIKELY TO BE BENEFICIAL

#### Carbamazepine

RCTs in people with bipolar type I disorder experiencing a manic episode found no significant difference in manic symptoms at 4–6 weeks between carbamazepine and lithium or valproate.

#### Clonazepam

We found no RCTs comparing clonazepam versus placebo in people with bipolar mania. RCTs in people with bipolar type I disorder experiencing a manic episode suggest that clonazepam may be as effective as lithium in improving manic symptoms at 1–4 weeks.

#### Haloperidol

We found no RCTs comparing haloperidol versus placebo in people with bipolar mania. RCTs in people with bipolar type I disorder experiencing a manic episode found no significant difference in manic symptoms at 1–3 weeks between haloperidol and lithium or valproate, although haloperidol was associated with more extrapyramidal adverse effects and sedation than valproate.

◄ **Risperidone**

We found no RCTs comparing risperidone versus placebo in people with bipolar mania. One RCT in people with bipolar type I disorder experiencing a manic episode found that risperidone reduced manic symptoms at 4 weeks compared with lithium. It gave no information on adverse effects.

**UNKNOWN EFFECTIVENESS**

**Chlorpromazine**

One very small RCT in people with mania found limited evidence that chlorpromazine may improve manic symptoms over 7 weeks more than placebo or imipramine. One systematic review found that fewer people had remission of symptoms at 3 weeks with chlorpromazine than with lithium.

**Lamotrigine**

We found no RCTs comparing lamotrigine versus placebo in people with bipolar mania. One RCT in people with bipolar type I disorder experiencing a manic episode found no significant difference in manic symptoms at 4 weeks between lamotrigine and lithium.

---

## What are the effects of treatments in bipolar depression? New

**LIKELY TO BE BENEFICIAL**

**Lamotrigine**

One RCT in people with bipolar type I disorder experiencing a major depressive episode found that lamotrigine increased the proportion of people who responded over 7 weeks compared with placebo.

**TRADE OFF BETWEEN BENEFITS AND HARMS**

**Antidepressants**

Systematic reviews found that antidepressants improved depressive symptoms at the end of the trial (unspecified) compared with placebo. They found limited evidence that selective serotonin reuptake inhibitors were more effective than tricyclic antidepressants, and found no significant difference in symptoms between monoamine oxidase inhibitors and tricyclic antidepressants or between selective serotonin reuptake inhibitors and serotonin noradrenaline reuptake inhibitors. The reviews provided insufficient evidence to assess whether antidepressants induce bipolar mania.

**UNKNOWN EFFECTIVENESS**

**Carbamazepine; lithium**

One systematic review identified no RCTs of sufficient quality to assess these treatments in people with bipolar depression.

**Psychological treatments; valproate**

We found no RCTs of these treatments in people with bipolar depression.

# Bipolar disorder

## What are the effects of interventions to prevent relapse of mania or bipolar depression? New

### BENEFICIAL

#### Lithium

RCTs have found that lithium reduces relapse⊕ over 2 years compared with placebo, and have found no significant difference in relapse between lithium and valproate, carbamazepine or lamotrigine.

### LIKELY TO BE BENEFICIAL

#### Carbamazepine

We found no RCTs comparing carbamazepine versus placebo in preventing relapse. One systematic review found no significant difference between carbamazepine and lithium in the proportion of people who relapsed over 1–3 years.

#### Education to recognise symptoms of relapse

One RCT found limited evidence that an educational programme to recognise symptoms of relapse reduced manic relapse over 18 months, but that it may increase depressive episodes.

#### Lamotrigine (bipolar depressive episodes)

Three RCTs have found that lamotrigine reduces relapse compared with placebo. However, secondary analyses in two of the RCT suggested that lamotrigine protected against depressive relapse, but not manic relapse. RCTs have found no significant difference between lamotrigine and lithium in the proportion of people who relapse.

#### Valproate

One RCT found that valproate reduced relapse over 12 months compared with placebo. One systematic review found no significant difference between lithium and valproate in relapse over 12 months.

### UNKNOWN EFFECTIVENESS

#### Antidepressant drugs

One systematic review provided insufficient evidence to assess antidepressants in preventing relapse of bipolar disorder.

#### Family focused psychoeducation

One RCT found that 21 sessions of family focused psychoeducation reduced relapse over 12 months compared with two family sessions plus crisis management.

**DEFINITION**    Bipolar disorder (bipolar affective disorder, manic depressive disorder) is characterised by marked mood swings between mania (mood elevation) and bipolar depression that cause significant personal distress or social dysfunction, and are not caused by drugs or known physical disorder. **Bipolar type I disorder** is diagnosed when episodes of depression are interspersed with mania or mixed episodes. **Bipolar type II disorder** is diagnosed when depression is interspersed with less severe episodes of elevated mood that do not lead to dysfunction or disability (hypomania). Bipolar disorder has been subdivided in several further ways❶.[1]

**INCIDENCE/ PREVALENCE** One 1996 cross-national community based study (38 000 people) found lifetime prevalence rates of bipolar disorder ranging from 0.3% in Taiwan to 1.5% in New Zealand.[2] It found that men and women were at similar risk, and that the age at first onset ranged from 19–29 years (average of 6 years earlier than first onset of major depression).

**AETIOLOGY/ RISK FACTORS** The cause of bipolar disorder is uncertain, although family and twin studies suggest a genetic basis.[3] The lifetime risk of bipolar disorder is increased in first degree relatives of a person with bipolar disorder (40–70% for a monozygotic twin; 5–10% for other first degree relatives). If the first episode of mania occurs in an older adult, it may be secondary mania due to underlying medical or substance induced factors.[4]

**PROGNOSIS** Bipolar disorder is a recurring illness and is one of the leading causes of worldwide disability, especially in the 15–44 year age group.[5] One 4 year inception cohort study (173 people treated for a first episode of mania or mixed affective disorder) found that 93% of people no longer met criteria for mania at 2 years (median time to recover from a syndrome 4.6 weeks), but that only 36% had recovered to premorbid function.[6] It found that 40% of people had a recurrent manic (20%) or depressive (20%) episode within 2 years of recovering from the first episode. A meta-analysis, comparing observed suicide versus expected rates of suicide in an age and sex matched sample of the general population, found that the lifetime prevalence of suicide was about 2%, or 15 times greater than expected, in people with bipolar disorder.[7]

---

Please refer to CD-ROM for full text and references.

# Bulimia nervosa

**Search date December 2002**

*Phillipa Hay and Josue Bacaltchuk*

## What are the effects of treatments?

**LIKELY TO BE BENEFICIAL**

### Antidepressant medication (tricyclic antidepressants, monoamine oxidase inhibitors, and fluoxetine)

Systematic reviews and one subsequent RCT have found short term reduction in bulimic symptoms with tricyclic antidepressants, monoamine oxidase inhibitors, and fluoxetine. A further subsequent RCT found no significant difference in symptoms between moclobemide and placebo. One systematic review and one subsequent RCT found no significant difference in symptoms with antidepressants versus cognitive behavioural therapy.

### Cognitive behavioural therapy

One systematic review has found that cognitive behavioural therapy⊕ compared with remaining on a waiting list reduces specific symptoms of bulimia nervosa and improves non-specific symptoms such as depression. One systematic review found cognitive behavioural therapy compared with other psychotherapies improved abstinence from binge eating and depression scores at the end of treatment. One RCT in the review found that cognitive behavioural therapy compared with interpersonal psychotherapy reduced binge eating in the short term, but there was no significant difference in the longer term. One systematic review and one RCT found no significant difference in symptoms with cognitive behavioural therapy compared with antidepressants.

### Other psychotherapies

One systematic review has found that non-cognitive behavioural psychotherapy increases abstinence from binge eating compared with waiting list controls. The systematic review found that the combined result for four specific psychotherapies, other than cognitive behavioural therapy, reduced bulimic symptoms compared with specified control psychotherapies, but the review included RCTs with weak methods, and the result was significant in only one of the four individual results. One systematic review found cognitive behavioural therapy compared with other psychotherapies improved abstinence from binge eating and depression scores at the end of treatment. One RCT in the review found that cognitive behavioural therapy compared with interpersonal psychotherapy⊕ reduced binge eating in the short term, but there was no significant difference in the longer term.

### Combination treatment (antidepressants plus psychotherapy)

One systematic review and one subsequent RCT found no significant difference between combination treatment (antidepressants plus psychotherapy) and antidepressants alone in binge frequency, depressive symptoms, and remission rates. The systematic review found that, compared with psychotherapy alone, combination treatment improved short term remission, but there was no significant difference in binge frequency and depressive symptoms. The systematic review found that combination treatment was with psychotherapy were associated with higher withdrawal rates compared with psychotherapy alone. One subsequent RCT of cognitive behavioural therapy in a self help form plus fluoxetine found limited evidence that combined treatment reduced bulimic symptoms compared with cognitive behavioural therapy alone. A second subsequent RCT found no significant difference in symptoms between group based CBT, fluoxetine, and their combination.

◀ **UNKNOWN EFFECTIVENESS**

### Antidepressants as maintenance
We found insufficient evidence to assess the effects of antidepresssants for maintenance.

### Other antidepressants (venlafaxine, mirtazapine, and reboxetine)
We found no RCTs on the effects of venlafaxine, mirtazapine, and reboxetine.

### Selective serotonin reuptake inhibitors (other than fluoxetine)
We found no good evidence on selective serotonin reuptake inhibitors other than fluoxetine.

**DEFINITION**  Bulimia nervosa⑥ is an intense preoccupation with body weight and shape, with regular episodes of uncontrolled overeating of large amounts of food (binge eating⑥) associated with use of extreme methods to counteract the feared effects of overeating. If a person also meets the diagnostic criteria for anorexia nervosa, then the diagnosis of anorexia nervosa takes precedence.[1] Bulimia nervosa can be difficult to identify because of extreme secrecy about binge eating and purgative behaviour. Weight may be normal but there is often a history of anorexia nervosa or restrictive dieting. Some people alternate between anorexia nervosa and bulimia nervosa. Some RCTs included participants with subthreshold bulimia nervosa or a related eating disorder, binge eating disorder. Where possible, only results relevant to bulimia nervosa are reported in the review.

**INCIDENCE/ PREVALENCE**  In community based studies, the prevalence of bulimia nervosa is between 0.5% and 1.0% in young women, with an even social class distribution.[2–4] About 90% of people diagnosed with bulimia nervosa are women. The numbers presenting with bulimia nervosa in industrialised countries increased during the decade that followed its recognition in the late 1970s and "a cohort effect" is reported in community surveys,[2,5,6] implying an increase in incidence. The prevalence of eating disorders such as bulimia nervosa is lower in non-industrialised populations[7] and varies across ethnic groups. African-American women have a lower rate of restrictive dieting than white American women, but have a similar rate of recurrent binge eating.[8]

**AETIOLOGY/ RISK FACTORS**  Young women from the developed world who restrict their dietary intake are at greatest risk of developing bulimia nervosa and other eating disorders. One community based case control study compared 102 people with bulimia nervosa with 204 healthy controls and found higher rates of the following in people with the eating disorder: obesity, mood disorder, sexual and physical abuse, parental obesity, substance misuse, low self esteem, perfectionism, disturbed family dynamics, parental weight/shape concern, and early menarche.[9] Compared with a control group of 102 women who had other psychiatric disorders, women with bulimia nervosa had higher rates of parental problems and obesity.

**PROGNOSIS**  A 10 year follow up study (50 people with bulimia nervosa from a former trial of mianserin treatment) found that 52% had fully recovered, and only 9% continued to experience full symptoms of bulimia nervosa.[10] A larger study (222 people from a trial of antidepressants and structured, intensive group psychotherapy) found that, after a mean follow up of 11.5 years, 11% still met criteria for bulimia nervosa, whereas 70% were in full or partial remission.[11] Short term studies found similar results: about 50% of people made a full recovery, 30% made a partial recovery, and 20% continued to be symptomatic.[12] There are few consistent predictors of longer term outcome. Good prognosis has been associated with shorter illness duration, a younger age of onset, higher social class, and a family history of alcohol abuse.[10] Poor prognosis has been associated with a history of substance misuse,[13] premorbid ▶

# Bulimia nervosa

and paternal obesity,[14] and, in some studies, personality disorder.[15-18] One study (102 people) of the natural course of bulimia nervosa found that 31% still had the disorder at 15 months and 15% at 5 years.[19] Only 28% received treatment during the follow up period. In an evaluation of response to cognitive behavioural therapy, early progress (by session 6) best predicted outcome.[20] A subsequent systematic review of the outcome literature found no consistent evidence to support early intervention and a better prognosis.[21]

Please refer to CD-ROM for full text and references.

### Search date April 2003

*G Mustafa Soomro*

## What are the effects of treatments for deliberate self harm in adults? New

We found little RCT evidence for any intervention in people with deliberate self harm. Most RCTs and meta-analyses of small RCTs are likely to have been underpowered to detect clinically important outcomes of interventions.

### UNKNOWN EFFECTIVENESS

**Continuity of care**

One systematic review of one RCT found limited evidence that follow up after hospital treatment with the same compared with a different therapist may increase repetition of deliberate self harm over 3 months, although this may be explained by a higher level of risk factors for repetition in the group receiving same therapist follow up, despite randomisation.

**Dialectal behaviour therapy**

One RCT found limited and equivocal evidence that dialectical behaviour therapy⊕ may reduce the proportion of people with repetition of self harm over 12 months compared with usual care.

**Emergency card**

One systematic review found no significant difference in the proportion of people who repeated deliberate self harm over 12 months between emergency card (allowing emergency admission or contact with a doctor) and usual care.

**Flupentixol depot injection**

One small RCT found that flupentixol depot injection reduced the proportion of people who repeated deliberate self harm over 6 months compared with placebo. However, we were unable to draw reliable conclusions from this small study. Typical antipsychotics such as flupentixol are associated with a wide range of adverse effects.

**Hospital admission**

One RCT found no significant difference between hospital admission and immediate discharge in the proportion of people who repeated deliberate self harm over 16 weeks, but it is likely to have been too small to exclude a clinically important difference.

**Intensive outpatient follow up plus outreach**

One systematic review found no significant difference in the proportion of people who repeated deliberate self harm over 4–12 months between intensive intervention plus outreach and usual care.

**Mianserin**

RCTs provided insufficient evidence to assess mianserin.

**Nurse led case management**

One RCT found no significant difference between nurse led case management⊕ and usual care in the proportion of people who were admitted to emergency departments for episodes of deliberate self harm over 12 months.

### Paroxetine

One RCT in people with deliberate self harm receiving psychotherapy found no significant difference between paroxetine and placebo in the proportion of people who repeated self harm over 12 months. It found that paroxetine increased diarrhoea and tremor compared with placebo.

### Problem solving therapy

One systematic review of small RCTs found no significant difference between problem solving therapy⊙ and usual care in the proportion of people who repeated deliberate self harm over 6-12 months. Another systematic review found that problem solving therapy reduced depression, anxiety, and hopelessness, and improved problems compared with usual care.

### Psychodynamic interpersonal therapy

One RCT found that psychodynamic interpersonal therapy⊙ for 4 weeks reduced repetition of deliberate self harm, depression, and suicidal ideation over 6 months compared with usual care. However, we were unable to draw reliable conclusions from one RCT.

### Same number of therapy sessions given over long term versus over short term

One systematic review of one RCT found no significant difference in the proportion of people who repeated deliberate self harm at 12 months with therapy given over 3 months compared with 12 months.

### Telephone contact

One RCT found no significant difference between telephone contact at 4 and 8 months and usual care in repetition of deliberate self harm, global functioning, and suicidal ideation over 12 months.

## UNLIKELY TO BE BENEFICIAL

### General practice based guidelines

One large cluster randomised trial comparing the use of general practitioner guidelines for management of deliberate self harm versus usual care found no significant difference in the proportion of people who repeated self harm over 12 months or in the time to repetition of self harm.

**DEFINITION**  Deliberate self harm is an acute non-fatal act of self harm carried out deliberately in the form of an acute episode of behaviour by an individual with variable motivation.[1] The intention to end life may be absent or present to a variable degree. Other terms used to describe this phenomenon are "attempted suicide" and "parasuicide". The terms are not entirely satisfactory. Common methods of deliberate self harm include self cutting and self poisoning, such as overdosing on medicines. Some acts of deliberate self harm are characterised by high suicidal intent, meticulous planning (including precautions against being found out), and severe lethality. Other acts of deliberate self harm are characterised by no or low intention of suicide, lack of planning and concealing of the act, and low lethality of the method used. The related term of "suicide" is defined as an act with a fatal outcome that is deliberately initiated and performed by the person with the knowledge or expectation of its fatal outcome.[1] This review focuses on recent deliberate self harm as the main presenting problem and excludes RCTs in which deliberate self harm is assessed as an outcome associated with other disorders, such as depression or borderline personality disorder. Deliberate self harm is not defined in the *Diagnostic and statistical manual of mental disorders* (DSM IV)[2] or the *International classification of mental and behavioural disorders* (ICD-10).[3]

◄ **INCIDENCE/**
**PREVALENCE**
Based on data from 16 European countries between 1989–1992, the lifetime prevalence of deliberate self harm in people treated in hospital and other medical facilities, including general practice settings, is estimated at about 3% for women and 2% for men.[4] Over the last 50 years there has been a rise in the incidence of deliberate self harm in the UK.[4] A reasonable current estimate is about 400/100 000 population a year.[5] In two community studies in the USA, 3–5% of responders said that they had made an attempt at deliberate self harm at some time.[6] Self poisoning using organophosphates is particularly common in developing countries.[7] A large hospital (catering for 900 000 people) in Sri Lanka, reported 2559 adult hospital admissions and 41% occupancy of medical intensive care beds for deliberate self harm with organophosphates over 2 years.[8] An international survey using representative community samples of adults (aged 18–64 years) reported lifetime prevalence of self reported suicide attempts of 3.82% in Canada, 5.93% in Puerto Rico, 4.95% in France, 3.44% in West Germany, 0.72% in Lebanon, 0.75% in Taiwan, 3.2% in Korea, and 4.43% in New Zealand.[6]

**AETIOLOGY/**
**RISK FACTORS**
Familial, biological, and psychosocial factors may contribute to deliberate self harm. Evidence for genetic factors includes a higher risk of familial suicide and greater concordance in monozygotic than dizygotic twins for deliberate self harm and suicide.[9] Evidence for biological factors includes reduced cerebrospinal fluid 5-hydroxyindole acetic acid (5-HIAA) levels and blunted prolactin response to fenfluramine challenge test, indicating a reduction in the function of serotonin in the central nervous system.[10] People who deliberately self harm also show traits of impulsiveness and aggression, inflexible and impulsive cognitive style, and impaired decision making and problem solving🄖.[11] Deliberate self harm is more likely in women, young adults, and people who are single or divorced, of low education level, unemployed, disabled, or suffering from a psychiatric disorder[12] particularly depression,[13] substance misuse,[14] borderline and antisocial personality disorders,[15] severe anxiety disorders,[16] and physical illness.[17]

**PROGNOSIS**
Suicide is highest during the first year after deliberate self harm.[18] One systematic review found median rates of repetition of deliberate self harm of 16.0% (interquartile range [IQR] 12.0% to 25.0%) within the first year, 21.0% (IQR 12.0% to 30.0%) within 1–4 years, and 23% (IQR 11% to 32%) within 4 years or longer. It found median mortality from suicide after deliberate self harm of 1.8% (IQR 0.8% to 2.6%) within the first year, 3.0% (IQR 2.0% to 4.4%) within 1–4 years, 3.4% (IQR 2.5% to 6.0%) within 5–10 years, and 6.7% (IQR 5.0% to 11.0%) within 9 years or longer.[18] Repetition of deliberate self harm is more likely in people aged 25–49 years, who are unemployed, divorced, from lower social class, or who suffer from substance misuse, depression, hopelessness, powerlessness, personality disorders, have unstable living conditions or live alone, have a criminal record, previous psychiatric treatment, a history of stressful traumatic life events, or a history of coming from broken home or of family violence.[12] Factor associated with risk of suicide after deliberate self harm are age over 45 years, male gender, unemployed or retired, separated, divorced, widowed, living alone, poor physical health, psychiatric disorder (particularly depression, alcoholism, schizophrenia, and sociopathic personality disorder), high suicidal intent in current episode including leaving a written note, violent method used in current attempt, and previous history of deliberate self harm.[19]

Please refer to CD-ROM for full text and references.

# Dementia

**Search date October 2002**

*James Warner, Rob Butler, and Pramod Prabhakaran*

## What are the effects of treatments on cognitive symptoms of dementia?

People in dementia RCTs are often not representative of people in routine settings. Few RCTs are conducted in primary care and few are conducted in people with types of dementia other than Alzheimer's disease.

### BENEFICIAL

**Donepezil**

One systematic review and two subsequent RCTs have found that, compared with placebo, donepezil improves cognitive function and global clinical state at up to 52 weeks in people with mild to moderate Alzheimer's disease. The review found no significant difference in patient rated quality of life at 12 or 24 weeks between donepezil and placebo. One RCT in people with mild to moderate Alzheimer's disease found no significant difference in cognitive function at 12 weeks between donepezil and rivastigmine, although significantly fewer people taking donepezil withdrew from the trial for any cause.

**Galantamine**

RCTs identified by a systematic review, and one additional RCT, have found that galantamine improves cognitive function compared with placebo in people with Alzheimer's disease or vascular dementia.

### LIKELY TO BE BENEFICIAL

**Ginkgo biloba**

RCTs found limited evidence that ginkgo biloba improved cognitive function compared with placebo in people with Alzheimer's disease.

**Oestrogen (in women)**

One systematic review has found that, in women with mild to moderate Alzheimer's disease, oestrogen improves cognition over 7–12 months treatment compared with no oestrogen.

**Reality orientation**

One systematic review of small RCTs found that reality orientation⊕ improved cognitive function compared with no treatment in people with various types of dementia.

**Selegiline**

One systematic review has found that, in people with mild to moderate Alzheimer's disease, selegiline improves cognitive function, behavioural disturbance, and mood compared with placebo, but has found no significant difference in global clinical state.

### TRADE OFF BETWEEN BENEFITS AND HARMS

**Physostigmine**

One systematic review in people with Alzheimer's disease found limited evidence that slow release physostigmine improved cognitive function compared with placebo, but adverse effects, including nausea, vomiting, diarrhoea, dizziness, and stomach pain, were common. ▶

◀ ## Rivastigmine

One systematic review and one additional RCT have found that rivastigmine improves cognitive function compared with placebo in people with Alzheimers disease or Lewy body dementia, but adverse effects such as nausea, vomiting, and anorexia are common. Subgroup analysis from one RCT in people with Alzheimer's disease suggests that people with vascular risk factors may respond better to rivastigmine than those without. One RCT in people with mild to moderate Alzheimer's disease found no significant difference in cognitive function at 12 weeks between donepezil and rivastigmine, although rivastigmine significantly increased the proportion of people who withdrew from the trial for any cause.

### UNKNOWN EFFECTIVENESS

### Lecithin

Small, poor RCTs identified by a systematic review provided insufficient evidence to assess lecithin in people with Alzheimer's disease.

### Music therapy

Poor studies identified by a systematic review provided insufficient evidence to assess music therapy.

### Nicotine

One systematic review found no RCTs of adequate quality on the effects of nicotine.

### Non-steroidal anti-inflammatory drugs

One RCT in people with Alzheimer's disease found no significant difference in cognitive function after 25 weeks' treatment with diclofenac plus misoprostol compared with placebo. Another RCT in people with Alzheimer's disease found that indometacin (indomethacin) improved cognitive function after 6 months' treatment compared with placebo.

### Reminiscence therapy

One systematic review provided insufficient evidence to assess reminiscence therapy☺.

### Tacrine

Systematic reviews found limited evidence that tacrine improved cognitive function and global state in Alzheimer's disease compared with placebo, but adverse effects, including nausea and vomiting, diarrhoea, anorexia, and abdominal pain, were common.

### Vitamin E

One RCT in people with moderate to severe Alzheimer's disease found no significant difference in cognitive function after 2 years' treatment with vitamin E compared with placebo. However, it found that vitamin E reduced mortality, institutionalisation, loss of ability to perform activities of daily living, and the proportion of people who developed severe dementia.

## What are the effects of treatments on behavioural and psychological symptoms of dementia?

### LIKELY TO BE BENEFICIAL

### Carbamazepine

One RCT found that carbamazepine reduced agitation and aggression compared with placebo in people with various types of dementia.

# Dementia

### Olanzapine

One RCT in people with Alzheimer's disease found that olanzapine (5–10 mg daily) reduced agitation, hallucinations, and delusions compared with placebo.

### Reality orientation

One systematic review of small RCTs found that reality orientation significantly improved behaviour compared with no treatment in people with various types of dementia.

### Risperidone

One RCT in people with moderate to severe dementia, including Alzheimer's disease and vascular dementia, found that risperidone significantly improved behavioural and psychological symptoms over 12 weeks compared with placebo, but another RCT in people with severe dementia and agitation found no significant difference in symptoms over 13 weeks.

## UNKNOWN EFFECTIVENESS

### Cholinesterase inhibitors

One RCT in people with mild to moderate Alzheimer's disease found no significant difference in psychiatric symptoms at 3 months between galantamine and placebo, but another RCT found that galantamine significantly improved psychiatric symptoms at 6 months compared with placebo. One RCT in people with moderate to severe Alzheimer's disease found that donepezil significantly improved functional and behavioural symptoms at 24 weeks compared with placebo, but another RCT in people with mild to moderate Alzheimer's disease found no significant difference in psychiatric symptoms at 24 weeks between donepezil and placebo.

### Haloperidol

One systematic review in people with various types of dementia found no significant difference in agitation between haloperidol and placebo, but found limited evidence that haloperidol may reduce aggression.

### Sodium valproate

One RCT found that sodium valproate reduced agitation over 6 weeks in people with dementia, but another RCT found no significant difference in aggressive behaviour over 8 weeks between sodium valproate and placebo.

### Trazodone

One RCT in people with Alzheimer's disease found no significant difference between trazodone and haloperidol in reducing agitation. Another RCT in people with dementia and agitated behaviour found no significant difference in agitation among trazodone, haloperidol, behavioural management techniques, and placebo. The RCTs may have been too small to exclude a clinically important difference.

**DEFINITION** **Dementia** is characterised by chronic, global, non-reversible impairment of cerebral function. It usually results in loss of memory (initially of recent events), loss of executive function (such as the ability to make decisions or sequence complex tasks), and changes in personality. **Alzheimer's disease** is a type of dementia characterised by an insidious onset and slow deterioration, and involves speech, motor, personality, and executive function impairment. It should be diagnosed after other systemic, psychiatric, and neurological causes of dementia have been excluded clinically and by laboratory investigation. **Vascular dementia** is multi-infarct dementia involving a step-wise deterioration of executive function with or without language and motor dysfunction occurring as a result of cerebral arterial occlusion. It usually occurs in the presence of vascular risk factors (diabetes, hypertension, and smoking). Characteristically, it has a more sudden onset and stepwise progression than Alzheimer's disease. **Lewy body dementia** is a type of dementia involving insidious impairment of executive functions with (1) Parkinsonism, (2) visual hallucinations, and (3) fluctuating cognitive abilities and increased risk of falls or autonomic failure.[1,2] Careful clinical examination of people with mild to moderate dementia, and the use of established diagnostic criteria, has an antemortem positive predictive value of 70–90% compared with the gold standard of postmortem diagnosis.[3,4]

**INCIDENCE/ PREVALENCE** About 6% of people aged over 65 years and 30% of people aged over 90 years have some form of dementia.[5] Dementia is rare before the age of 60 years. The most common types of dementia are Alzheimer's disease, vascular dementia, mixed vascular and Alzheimer's disease, and Lewy body dementia. Alzheimer's disease and vascular dementia (including mixed dementia) are each estimated to account for 35–50% of dementia, and Lewy body dementia is estimated to account for up to 20% of dementia in the elderly, varying with geographical, cultural, and racial factors.[1,5–10]

**AETIOLOGY/ RISK FACTORS** **Alzheimer's disease:** The cause of Alzheimer's disease is unclear. A key pathological process is deposition of abnormal amyloid in the central nervous system.[11] Most people with the relatively rare condition of early onset Alzheimer's disease (before age 60 years) show an autosomal dominant inheritance due to mutations on presenelin or amyloid precursor protein genes. Several genes (*APP*, *PS-1*, and *PS-2*) have been identified. Later onset dementia is sometimes clustered in families, but specific gene mutations have not been identified. Head injury, Down's syndrome, and lower premorbid intellect may be risk factors for Alzheimer's disease. **Vascular dementia** is related to cardiovascular risk factors, such as smoking, hypertension, and diabetes. **Lewy body dementia:** The aetiology of Lewy body dementia is unknown. Brain acetylcholine activity is reduced in many forms of dementia, and the level of reduction correlates with cognitive impairment. Many treatments for Alzheimer's disease enhance cholinergic activity.[1,6]

**PROGNOSIS** **Alzheimer's disease:** Alzheimer's disease usually has an insidious onset with progressive reduction in cerebral function. Diagnosis is difficult in the early stages. Average life expectancy after diagnosis is 7–10 years.[10] **Lewy body dementia:** People with Lewy body dementia have an average life expectancy of around 6 years after diagnosis.[5] Behavioural problems, depression, and psychotic symptoms are common in all types of dementia.[12,13] Eventually, most people with dementia find it difficult to perform simple tasks without help.

Please refer to CD-ROM for full text and references.

# Depressive disorders

**Search date July 2002**

*John Geddes, Rob Butler, and Simon Hatcher*

## What are the effects of treatments?

We found no reliable direct evidence that one type of treatment (drug or non-drug) is superior to another in improving symptoms of depression. However, we found strong evidence that some treatments are effective, whereas the effectiveness of others remains uncertain. Of the interventions examined, prescription antidepressant drugs and electroconvulsive therapy are the only treatments for which there is good evidence of effectiveness in severe and psychotic depressive disorders. We found no RCTs comparing drug and non-drug treatments in severe depressive disorders.

### BENEFICIAL

**Cognitive therapy (in mild to moderate depression)**

One systematic review in younger and older adults has found that cognitive therapy❸ significantly improves the symptoms of depression compared with no treatment.

**Continuation drug treatment in mild to moderate depression (reduces risk of relapse in mild to moderate depression)**

One systematic review and subsequent RCTs in younger and older adults have found that continuation treatment❸ with antidepressant drugs compared with placebo for 4–6 months after recovery significantly reduces the risk of relapse. One RCT in people aged over 60 years has found that continuation treatment with dosulepin (dothiepin) significantly reduces the risk of relapse over 2 years compared with placebo.

**Electroconvulsive therapy (in severe depression)**

Two systematic reviews and additional RCTs in people aged over 16 years have found that electroconvulsive therapy significantly improves symptoms in severe depression compared with simulated electroconvulsive therapy.

**Interpersonal psychotherapy (in mild to moderate depression)**

One large RCT has found that interpersonal psychotherapy❸ significantly improves rates of recovery from depression after 16 weeks compared with antidepressants or standard care.

**Prescription antidepressant drugs (in mild to moderate and severe depression)**

Systematic reviews in people aged 16 years or over have found that antidepressant drugs are effective in acute treatment of all grades of depressive disorders compared with placebo. Systematic reviews have found no significant difference in outcomes with different kinds of antidepressant drug. One systematic review in people aged 55 years or over with all grades of depressive disorder has found that tricyclic antidepressants, selective serotonin reuptake inhibitors, or monoamine oxidase inhibitors significantly reduce the proportion of people who fail to recover over 26–49 days compared with placebo. We found no specific evidence on adverse effects in older adults. However, the drugs differ in their adverse event profiles.

One systematic review found that monoamine oxidase inhibitors were less effective than tricyclic antidepressants in people with severe depressive disorders, but may be more effective in atypical depressive disorders with biological features such as increased sleep, increased appetite, mood reactivity, and rejection sensitivity. ▶

◄ One systematic review found that selective serotonin reuptake inhibitors were associated with a lower rate of adverse effects compared with tricyclic antidepressants, but the difference was small. Another systematic review and one retrospective cohort study found no strong evidence that fluoxetine was associated with increased risk of suicide compared with tricyclic antidepressants or placebo. One RCT and observational data suggest that abrupt withdrawal of selective serotonin reuptake inhibitors is associated with symptoms including dizziness, nausea, paraesthesia, headache, and vertigo, and that these symptoms are more likely with drugs with a short half life, such as paroxetine.

### Tricyclic antidepressants
One systematic review found that tricyclic antidepressants were associated with higher rates of adverse effects compared with selective serotonin reuptake inhibitors, but the difference was small.

## LIKELY TO BE BENEFICIAL

### Care pathways (in mild to moderate depression)
Five RCTs in people aged over 18 years found limited evidence that the effectiveness of antidepressant treatment may be improved by several approaches, including collaborative working between primary care clinicians and psychiatrists plus intensive patient education, case management, telephone support, and relapse prevention programmes. One RCT found that a clinical practice guideline and practice based education did not improve either detection or outcome of depression compared with usual care.

### Combining prescription antidepressant drug and psychological treatment (in mild to moderate and severe depression)
One non-systematic review of RCTs in people aged 18–80 years has found that, in people with severe depression, adding drug treatment to interpersonal psychotherapy or to cognitive therapy compared with either psychological treatment alone improves symptoms, but found no significant difference in symptoms in people with mild to moderate depression. Subsequent RCTs in younger and older adults with mild to moderate depression have found that combining antidepressants plus psychotherapy improves symptoms significantly more than either antidepressants or psychotherapy alone. One RCT in older adults with mild to moderate depression found that cognitive behavioural therapy⊙ plus desipramine improved symptoms significantly more than desipramine alone.

### Non-directive counselling (in mild to moderate depression)
One systematic review in people aged over 18 years with recent onset psychological problems, including depression, found that brief, non-directive counselling⊙ significantly reduced symptom scores in the short term (< 6 months) compared with usual care, but found no significant difference in scores in the long term (> 6 months).

### Problem solving treatment (in mild to moderate depression)
RCTs have found that problem solving treatment⊙ significantly improves symptoms over 3–6 months compared with placebo or control, and have found no significant difference in symptoms between problem solving treatment and drug treatment.

### St John's Wort (in mild to moderate depression)
Systematic reviews in people with mild to moderate depressive disorders have found that St John's Wort (Hypericum perforatum) significantly improves depressive symptoms over 4–12 weeks compared with placebo, and have found no significant difference in symptoms with St John's Wort compared with prescription antidepressant drugs. The results of the reviews should be interpreted with caution ►

# Depressive disorders

because the RCTs did not use standardised preparations of St John's Wort, and doses of antidepressants varied. One large subsequent RCT in people aged over 18 with major depressive disorder found no significant difference in depressive symptoms at 8 weeks between a standardised preparation of St John's Wort and placebo or sertraline, but it is likely to have been underpowered to detect a clinically important difference.

## UNKNOWN EFFECTIVENESS

### Befriending (in mild to moderate depression)
One small RCT provided insufficient evidence to assess befriending🔾.

### Bibliotherapy (in mild to moderate depression)
One systematic review of RCTs in younger and older adults recruited by advertisement found limited evidence that bibliotherapy🔾 may reduce mild depressive symptoms compared with waiting list control or standard care. Another systematic review in people with combined anxiety and depression, anxiety, or chronic fatigue found that bibliotherapy may improve symptoms over 2–6 months compared with standard care. It is unclear whether people in the RCTs identified by the reviews are clinically representative of people with depressive disorders.

### Care pathways versus usual care for long term outcomes (in mild to moderate depression)
One RCT found that a multifaceted "quality improvement programme" significantly improved symptoms and increased the proportion of people who returned to work over 1 year compared with usual care, but found no significant difference in outcomes at 2 years.

### Cognitive therapy versus antidepressants for long term outcomes (in mild to moderate depression)
One systematic review and one additional RCT in younger and older adults found limited evidence by combining relapse rates across different RCTs that cognitive therapy may reduce the risk of relapse over 2 years compared with antidepressants.

### Exercise (in mild to moderate depression)
One systematic review found limited evidence from poor RCTs that exercise may improve symptoms compared with placebo, and may be as effective as cognitive therapy or anitdepressants.

### Psychological treatments (cognitive therapy, interpersonal psychotherapy, and problem solving treatment) in severe depression
RCTs provided insufficient evidence to assess psychological treatments in severe depression.

**DEFINITION**    **Depressive disorders** are characterised by persistent low mood, loss of interest and enjoyment, and reduced energy. They often impair day to day functioning. Most of the RCTs assessed in this review classify depression using the *Diagnostic and statistical manual of mental disorders* (DSM IV)[1] or the *International classification of mental and behavioural disorders* (ICD-10).[2] DSM IV divides depression into major depressive disorder or dysthymic disorder. **Major depressive disorder** is characterised by one or more major depressive episodes (i.e. at least 2 wks of depressed mood or loss of interest accompanied by at least 4 additional symptoms of depression). **Dysthymic disorder** is characterised by at least 2 years of depressed mood for more days than not, accompanied by additional symptoms that do not reach the criteria for major depressive disorder.[1] ICD-10 divides depression into mild to moderate or severe depressive episodes.[2] **Mild to moderate depression** is characterised by depressive symptoms and some functional impairment. ▶

Severe depression is characterised by additional agitation or psychomotor retardation with marked somatic symptoms.[2] In this review, we use both DSM IV and ICD-10 classifications, but treatments are considered to have been assessed in severe depression if the RCT included inpatients. **Older adults:** Older adults are generally defined as people aged 65 years or older. However, some of the RCTs of older people in this review included people aged 55 years or over. The presentation of depression in older adults may be atypical: low mood may be masked and anxiety or memory impairment may be the principal presenting symptoms. Dementia should be considered in the differential diagnosis of depression in older adults.[3]

**INCIDENCE/ PREVALENCE** Depressive disorders are common, with a prevalence of major depression between 5% and 10% of people seen in primary care settings.[4] Two to three times as many people may have depressive symptoms but do not meet DSM IV criteria for major depression. Women are affected twice as often as men. Depressive disorders are the fourth most important cause of disability worldwide and they are expected to become the second most important cause by the year 2020.[5,6] **Older adults:** Between 10% and 15% of older people have depressive symptoms, although major depression is relatively rare in older adults.[7]

**AETIOLOGY/ RISK FACTORS** The causes are uncertain but include both childhood events and current psychosocial adversity.

**PROGNOSIS** About half of people suffering a first episode of major depressive disorder experience further symptoms in the next 10 years.[8] **Older adults:** One systematic review (search date 1996, 12 prospective cohort studies, 1268 people, mean age 60 years) found that the prognosis may be especially poor in elderly people with a chronic or relapsing course of depression.[9] Another systematic review (search date 1999, 23 prospective cohort studies in people aged > 65 years, including 5 identified by the first review) found that depression in older people was associated with increased mortality (15 studies; pooled OR 1.73, 95% CI 1.53 to 1.95).[10]

---

Please refer to CD-ROM for full text and references.

# Domestic violence

**Search date November 2002**

*Joanne Klevens and Laura Sadowski*

## What are the effects of interventions initiated by health care professionals, aimed at female victims of domestic violence, on the risk of reoccurrence? *New*

### LIKELY TO BE BENEFICIAL

**Advocacy**

One RCT and one non-randomised controlled trial found a reduction in reabuse with advocacy compared with no treatment. The RCT also found an improvement in women's quality of life with advocacy compared with no treatment. A controlled trial conducted in pregnant Hispanic women combining counselling with mentoring (similar to advocacy) found no significant differences in reabuse rates compared with a resource card, but found a small reduction in abuse when compared with unlimited counselling. A small RCT and a non-randomised controlled trial found no effects of advocacy on the reoccurrence of abuse but reported increased use of intimate partner violence services and resources by women assigned to advocates.

### UNKNOWN EFFECTIVENESS

**Cognitive behaviour orientated counselling**

One controlled trial found cognitive behaviour orientated therapy to be better than non-specific support in improving women's assertiveness and reducing exposure to abuse.

**Couple counselling**

One RCT and one non-randomised controlled trial comparing gender specific counselling versus couples counselling found a reduction in levels of physical aggression. In addition, the non-randomised controlled trial found reductions in psychological aggression and depression in wives compared with baseline values. No differences were found between treatments. One controlled trial found no difference between group and individual couple counselling on reduction in physical violence or on psychological wellbeing.

**Grief resolution orientated counselling**

One controlled trial found grief resolution orientated counselling to be better than feminist orientated counselling in improving self esteem and self efficacy.

**Peer support groups**

We found no systematic reviews or controlled trials on the effect of peer support groups.

**Safety planning**

We found no comparisons of safety planning in isolation versus other types of interventions. One controlled trial conducted in pregnant women that included safety planning along with advocacy, counselling, and a brochure found a decrease in spouse abuse and an increase in safety behaviours among the women receiving the intervention compared with women receiving a wallet sized card with information on community resources.

**Shelters for women engaged in help seeking behaviour**

We found evidence from a comparative cohort study on the utility of shelters but only in women who engage in other types of help seeking behaviour.

◀ **UNLIKELY TO BE BENEFICIAL**

### Unspecified orientation of counselling

Two controlled trials and one comparative cohort study found no effect of counselling compared with no treatment on medical care utilisation rates, reported exposure to violence and threats of violence, or depression, anxiety, and self esteem.

**DEFINITION** Domestic violence, also called intimate partner violence, is actual or threatened physical or sexual violence, or emotional or psychological abuse (including coercive tactics) by a current or former spouse or dating partner (including same sex partners).[1] Other terms commonly used to describe intimate partner violence include domestic violence or abuse, spouse abuse, marital violence, and battering.

**INCIDENCE/ PREVALENCE** Between 10% and 69% of women participating in population based surveys in 48 countries from around the world reported being physically assaulted by a partner during their lifetime.[2] Rates of assault by a partner are 4.3 times higher among women than men.[3] Nearly 25% of surveyed women in the USA reported being physically and/or sexually assaulted by a current or former partner at some time during their lives and 1.5% were victimised during the previous 12 months.[3] Rates of violence against pregnant women range from 0.9% to 20%.[4] Between 11.7–24.5% of women in prenatal clinics[5–8] and 5.5–17% of women in primary or ambulatory care reported being abused by a partner in the past year.[9–12]

**AETIOLOGY/ RISK FACTORS** A recent systematic review found that physical domestic violence in women is associated with lower levels of education and unemployment, low family income, marital discord, and with the partner's lower level of occupation, childhood experiences of abuse, witnessing interparental violence, higher levels of anger, depression, heavy or problem drinking, drug use, jealousy, and lack of assertiveness with spouse.[13] A similar review of research on psychological aggression found that the few demographic and psychological variables assessed either were inconsistently associated with psychological domestic violence or were found to be associated with psychological domestic violence in studies with serious methodological limitations.[14]

**PROGNOSIS** There are few prospective studies documenting the course of domestic violence and its outcomes. Cross-sectional surveys suggest that domestic violence is a repetitive event for at least two thirds of women.[15,16] Among black and Hispanic people persistence of domestic violence appears to be dependent on initial severity.[17] For all ethnic groups, half of those reporting moderate domestic violence have remission, but for people of black or Hispanic origin reporting severe domestic violence only a third reach remission. A case control study conducted in middle class working women found that, compared with non-abused women, women abused by their partners during the previous 9 years were significantly more likely to have or report headaches (48% v 35%), back pain (40% v 25%), sexually transmitted diseases (6% v 2%), vaginal bleeding (17% v 6%), vaginal infections (30% v 21%), pelvic pain (17% v 9%), painful intercourse (13% v 7%), urinary tract infections (22% v 12%), appetite loss (9% v 3%), digestive problems (35% v 19%), abdominal pain (22% v 11%), and facial injuries (8% v 1%).[18] After adjusting for age, race, insurance status, and cigarette smoking, a cross-sectional survey found that women experiencing psychological abuse are also more likely to report poor physical and mental health, disability preventing work, arthritis, chronic pain, migraine and other frequent headaches, sexually transmitted infections, chronic pelvic pain, stomach ulcers, spastic colon, frequent indigestion, diarrhoea, or constipation 🜚.[19]

---

Please refer to CD-ROM for full text and references.

# Generalised anxiety disorder

**Search date October 2002**

*Christopher Gale and Mark Oakley-Browne*

Mental health

---

## What are the effects of treatments?

### LIKELY TO BE BENEFICIAL

#### Buspirone

RCTs have found that buspirone versus placebo significantly improves symptoms compared with placebo over 4–9 weeks. RCTs found no significant difference in symptoms over 6–8 weeks with buspirone versus antidepressants, diazepam, or hydroxyzine, but the studies may have lacked power to detect clinically important differences among treatment.

#### Certain antidepressants (imipramine, opipramol, paroxetine, trazodone, venlafaxine)

One systematic review and four additional RCTs have found that antidepressants (imipramine, opipramol, paroxetine, trazodone, and venlafaxine) versus placebo significantly improve symptoms over 4–8 weeks. RCTs found no significant difference among these antidepressants or between antidepressants and benzodiazepines or buspirone. RCTs and observational studies have found that antidepressants are associated with sedation, dizziness, nausea, falls, and sexual dysfunction.

#### Cognitive therapy

Two systematic reviews have found limited evidence that cognitive behavioural therapy❻, using a combination of interventions, such as exposure, relaxation, and cognitive restructuring, improves anxiety and depression over 4–12 weeks compared with waiting list control, anxiety management training alone, relaxation training alone, or non-directive psychotherapy. Two subsequent RCTs found no significant difference in symptoms for cognitive therapy❻ versus applied relaxation at 13 weeks and 24 months.

### TRADE OFF BETWEEN BENEFITS AND HARMS

#### Benzodiazepines

One systematic review and one subsequent RCT found limited evidence that benzodiazepines versus placebo reduced symptoms over 2–9 weeks. However, RCTs and observational studies found that benzodiazepines increased the risk of dependence, sedation, industrial accidents, and road traffic accidents. One non-systematic review found that, if used in late pregnancy or while breast feeding, benzodiazepines may cause adverse effects in neonates. One RCT found no significant difference in symptoms of anxiety with sustained release alprazolam versus bromazepam, and another RCT found no significant difference in overall symptoms with mexazolam versus alprazolam. Limited evidence from RCTs found no significant difference in symptoms over 6–8 weeks with benzodiazepines versus buspirone, abecarnil, or antidepressants. One systematic review of poor quality RCTs found insufficient evidence about the effects of long term treatment with benzodiazepines.

#### Kava

One systematic review in people with anxiety, including generalised anxiety disorder (GAD), found that kava versus placebo significantly reduced symptoms of anxiety over 4 weeks. Observational evidence suggests that kava may be associated with hepatotoxicity.

### UNKNOWN EFFECTIVENESS

#### Abecarnil

RCTs found conflicting evidence of the effects of abecarnil versus placebo in improving symptoms.

#### Antipsychotic drugs

We found limited evidence from one RCT that trifluoperazine significantly reduced anxiety compared with placebo after 4 weeks, but caused more drowsiness, extrapyramidal reactions, and other movement disorders.

#### Applied relaxation

We found no RCTs of applied relaxation⊕ versus placebo or no treatment. One RCT found no significant difference in symptoms at 13 weeks for applied relaxation versus cognitive behaviour therapy.

#### β Blockers

We found no RCTs on the effects of β blockers.

#### Hydroxyzine

Two RCTs compared hydroxyzine versus placebo and found different results. After about 1 month, one RCT found that hydroxyzine versus placebo significantly improved symptoms of anxiety, but the other found no significant difference between treatments. One further RCT found no significant difference for hydroxyzine versus buspirone after 28 days. We found no RCTs of longer term treatment.

**DEFINITION**   GAD is defined as excessive worry and tension about every day events and problems, on most days, for at least 6 months, to the point where the person experiences distress or has marked difficulty in performing day-to-day tasks.[1] It may be characterised by the following symptoms and signs: increased motor tension (fatigability, trembling, restlessness, and muscle tension); autonomic hyperactivity (shortness of breath, rapid heart rate, dry mouth, cold hands, and dizziness); and increased vigilance and scanning (feeling keyed up, increased startling, and impaired concentration), but not panic attacks.[1] One non-systematic review of epidemiological and clinical studies found marked reduction of quality of life and psychosocial functioning in people with anxiety disorders (including GAD).[2] It also found that people with GAD have low overall life satisfaction and some impairment in ability to fulfil roles, social tasks, or both.[2]

**INCIDENCE/**   One overview found that the prevalence of GAD among adults in the commu-
**PREVALENCE**   nity is 1.5–3.0%.[3] It found that 3–5% of adults have had GAD in the past year and 4–7% have had GAD during their life. One non-systematic review identified the US National Comorbidity Survey, which found that over 90% of people diagnosed with GAD had a co-morbid diagnosis, including dysthymia (22%), depression (39–69%), somatisation, other anxiety disorders, bipolar disorder, or substance abuse.[4] The reliability of the measures used to diagnose GAD in epidemiological studies is unsatisfactory.[5,6] One US study, with explicit diagnostic criteria (DSM-III-R), estimated that 5% of people will develop GAD at some time during their lives.[6] A recent cohort study of people with depressive and anxiety disorders found that 49% of people initially diagnosed with GAD retained this diagnosis over 2 years.[7] One non-systematic review found that the incidence of GAD in men is only half the incidence in women.[8] One non-systematic review of seven epidemiological studies found reduced prevalence of anxiety disorders in older people.[9] Another non-systematic review of 20 observational studies in younger and older adults suggested that autonomic arousal to stressful tasks is decreased in older people, and that older people become accustomed to stressful tasks more quickly than younger people.[10]

# Generalised anxiety disorder

**AETIOLOGY/ RISK FACTORS**

One community study and a clinical study have found that GAD is associated with an increase in the number of minor stressors, independent of demographic factors,[11,12] but this finding was common in people with other diagnoses in the clinical population.[7] One non-systematic review (5 case control studies) of psychological sequelae to civilian trauma found that rates of GAD reported in four of the five studies were increased significantly compared with a control population (rate ratio 3.3, 95% CI 2.0 to 5.5).[13] One systematic review of cross-sectional studies found that bullying (or peer victimisation) was associated with a significant increase in the incidence of GAD (effect size 0.21).[14] One systematic review (search date not stated) of the genetic epidemiology of anxiety disorders (including GAD) identified two family studies and three twin studies.[15] The family studies (45 index cases, 225 first degree relatives) found a significant association between GAD in the index cases and in their first degree relatives (OR 6.1, 95% CI 2.5 to 14.9). The twin studies (13 305 people) estimated that 32% (95% CI 24% to 39%) of the variance to liability to GAD was explained by genetic factors.[15]

**PROGNOSIS**

One systematic review found that 25% of adults with GAD will be in full remission after 2 years, and 38% will have a remission after 5 years.[3]

Please refer to CD-ROM for full text and references.

### Search date January 2003
*G Mustafa Soomro*

## What are the effects of initial treatments in adults?

### BENEFICIAL

#### Behavioural therapy

We found no RCTs comparing behaviourla therapy versus no treatment. One systematic review and subsequent RCTs have found that behavioural therapy❶ improves symptoms compared with relaxation. The review and one subsequent RCT found no significant difference in symptoms over 4–13 weeks between behavioural therapy and cognitive therapy❶. One additional RCT found limited evidence that group behavioural therapy improved symptoms after 12 weeks compared with group cognitive therapy.

#### Cognitive therapy

We found no RCTs comparing cognitive therapy versus no treatment. One systematic review and one subsequent RCT found no significant difference in symptoms over 4–13 weeks between behavioural therapy and cognitive therapy. Another subsequent RCT found limited evidence that group cognitive therapy was less effective in reducing symptoms over 12 weeks than group behavioural therapy.

#### Serotonin reuptake inhibitors (citalopram, clomipramine, fluoxetine, fluvoxamine, paroxetine, sertraline)

RCTs have found that selective and non-selective serotonin reuptake inhibitors (citalopram, clomipramine, fluoxetine, fluvoxamine, paroxetine) reduce symptoms compared with placebo. Two systematic reviews found inconsistent results about the effects of sertraline compared with placebo. RCTs have found that selective and non-selective serotonin reuptake inhibitors (citalopram, clomipramine, fluoxetine, fluvoxamine, paroxetine, sertraline) reduce symptoms compared with tricyclic antidepressants or monoamine oxidase inhibitors. RCTs have found no consistent evidence of a difference in efficacy among serotonin reuptake inhibitors, but have found that the non-selective serotonin reuptake inhibitor clomipramine is associated with more adverse effects than selective serotonin reuptake inhibitors.

### UNKNOWN EFFECTIVENESS

#### Behavioural or cognitive therapy plus selective and non-selective serotonin serotonin reuptake inhibitors (compared with behavioural or cognitive therapy alone)

RCTs provided insufficient evidence to assess the effects of adding serotonin reuptake inhibitors to behavioural or cognitive therapy.

#### Electroconvulsive therapy

We found no RCTs of electroconvulsive therapy in people with obsessive compulsive disorder.

#### Venlafaxine

One RCT provided insufficient evidence to compare vanlafaxine versus clomipramine.

# Obsessive compulsive disorder

## What is the optimum duration of maintenance treatment with selective and non-selective reuptake inhibitors?

### UNKNOWN EFFECTIVENESS

**Optimum duration of treatment with selective and non-selective serotonin reuptake inhibitors**

RCTs provided insufficient evidence to define the optimum duration of treatment with serotonin reuptake inhibitors.

## What are the effects of treatments in adults who have not responded to initial treatment with serotonin reuptake inhibitors?

### LIKELY TO BE BENEFICIAL

**Addition of antipsychotics in people who have not responded to serotonin reuptake inhibitors**

Three small RCTs in people unresponsive to serotonin reuptake inhibitors found that the addition of antipsychotics improved symptoms compared with placebo.

**DEFINITION**  Obsessive compulsive disorder involves obsessions and/or compulsions that are not caused by drugs or a physical disorder, and which cause significant personal distress or social dysfunction.[1,2] The disorder may have a chronic🅖 or an episodic🅖 course. **Obsessions** are recurrent and persistent ideas, images, or impulses that cause pronounced anxiety and that the person perceives to be self produced. **Compulsions** are repetitive behaviours or mental acts performed in response to obsessions or according to certain rules, which are aimed at reducing distress or preventing certain imagined dreaded events. People with obsessive compulsive disorder may have insight into their condition, in that obsessions and compulsions are usually recognised and resisted. There are minor differences in the criteria for obsessive compulsive disorder between the third, revised third, and fourth editions of the *Diagnostic and Statistical Manual*: DSM-III, DSM-III-R, and DSM-IV[1] and *The ICD-10 classification of mental and behavioural disorders*.[2]

**INCIDENCE/ PREVALENCE**  One national, community based survey of obsessive compulsive disorder in the UK (1993, 10 000 people) found that 1% of men and 1.5% of women reported symptoms in the last month.[3] A survey in the USA (18 500 people) found a lifetime prevalence of obsessive compulsive disorder of between 1.9 and 3.3% in 1984.[4] An international study found a lifetime prevalence of 3% in Canada, 3.1% in Puerto Rico, 0.3–0.9% in Taiwan, and 2.2% in New Zealand.[3]

**AETIOLOGY/ RISK FACTORS**  The aetiology of obsessive compulsive disorder is uncertain. Behavioural, cognitive, genetic, and neurobiological factors have been implicated.[5–11] Risk factors include a family history of obsessive compulsive disorder, being single (which could be consequence of the disorder), and belonging to a higher socioeconomic class.[12]

**PROGNOSIS**  One study (144 people followed for a mean of 47 years) found that an episodic course of obsessive compulsive disorder was more common during the initial years (about 1–9 years), but a chronic course was more common afterwards.[13] Over time, the study found that 39–48% of people had symptomatic improvement. A 1 year prospective cohort study found 46% of people had an episodic course and 54% had a chronic course.[14]

Please refer to CD-ROM for full text and references.

Search date January 2003

*Shailesh Kumar and Mark Oakley Browne*

## What are the effects of drug treatments?

### BENEFICIAL

#### Selective serotonin reuptake inhibitors

Systematic reviews and one additional RCT have found that selective serotonin reuptake inhibitors improve symptoms in panic disorder compared with placebo. One subsequent RCT found that discontinuation of sertraline in people with a good response increased exacerbation of symptoms. A second subsequent RCT found that paroxetine plus cognitive behavioural therapy⊙ improved symptoms compared with placebo plus cognitive behavioural therapy.

#### Tricyclic antidepressants (imipramine)

One systematic review, one subsequent RCT and one additional RCT have found that imipramine improves symptoms compared with placebo. One subsequent RCT found that imipramine reduced relapse rates over 12 months.

### TRADE OFF BETWEEN BENEFITS AND HARMS

#### Benzodiazepines

One systematic review and one additional RCT have found that alprazolam reduces the number of panic attacks and improves symptoms compared with placebo. However, benzodiazepines are associated with a wide range of adverse effects both during and after treatment.

### UNKNOWN EFFECTIVENESS

#### Buspirone

We found insufficient evidence to assess the effects of buspirone compared with placebo.

#### Monoamine oxidase inhibitors

We found no RCTs on the effects of monoamine oxidase inhibitors.

**DEFINITION**
A panic attack is a period in which there is sudden onset of intense apprehension, fearfulness, or terror often associated with feelings of impending doom. Panic disorder occurs when there are recurrent, unpredictable attacks followed by at least 1 month of persistent concern about having another panic attack, worry about the possible implications or consequences of the panic attacks, or a significant behavioural change related to the attacks.[1] The term panic disorder excludes panic attacks attributable to the direct physiological effects of a general medical condition, substance, or another mental disorder. Panic disorder is sometimes categorised as with or without agoraphobia.[1] Alternative categorisations focus on phobic anxiety disorders and specify agoraphobia with or without panic disorder.[2]

**INCIDENCE/ PREVALENCE**
Panic disorder often starts at around 20 years of age (between late adolescence and the mid 30s).[3] Lifetime prevalence is between 1–3%, and panic disorder is more common in women than in men.[4] An Australian community study found 1 month prevalence rates for panic disorder (with or without agoraphobia) of 0.4% using International Classification of Diseases (ICD)-10 diagnostic criteria and of 0.5% using Diagnostic and Statistical Manual (DSM)-IV diagnostic criteria.[5]

# Panic disorder

**AETIOLOGY/ RISK FACTORS** Stressful life events tend to precede the onset of panic disorder,[6,7] although a negative interpretation of these events in addition to their occurrence has been suggested as an important casual factor.[8] Panic disorder is associated with major depression,[9] social phobia, generalised anxiety disorder, obsessive compulsive disorder,[10] and a substantial risk of drug and alcohol abuse.[11] It is also associated with avoidant, histrionic, and dependent personality disorders.[10]

**PROGNOSIS** The severity of symptoms in people with panic disorder fluctuates considerably, with periods of no attacks, or only mild attacks with few symptoms, being common. There is often a long delay between the initial onset of symptoms and presentation for treatment. Recurrent attacks may continue for a number of years, especially if associated with agoraphobia. Reduced social or occupational functioning varies among people with panic disorder and is worse in people with associated agoraphobia. Panic disorder is also associated with an increased rate of attempted but unsuccessful suicide.[12] One study analysing RCT and systematic review data found that co-existence of anxiety and depressive features adversely affects treatment response at 12 years compared with panic disorder alone.[13]

Please refer to CD-ROM for full text and references.

Search date September 2002

*Jonathan Bisson*

## What are the effects of preventive psychological interventions?

### LIKELY TO BE BENEFICIAL

**Multiple episode cognitive behavioural therapy in people with acute stress disorder**

Two small RCTs in people with acute stress disorder after a traumatic event (accident or non-sexual assault) found that five sessions of cognitive behavioural therapy⊙ significantly reduces the proportion of people with post-traumatic stress disorder after 6 months compared with supportive counselling⊙.

### UNKNOWN EFFECTIVENESS

**Multiple episode cognitive behavioural therapy in all people exposed to a traumatic event**

One RCT in bus drivers who had been attacked in the past 5 months found that cognitive behavioural therapy significantly improved measures of anxiety and intrusive symptoms at 6 months compared with usual care, but found no significant difference in measures of depression or avoidance symptoms. Another RCT comparing cognitive behavioural therapy versus standard care in people who had been exposed to a traumatic event in the past 5–12 months found no significant difference in overall symptoms of post-traumatic stress disorder at 6 months.

**Multiple episode memory restructuring**

One RCT provided insufficient evidence to assess memory restructuring compared with supportive care in people exposed to a traumatic event in the past 24 hours.

**Multiple episode trauma support**

Two RCTs provided insufficient evidence to assess collaborative care⊙ interventions involving emotional, social, and practical support in people exposed to a traumatic event in the past 1 day to 1 week.

### UNLIKELY TO BE BENEFICIAL

**Single episode psychological interventions ("debriefing") in all people exposed to a traumatic event**

RCTs in people who had been exposed to a traumatic event in the previous month found no significant difference between a single session of psychological debriefing⊙ and no debriefing in the incidence of post-traumatic stress disorder at 3 months or 1 year.

## What are the effects of treatments?

### BENEFICIAL

**Cognitive behavioural therapy**

RCTs have found that cognitive behavioural therapy significantly improves post-traumatic stress disorder symptoms, anxiety, and depression compared with no treatment or supportive counselling.

▶

# Post-traumatic stress disorder

### Eye movement desensitisation and reprocessing

RCTs have found that eye movement desensitisation and reprocessing ⊕ improves symptoms compared with waiting list control or relaxation treatment debriefing⊕. Two RCTs found no significant difference in symptoms between eye movement desensitisation and reprocessing compared with exposure therapy.

### Paroxetine

One systematic review and subsequent RCTs found that paroxetine reduced symptoms at 3 months compared with placebo.

### Sertraline

One systematic review and subsequent RCTs found that sertraline significantly reduced symptoms at 3–7months compared with placebo.

## LIKELY TO BE BENEFICIAL

### Fluoxetine

Two RCTs found that fluoxetine may reduce symptoms at 3 months compared with placebo.

## UNKNOWN EFFECTIVENESS

**Affect management⊕; drama therapy⊕; hypnotherapy⊕; inpatient programmes; other drug treatments (brofaromine, amitriptyline, lamotrigine, imipramine, phenelzine, nefazodone, carbamazepine, antipsychotics, benzodiazepines); psychodynamic psychotherapy⊕; supportive counselling**

We found insufficient evidence about the effects of these interventions in improving symptoms.

**DEFINITION**     Post-traumatic stress disorder can occur after a major traumatic event. Symptoms include upsetting thoughts and nightmares about the traumatic event, avoidance behaviour, numbing of general responsiveness, increased irritability, and hypervigilance for at least 1 month.[1] Acute stress disorder occurs within the first month after a major traumatic event and requires the presence of symptoms for at least 2 days. It is similar to post-traumatic stress disorder but more dissociative symptoms are required to make the diagnosis.

**INCIDENCE/**     One large cross-sectional study in the USA found that 1/10 women and 1/20
**PREVALENCE**     men experience post-traumatic stress disorder at some stage in their lives.[2]

**AETIOLOGY/**     Risk factors include major trauma, such as rape, a history of psychiatric
**RISK FACTORS**  disorders, acute distress and depression after the trauma, lack of social support, and personality factors (such as neuroticism).[3]

**PROGNOSIS**     One large cross-sectional study in the USA found that over a third of sufferers continued to satisfy the criteria for a diagnosis of post-traumatic stress disorder 6 years after diagnosis.[2] However, cross-sectional studies provide weak evidence about prognosis.

Please refer to CD-ROM for full text and references.

### Search date December 2002

*Zia Nadeem, Andrew McIntosh, and Stephen Lawrie*

## What are the effects of treatments?

Most evidence is from systematic reviews of RCTs that report disparate outcomes. There is a need for larger RCTs, over longer periods, with well designed end points, including standardised, validated symptom scales. No intervention has been found to consistently reduce negative symptoms.

### BENEFICIAL

**Continuation of antipsychotic drugs for 6–9 months after an acute episode to reduce relapse rates**

Systematic reviews have found that continuing antipsychotic drugs for at least 6 months after an acute episode reduces relapse rates compared with no treatment or placebo, and that some benefit of continuing antipsychotics is apparent for up to 2 years.

**Multiple session family interventions to reduce relapse rates**

One systematic review found that multiple session family interventions reduced relapse rates at 12 months compared with usual care, single session family interventions, or psychoeducational interventions.

**Psychoeducational interventions to reduce relapse rates**

One systematic review has found that psychoeducation reduces relapse rates at 9–18 months compared with a control intervention.

### LIKELY TO BE BENEFICIAL

**Behavioural therapy to improve adherence**

One RCT found that behavioural interventions improved adherence to antipsychotic medication over 3 months compared with usual treatment. Two RCTs found limited evidence that behavioural interventions may improve adherence more than psychoeducational therapy.

**Compliance therapy to improve adherence**

Two RCTs found limited evidence that compliance therapy **G** may increase adherence to antipsychotic drugs at 6 and 18 months compared with non-specific counselling.

**Psychoeducational interventions to improve adherence**

One systematic review found limited evidence that psychoeducation improved adherence to antipsychotic medication compared with usual care. Two RCTs found limited evidence that psychoeducational therapy may improve adherence less than behavioural therapy.

### TRADE OFF BETWEEN BENEFITS AND HARMS

### Chlorpromazine

One systematic review has found that, compared with placebo, chlorpromazine reduces the proportion of people who have no improvement, or have marked or worse severity of illness at 6 months on a psychiatrist rated scale. The review found that chlorpromazine caused more adverse effects, such as sedation, acute dystonia, and parkinsonism, than placebo.

# Schizophrenia

### Clozapine
Two systematic reviews found that clozapine improved symptoms over 4–10 weeks compared with standard antipsychotic drugs. However, RCTs found that clozapine may be associated with blood dyscrasias. Three systematic reviews of small RCTs provided insufficient evidence to compare clozapine versus other new antipsychotic drugs. One systematic review in people resistant to standard treatment found that clozapine improved symptoms after 12 weeks and after 2 years compared with standard antipsychotic drugs. RCTs provided insufficient evidence to compare clozapine versus other newer antipsychotics in people resistant to standard antipsychotic drugs.

### Depot bromperidol decanoate
RCTs found no significant difference in the proportion of people who needed additional medication, left the trial early, or had movement disorders over 6–12 months between depot bromperidol decanoate and haloperidol or fluphenazine decanoate.

### Depot haloperidol decanoate
One systematic review of one small RCT found no significant difference in global clinical state at 4 months between depot haloperidol decanoate and oral haloperidol, but it may have been too small to exclude a clinically important difference. Haloperidol is associated with acute dystonia, akathisia, and parkinsonism.

### Haloperidol
One systematic review has found that haloperidol increases physician rated global improvement at 6 and 24 weeks compared with placebo but is associated with acute dystonia, akathisia, and parkinsonism.

### Thioridazine
One systematic review has found that thioridazine improves global mental state over 3–12 months compared with placebo.

### Amisulpride; loxapine; molindone; olanzapine; pimozide; quetiapine; risperidone; sulpiride; ziprasidone; zotepine
Systematic reviews have found that these newer antipsychotic drugs are as effective in improving symptoms as standard antipsychotic drugs, and have different profiles of adverse effects.

## UNKNOWN EFFECTIVENESS

### Cognitive behavioural therapy to reduce relapse rates
Limited evidence from a systematic review of two RCTs found no significant difference in relapse rates between cognitive behavioural therapy plus standard care and standard care alone.

### Multiple session family interventions to improve adherence
One systematic review found that "compliance with medication" over 9–24 months was higher in people who received multiple family interventions compared with usual care, single family interventions, or psychoeducational interventions, but the difference did not quite reach significance.

### Perazine
RCTs provided insufficient evidence to assess perazine.

### Social skills training to reduce relapse rates
One systematic review of small RCTs provided insufficient evidence to assess social skills training.

◄ **DEFINITION** Schizophrenia is characterised by the positive symptoms**ⓖ** of auditory hallu-cinations, delusions, and thought disorder, and by the negative symptoms**ⓖ** of demotivation, self neglect, and reduced emotion.[1] People are defined as being resistant to standard antipsychotic drugs if, over the preceding 5 years, they have not had a clinically important improvement in symptoms after 2–3 regimens of treatment with standard antipsychotic drugs for at least 6 weeks (from at least 2 classes at doses equivalent to or greater than 1000 mg/day chlorpromazine) and they have had no period of good functioning.[2,3] Approxi-mately 30% (10–45%) of people with schizophrenia meet these criteria.[3]

**INCIDENCE/** Onset of symptoms typically occurs in early adult life (average age 25 years) **PREVALENCE** and is earlier in men than women.[4,5] Prevalence worldwide is 2–4/1000. One in 100 people will develop schizophrenia in their lifetime.

**AETIOLOGY/** Risk factors include a family history (although no major genes have been **RISK FACTORS** identified); obstetric complications; developmental difficulties; central nervous system infections in childhood; cannabis use; and acute life events.[4] The precise contributions of these factors and ways in which they may interact are unclear.

**PROGNOSIS** About three quarters of people suffer recurrent relapse and continued disability, although the proportion of people who improved significantly increased after the mid-1950s (mean 48.5% from 1956–1985 v 35.4% from 1895–1956).[6] Outcome may be worse in people with insidious onset and delayed initial treatment, social isolation, or a strong family history; in people living in industrialised countries; in men; and in people who misuse drugs.[5] Drug treatment is generally successful in treating positive symptoms, but up to a third of people derive little benefit and negative symptoms are notoriously difficult to treat. About half of people with schizophrenia do not adhere to treatment in the short term. The figure is even higher in the longer term.[7]

Please refer to CD-ROM for full text and references.

# Acute gout

**Search date December 2002**

*Martin Underwood*

---

## What are the effects of treatments for acute gout? New

**UNKNOWN EFFECTIVENESS**

### Non-steroidal anti-inflammatory drugs

We found limited evidence from one RCT that tenoxicam reduced short term pain and tenderness in acute gout compared with placebo. However, we were unable to draw reliable conclusions from this small study. We found no evidence of the effects of other non-steroidal anti-inflammatory drugs compared with placebo in acute gout. We found insufficient evidence on the relative benefits and harms of different non-steroidal anti-inflammatory drugs.

### Oral colchicine

We found limited evidence from one small RCT that colchicine improved pain in acute gout. However, we were unable to draw reliable conclusions from this small study.

### Intra-articular corticosteroids; oral corticosteroids; parenteral corticosteroids

We found no evidence on the effects of intra-articular, parenteral, or oral corticosteroids for acute gout.

---

## What are the effects of treatments to prevent recurrent gout? New

**UNKNOWN EFFECTIVENESS**

### Advice to reduce alcohol intake; advice to reduce dietary intake of purines; allopurinol; benzbromarone; colchicine; probenecid; sulphinpyrazone; weight reduction advice

We found insufficient evidence on effects of these treatments to prevent attacks of recurrent gout.

**DEFINITION**  Gout is a syndrome caused by deposition of urate crystals.[1] It typically presents as an acute monoarthritis of rapid onset. The first metatarsal phalangeal joint is the most commonly affected joint (podagra). Acute gout also affects other joints: joints in the foot, ankle, knee, wrist, finger, and elbow are the most frequently affected. Crystal deposits (tophi) may develop around hands, feet, elbows, and ears. The diagnosis is usually made clinically. The American College of Rheumatology (ACR) criteria for diagnosing gout are a) characteristic urate crystals in joint fluid, b) a tophus proved to contain urate crystals, or c) the presence of six or more defined clinical laboratory and x ray phenomena❶.[2] We have included studies of people meeting the ACR classification criteria for acute gout and studies that used other criteria or where the diagnosis was made clinically.

**INCIDENCE/ PREVALENCE**  Prevalence data from general practice records suggest that gout is more common in older people and men.[3] In people aged 65–74 years in the UK, the prevalence is about 50/1000 in men and about 9/1000 in women.[3] The annual incidence of gout in the USA is 1.6/1000 men and 0.3/1000 for women aged over 50 years.[4] Gout may be more common in some non-white ▶

ethnic groups. Cohort studies of male former medical students found the annual incidence of gout to be 3.1/1000 person-years in black people and 1.8/1000 person-years in white people. After correcting for incident hypertension, the relative risk of gout was 1.3 (95% CI 0.77 to 2.19).[5]

**AETIOLOGY/ RISK FACTORS**
Urate crystals form when serum urate concentration exceeds 0.42 mmol/L.[6] Serum urate concentration is the principal risk factor for a first attack of gout,[7] although the concentration may be normal in 40% of people if measured during an attack of gout.[6,8–10] A cohort study of 2046 men followed for about 15 years found that the annual incidence is about 0.4% in men with a urate concentration of 0.42–0.47 mmol/L, rising to 4.3% when serum urate concentration is 0.45–0.59 mmol/L.[11] A 5 year longitudinal study of 223 asymptomatic men with hyperuricaemia estimated 5 year cumulative incidence of gout to be 10.8% for those with baseline serum urate of 0.42–0.47 mmol/L, 27.7% for baseline urate 0.48–0.53 mmol/L, and 61.1% for baseline urate levels of 0.54 mmol/L or more.[7] The study found that a 0.6 mmol/L difference in baseline serum urate increased the odds of an acute attack of gout by a factor of 1.8 (OR adjusted for other risk factors for gout: 1.84, 95% CI 1.24 to 2.72). It also found that alcohol and diuretics were risk factors for gout (adjusted OR for any alcohol intake v no alcohol intake: 3.45, 95% CI 1.58 to 7.56; adjusted OR for diuretics v no diuretics: OR 6.55, 95% CI 2.98 to 14.35). Other suggested risk factors for gout include obesity, insulin resistance, dyslipidaemia, hypertension, and cardiovascular disorders.[12,13]

**PROGNOSIS**
We found few reliable data about prognosis or complications of acute gout. One study of untreated acute gout found that 3/11 (27%) people with podagra experienced spontaneous resolution after 7 days.[14] A case series of 614 people with gout who had not had treatment to reduce urate levels and could recall the interval between first and second attacks reported recurrence rates of 62% after 1 year, 78% after 2 years, and 84% by 3 years.[15] An analysis of two prospective cohort studies of 371 black and 1181 white male former medical students followed up for about 30 years found no significant difference in risk of coronary heart disease in men who had developed gout compared with men who had not (RR 0.85, 95% CI 0.40 to 1.81).[16]

Please refer to CD-ROM for full text and references.

# Ankle sprain

**Search date November 2002**

*Peter Struijs and Gino Kerkhoffs*

## What are the effects of treatments for acute ankle ligament rupture?

### BENEFICIAL

#### Functional treatment

One systematic review and one subsequent RCT found limited evidence that functional treatment⊙ reduced the risk of the ankle giving way compared with minimal treatment. One systematic review found that, compared with immobilisation, functional treatment improved seven outcomes at either short (up to 6 weeks), intermediate (6 weeks to 1 year), or long term (over 1 year) follow up. However, effects were less marked at long term follow up, or if only results from high quality trials were analysed. Another systematic review found that, compared with immobilisation, functional treatment reduced persistent subjective instability, but found no significant difference in pain. Two systematic reviews found insufficient evidence to compare functional treatment versus surgery. One systematic review and three additional RCTs provided insufficient evidence to compare different functional treatments.

### LIKELY TO BE BENEFICIAL

#### Immobilisation

One systematic review found that, compared with functional treatment, immobilisation was associated with less improvement in seven outcomes at either short (up to 6 weeks), intermediate (6 weeks to 1 year), or long term (over 1 year) follow up. However, effects were less marked at long term follow up, or if only results from high quality trials were analysed. Another systematic review found that, compared with functional treatment immobilisation was less effective at reducing systematic instability, but found no significant difference in pain. One systematic review found no significant difference between immobilisation and surgery in pain or subjective instability. One systematic review found insufficient evidence to compare immobilisation versus physiotherapy.

#### Surgery

One systematic review found no significant difference between surgery and immobilisation in pain or subjective instability. One systematic review found insufficient evidence to compare surgery versus functional treatment. One systematic review found insufficient evidence to compare surgery versus conservative treatment (immobilisation or functional treatment).

### UNKNOWN EFFECTIVENESS

#### Diathermy

One systematic review found insufficient evidence on the effects of diathermy versus placebo on walking ability and reduction in swelling.

#### Homeopathic ointment

One systematic review of one small RCT found limited evidence that homeopathic ointment improved outcome on a "composite criteria" of treatment success compared with placebo.

## Cold pack compression

Two RCTs found no significant difference in symptoms between cold pack placement and placebo or control. One RCT found less oedema with cold pack placement compared with heat or a contrast bath at 3–5 days after injury.

## Ultrasound

One systematic review found no significant difference between ultrasound and sham ultrasound in the general improvement of symptoms or the ability to walk or bear weight at 7 days. Three RCTs provided insufficient evidence to compare ultrasound versus other treatments.

**DEFINITION**    Ankle sprain is an injury of the lateral ligament complex of the ankle joint. Such injury can range from mild to severe and is graded on the basis of severity.[1-5] Grade I is a mild stretching of the ligament complex without joint instability; grade II is a partial rupture of the ligament complex with mild instability of the joint (such as isolated rupture of the anterior talofibular ligament); grade III involves complete rupture of the ligament complex with instability of the joint.

**INCIDENCE/ PREVALENCE**    Ankle sprain is a common problem in acute medical care, occurring at a rate of about one injury/10 000 population/day.[6] Injuries of the lateral ligament complex of the ankle form a quarter of all sports injuries.[6]

**AETIOLOGY/ RISK FACTORS**    The usual mechanism of injury is inversion and adduction (usually referred to as supination) of the plantar flexed foot. Predisposing factors are a history of ankle sprains and specific malalignment, like crus varum and pes cavo-varus.

**PROGNOSIS**    Some sports (e.g. basketball, football/soccer, and volleyball) are associated with a particularly high incidence of ankle injuries. Pain is the most frequent residual problem, often localised on the medial side of the ankle.[4] Other residual complaints include mechanical instability, intermittent swelling, and stiffness. People with more extensive cartilage damage have a higher incidence of residual complaints.[4] Long term cartilage damage can lead to degenerative changes, especially if there is persistent or recurrent instability. Every further sprain has the potential to add new damage.

Please refer to CD-ROM for full text and references.

# Bunions

**Search date January 2003**

*Jill Ferrari*

---

## What are the effects of interventions?

### LIKELY TO BE BENEFICIAL

**Chevron osteotomy (compared with no treatment or with orthoses)**
One RCT found that chevron osteotomy◉ improved outcomes compared with orthoses or no treatment after 1 year.

**Different methods of bone fixation**
We found limited evidence on the effects of different methods of bone fixation. One small RCT found that screw fixation plus early weight bearing reduced time to return to work and social activity compared with suture fixation and later weight bearing.

### UNKNOWN EFFECTIVENESS

**Chevron osteotomy (compared with proximal osteotomy)**
We found conflicting evidence on the effects of chevron osteotomy compared with proximal osteotomy.

**Chevron osteotomy plus adductor tenotomy**
We found no evidence that adductor tenotomy plus chevron osteotomy improved outcomes compared with chevron osteotomy alone.

**Chevron osteotomy plus Akin osteotomy**
We found insufficient evidence to compare effects of chevron osteotomy plus Akin osteotomy◉ versus Akin osteotomy plus distal soft tissue reconstruction◉.

**Continuous passive motion**
One systematic review found insufficient evidence on the effects of continuous passive motion.

**Early weight bearing**
One systematic review found insufficient evidence on the effects of early weight bearing.

**Keller's arthroplasty**
One systematic review found insufficient evidence on the effects of Keller's arthroplasty◉ compared with other types of operation.

**Night splints**
We found insufficient evidence about the effects of night splints compared with other treatments.

**Orthoses to treat hallux valgus in adults**
We found limited evidence that orthoses reduced pain intensity compared with no treatment.

**Slipper casts**
One RCT found insufficient evidence on the effects of plaster slipper casts.

### UNLIKELY TO BE BENEFICIAL

**Orthoses to prevent hallux valgus in high risk adults**
One RCT in men with rheumatoid arthritis found no significant difference between orthoses and no treatment in rates of development of hallux valgus after 3 years. ▶

◀ **LIKELY TO BE INEFFECTIVE OR HARMFUL**

### Antipronatory orthoses in children

One RCT in children found limited evidence that antipronatory orthoses增 increased deterioration in metatarsophalangeal joint angles after 3 years compared with no treatment.

**DEFINITION**  **Hallux valgus** is a deformity of the great toe whereby the hallux (great toe) moves towards the second toe, overlying it in severe cases. This movement of the hallux is described as abduction (movement away from the midline of the body) and it is usually accompanied by some rotation of the toe so that the nail is facing the midline of the body (valgus rotation). With the deformity, the metatarsal head becomes more prominent and the metatarsal is said to be in an adducted position as it moves towards the midline of the body.[1] Radiological criteria for hallux valgus vary, but a commonly accepted criterion is to measure the angle formed between the metatarsal and the abducted hallux. This is called the metatarsophalangeal joint angle or hallux abductus angle and it is considered abnormal when it is greater than 14.5°.[2] **Bunion** is the lay term used to describe a prominent and often inflamed metatarsal head and overlying bursa. Symptoms include pain, limitation in walking, and problems with wearing normal shoes.

**INCIDENCE/**  The prevalence of hallux valgus varies in different populations. In a recent
**PREVALENCE**  study of 6000 UK school children aged 9–10 years, 2.5% had clinical evidence of hallux valgus, and 2% met both clinical and radiological criteria for hallux valgus. An earlier study found hallux valgus in 48% of adults.[2] Differences in prevalence may result from different methods of measurement, varying age groups, or different diagnostic criteria (e.g. metatarsal joint angle > 10° or > 15°).[3]

**AETIOLOGY/**  Nearly all population studies have found that hallux valgus is more common in
**RISK FACTORS**  women. Footwear may contribute to the deformity, but studies comparing people who wear shoes with those who do not have found contradictory results. Hypermobility of the first ray增 and excessive foot pronation are associated with hallux valgus.[4]

**PROGNOSIS**  We found no studies that looked at progression of hallux valgus. Progression of deformity and symptoms is rapid in some people, others remain asymptomatic. One study found that hallux valgus is often unilateral initially, but usually progresses to bilateral deformity.[2]

Please refer to CD-ROM for full text and references.

# Carpal tunnel syndrome

### Search date September 2002

*Shawn Marshall*

---

## What are the effects of treatments?

### Local corticosteroid injection (short term)

Two RCTs found local corticosteroid injection (methylprednisolone, hydrocortisone) versus placebo or no treatment significantly improved symptoms after 4–6 weeks. One small RCT found that local betamethasone injection versus betamethasone injection into the deltoid significantly improved symptoms after 1 month. One RCT found no significant difference with local methylprednisolone injection versus oral prednisolone in symptoms after 2 weeks, but found that local methylprednisolone injection versus oral prednisolone significantly improved symptoms after 8 and 12 weeks. One small RCT found that local methylprednisolone injection versus helium neon laser significantly improved symptoms after 20 days, but found no significant difference in symptoms between the two groups after 6 months. One small RCT found no significant difference with local methylprednisolone injection versus non-steroidal anti-inflammatory plus nocturnal neutral angle wrist splints in symptoms after 2 or 8 weeks.

### Oral corticosteroids (short term)

One small RCT found that oral prednisone versus placebo significantly improved the mean global symptom score after 2 weeks, but not after 4 or 8 weeks. One small RCT found that oral prednisolone versus placebo significantly improved the mean global symptom score after 2 and 4 weeks. One small RCT found that oral prednisolone versus placebo significantly improved the median global symptom score after 2 and 8 weeks. One RCT found no significant difference with local methylprednisolone injection versus oral prednisolone in symptoms after 2 weeks, but found that local methylprednisolone injection versus oral prednisolone significantly improved symptoms after 8 and 12 weeks.

### Endoscopic carpal tunnel release versus open carpal tunnel release

We found no RCTs comparing surgery versus placebo. One systematic review and subsequent RCTs found no clear evidence of a difference in symptoms with endoscopic carpal tunnel release versus open carpal tunnel release up to 12 months after the operation. RCTs found conflicting evidence on differences in the time taken to return to work between endoscopic carpal tunnel release versus open carpal tunnel release. Harms resulting from endoscopic carpal tunnel release and open carpal tunnel release vary between RCTs. One systematic review comparing the interventions suggests that endoscopic carpal tunnel release may cause more transient nerve problems whereas open carpal tunnel release may cause more wound problems.

### Nerve and tendon gliding exercises

One small RCT found no significant difference with nerve and tendon gliding exercises**ⓖ** plus neutral angle wrist splint versus neutral angle wrist splint alone in mean symptom severity score or mean functional status score assessed 8 weeks after the end of the treatment.

### Pyridoxine

One very small RCT found a similar improvement in symptoms with pyridoxine versus placebo or no treatment after 10 weeks. The RCT may have been too small to detect a clinically important difference between treatments. One small RCT found no significant difference with pyridoxine versus placebo in nocturnal pain, numbness, or tingling after 12 weeks.

### Surgery versus placebo or non-surgical intervention

We found no RCTs comparing surgery versus placebo. One very small RCT found limited evidence that surgical section of the anterior carpal ligament versus splinting of the hand, wrist, and arm for 1 month increased the proportion of people with clinical improvement after 1 year.

### Therapeutic ultrasound

One RCT found ultrasound versus placebo significantly increased the proportion of wrists with satisfactory improvement or complete remission of symptoms after 6 months. One RCT found no significant difference in mean symptom severity with high intensity or low intensity ultrasound versus placebo after 2 weeks. One RCT found no significant difference in symptom severity scores with ibuprofen plus nocturnal wrist splint versus chiropractic manipulation plus ultrasound plus nocturnal wrist splint after 9 weeks.

### Wrist splints

One RCT found a significant improvement in symptoms after 2 and 4 weeks with a nocturnal hand brace versus no treatment. RCTs found no significant difference in symptoms with neutral angle versus 20° extension wrist splinting, or with full time versus night time only neutral angle wrist splinting.

### Local corticosteroid injection (long term); oral corticosteroids (long term)

We found no RCTs on the effects of these interventions.

## UNLIKELY TO BE BENEFICIAL

### Diuretics

One small RCT found no significant difference with trichlormethiazide versus placebo in mean global symptom score after 2 or 4 weeks. One RCT found no significant difference with bendrofluazide versus placebo in the proportion of people with no improvement in symptoms after 4 weeks.

### Internal neurolysis in conjunction with open carpal tunnel release

Three RCTs found no significant difference with open carpal tunnel release alone versus open carpal tunnel release plus internal neurolysis in symptoms.

### Non-steroidal anti-inflammatory drugs

One small RCT found no significant difference with tenoxicam versus placebo in mean global symptom score after 2 or 4 weeks. One RCT found no significant difference in symptom severity scores with ibuprofen plus nocturnal wrist splint versus chiropractic manipulation plus ultrasound plus nocturnal wrist splint after 9 weeks.

## LIKELY TO BE INEFFECTIVE OR HARMFUL

### Wrist splinting after carpal tunnel release surgery

Two RCTs in people after carpal tunnel release surgery found no significant difference with wrist splinting versus no splinting in median grip strength or in the number of people who considered themselves "cured". Another RCT found that splinting versus no splinting significantly increased pain at 1 month and the number of days taken to return to work.

# Carpal tunnel syndrome

**DEFINITION**　　Carpal tunnel syndrome is a neuropathy caused by compression of the median nerve within the carpal tunnel.[1] Classical symptoms of carpal tunnel syndrome include numbness, tingling, burning, or pain in at least two of the three digits supplied by the median nerve (i.e. the thumb, index, and middle fingers).[2] The American Academy of Neurology has described diagnostic criteria◐ that rely on a combination of symptoms and physical examination findings.[3] Other diagnostic criteria include results from electrophysiological studies.[2]

**INCIDENCE/**　A general population survey in Rochester, Minnesota, found the age adjusted
**PREVALENCE**　incidence of carpal tunnel syndrome to be 105 (95% CI 99 to 112) cases per 100 000 person years.[4,5] Age adjusted incidence rates were 52 (95% CI 45 to 59) cases for men and 149 (95% CI 138 to 159) cases for women per 100 000 person years. The study found incidence rates increased from 88 (95% CI 75 to 101) cases per 100 000 person years in 1961–1965 to 125 (95% CI 112 to 138) cases per 100 000 person years in 1976–1980. Incidence rates of carpal tunnel syndrome increased with age for men, whereas for women they peaked between the ages of 45–54 years. A general population survey in the Netherlands found prevalence to be 1% for men and 7% for women.[6] A more comprehensive study in southern Sweden found the general population prevalence for carpal tunnel syndrome was 3% (95% CI 2% to 3%).[7] As in other studies, the overall prevalence in women was higher than in men (male to female ratio 1 : 1.4); however, among older people, the prevalence in women was almost four times that in men (age group 65–74 years: men 1%, 95% CI 0% to 4%; women 5%, 95% CI 3% to 8%).

**AETIOLOGY/**　Most cases of carpal tunnel syndrome have no easily identifiable cause
**RISK FACTORS**　(idiopathic).[4] Secondary causes of carpal tunnel syndrome include the following: space occupying lesions (tumours, hypertrophic synovial tissue, fracture callus, and osteophytes); metabolic and physiological (pregnancy, hypothyroidism, rheumatoid arthritis); infections; neuropathies (associated with diabetes mellitus or alcoholism); and familial disorders.[4] One case control study found that risk factors in the general population included repetitive activities requiring wrist extension or flexion, obesity, very rapid dieting, shorter height, hysterectomy without oopherectomy, and recent menopause.[8]

**PROGNOSIS**　　One observational study (carpal tunnel syndrome defined by symptoms and electrophysiological study results) found that 34% of people with idiopathic carpal tunnel syndrome without treatment had complete resolution of symptoms (remission) within 6 months of diagnosis.[9] Remission rates were higher for younger age groups, for women versus men, and for pregnant versus non-pregnant women. A more recent observational study of untreated idiopathic carpal tunnel syndrome also demonstrated that symptoms may spontaneously resolve in some people. The main positive prognostic indicators were short duration of symptoms and young age, whereas bilateral symptoms and a positive Phalen's test were indicators of a poorer prognosis.[10]

Please refer to CD-ROM for full text and references.

# Chronic fatigue syndrome

### Search date March 2003

*Steven Reid, Trudie Chalder, Anthony Cleare, Matthew Hotopf, and Simon Wessely*

## What are the effects of treatments?

### BENEFICIAL

#### Cognitive behavioural therapy

One systematic review found that cognitive behavioural therapy administered by highly skilled therapists in specialist centres improved quality of life and physical functioning compared with standard medical care or relaxation therapy. One additional multicentre RCT found that cognitive behavioural therapy administered by less experienced therapists may also be effective compared with guided support groups or no interventions.

#### Graded aerobic exercise

RCTs have found that a graded aerobic exercise programme improves measures of fatigue and physical functioning compared with flexibility and relaxation training or general advice. One RCT has found that an educational package to encourage graded exercise improved measures of physical functioning, fatigue, mood, and sleep at 1 year compared with written information alone.

### UNKNOWN EFFECTIVENESS

#### Dietary supplements *New*

One small RCT found no significant difference between a nutritional supplement (containing multivitamins, minerals, and coenzymes) and placebo in fatigue severity or functional impairment at 10 weeks.

#### Evening primrose oil

One small RCT found no significant difference between evening primrose oil and placebo in depression scores at 3 months.

#### Magnesium (intramuscular)

One small RCT found that intramuscular magnesium injections improved symptoms at 6 weeks compared with placebo. However, we were unable to draw reliable conclusions from this small study.

#### Antidepressants; corticosteroids; oral nicotinamide adenine dinucleotide

RCTs found insufficient evidence about the effects of these interventions in people with chronic fatigue syndrome.

### UNLIKELY TO BE BENEFICIAL

#### Immunotherapy

Small RCTs found limited evidence that immunoglobulin G modestly improved physical functioning and fatigue at 3–6 months compared with placebo, but it was associated with considerable adverse effects. Small RCTs found insufficient evidence on the effects of interferon alfa or aciclovir compared with placebo. One RCT found that staphylococcus toxoid improved symptoms at six months compared with placebo, although it is associated with local reaction and could cause anaphylaxis.

#### Prolonged rest

We found no RCTs on the effects of prolonged rest. Indirect observational evidence in healthy volunteers and in people recovering from a viral illness suggests that prolonged rest may perpetuate or worsen fatigue and symptoms.

# Chronic fatigue syndrome

**DEFINITION** Chronic fatigue syndrome (CFS) is characterised by severe, disabling fatigue and other symptoms, including musculoskeletal pain, sleep disturbance, impaired concentration, and headaches. Two widely used definitions of CFS, from the US Centers for Disease Control and Prevention[1] and from Oxford, UK,[2] were developed as operational criteria for research❶. There are important differences between these definitions. The UK criteria insist upon the presence of mental fatigue, whereas the US criteria include a requirement for several physical symptoms, reflecting the belief that CFS has an underlying immunological or infective pathology.

**INCIDENCE/ PREVALENCE** Community and primary care based studies have reported the prevalence of CFS to be 0–3%, depending on the criteria used.[3,4] Systematic population surveys have found similar prevalences of CFS in people of different socio-economic status and in all ethnic groups.[4,5]

**AETIOLOGY/ RISK FACTORS** The cause of CFS is poorly understood. Women are at higher risk than men (RR 1.3–1.7 depending on diagnostic criteria used).[6]

**PROGNOSIS** Studies have focused on people attending specialist clinics. A systematic review of studies of prognosis (search date 1996) found that children with CFS had better outcomes than adults: 54–94% of children showed definite improvement (after up to 6 years' follow up), whereas 20–50% of adults showed some improvement in the medium term and only 6% returned to premorbid levels of functioning.[7] Despite the considerable burden of morbidity associated with CFS, we found no evidence of increased mortality. The systematic review found that outcome was influenced by the presence of psychiatric disorders (depression and anxiety) and beliefs about causation and treatment.[7]

Please refer to CD-ROM for full text and references.

# Fracture prevention in postmenopausal women

## Search date May 2003

*Olivier Bruyere, John Edwards, and Jean-Yves Reginster*

Musculoskeletal disorders

## What are the effects of treatments to prevent fractures in postmenopausal women?

### BENEFICIAL

**Alendronate**

Two systematic reviews in postmenopausal women have found that alendronate reduces vertebral and non-vertebral fractures compared with placebo.

**Risedronate**

One systematic review in postmenopausal women has found that risedronate reduces vertebral and non-vertebral fractures compared with placebo.

### LIKELY TO BE BENEFICIAL

**Calcitonin**

One systematic review in postmenopausal women found that calcitonin reduced vertebral fractures compared with placebo, but found no significant difference between calcitonin and placebo in non-vertebral fractures.

**Calcium plus vitamin D**

One large RCT in women aged 69–106 years living in nursing homes found that calcium plus vitamin D3 reduced hip fractures and non-vertebral fractures over 18 months to 3 years compared with placebo. One smaller RCT in women and men aged 65 years or older found that calcium plus vitamin D3 reduced non-vertebral fractures compared with placebo, but found no significant difference in hip fractures. One smaller RCT in postmenopausal women found no significant difference between calcium plus vitamin D3 and placebo in hip fracture after 2 years. The two smaller RCTs may have lacked power to exclude a clinically important difference. One systematic review in postmenopausal women reporting a combined analysis (for vitamin D alone and vitamin D plus calcium) found that standard or hydroxylated vitamin D with or without calcium reduced vertebral fractures compared with control, but found no significant difference between groups in non-vertebral fractures.

**Etidronate**

One systematic review in postmenopausal women found that etidronate reduced vertebral fractures over 2 years compared with control (placebo, calcium, or calcium plus vitamin D), but found no significant difference in non-vertebral fractures.

**Hip protectors**

One systematic review in elderly residents of nursing homes and one subsequent RCT found that hip protectors reduced hip fractures over 9–19 months compared with no hip protectors, whereas four other subsequent RCTs found no significant difference in hip fractures between groups. One other subsequent RCT in men and women aged over 65 years in institutional care found that a multifactorial intervention (including staff education, environmental manipulation, exercise, walking aids, drug regimen reviews, and hip protectors for those considered at higher risk) reduced hip fractures over 34 weeks compared with usual care. RCTs found no significant difference between hip protectors and no hip protectors in the occurrence of pelvic fractures.

▶

# Fracture prevention in postmenopausal women

### Pamidronate

One RCT in men and postmenopausal women found that pamidronate reduced new vertebral fractures after 3 years compared with placebo. One small RCT in postmenopausal women found no significant difference between pamidronate and placebo in vertebral fracture rate, but it was too small to exclude a clinically important difference.

## UNKNOWN EFFECTIVENESS

### Environmental manipulation

We found no RCTs assessing environmental manipulation❶ alone. One RCT in men and women aged over 70 years found no significant difference in new fractures over 4 years between health visitor care (aimed at assessing nutritional deficiencies, reducing smoking and alcohol intake, improving muscle tone and fitness, assessing medical conditions, use of medication, improving home environment such as lighting) and control. Another RCT in men and women aged over 65 years in institutional care found that a multifactorial intervention (including staff education, environmental manipulation, exercise, walking aids, drug regimen reviews, and hip protectors for those considered at higher risk) reduced hip fractures over 34 weeks compared with usual care.

### Exercise

Three RCTs found no significant difference in falls resulting in fracture over 1 year between exercise (advice to walk briskly three times weekly or balance and strength exercises plus walking) and control. One small RCT in postmenopausal women found no significant difference between a 2 year back strengthening exercise programme and usual care in vertebral fractures over 10 years. Another RCT in men and women aged over 65 years in institutional care found that a multifactorial intervention (including staff education, environmental manipulation, exercise, walking aids, drug regimen reviews, and hip protectors for those considered at higher risk) reduced hip fractures over 34 weeks compared with usual care.

## UNLIKELY TO BE BENEFICIAL

### Calcium alone

One systematic review in postmenopausal women found no significant difference between calcium supplementation and placebo in vertebral or non-vertebral fractures.

### Vitamin D alone

One large RCT in postmenopausal women and two large RCTs in postmenopausal women and men found no significant difference between vitamin D3 and placebo in hip fractures or non-vertebral fractures. However, one systematic review found limited evidence from two small RCTs in postmenopausal women that calcitriol reduced vertebral fractures over 3 years compared with placebo.

## LIKELY TO BE INEFFECTIVE OR HARMFUL

### Hormone replacement therapy

We found insufficient evidence of benefit, but reliable evidence of harm. One systematic review in postmenopausal women found that hormone replacement therapy reduced vertebral fractures compared with control. However, another systematic review and one subsequent RCT in postmenopausal women found no significant difference in vertebral fractures. Two systematic reviews and two subsequent RCTs provided insufficient evidence on the effects of hormone ▶

replacement therapy on non-vertebral fractures. One large RCT of oestrogen plus progestin versus placebo for primary prevention of coronary heart disease in healthy postmenopausal women was stopped because hormonal treatment increased risks of invasive breast cancer, coronary events, stroke, and pulmonary embolism.

**DEFINITION** This topic covers interventions to prevent fractures in postmenopausal women. Fractures may be symptomatic or asymptomatic. A fracture is a break or disruption of bone or cartilage. Symptoms and signs may include immobility, pain, tenderness, numbness, bruising, joint deformity, joint swelling, limb deformity, and limb shortening.[1] Diagnosis is usually based on a typical clinical picture combined with results from an appropriate imaging technique. Usually in trials dealing with osteoporosis, menopause is considered to be present 12 months after the last menstruation.

**INCIDENCE/ PREVALENCE** The lifetime risk of fracture in white women is 20% for the spine, 15% for the wrist, and 18% for the hip.[2] The incidence of postmenopausal fracture increases with age.[3] One observational study found that age specific incidence rates for postmenopausal fracture of the hip increased exponentially beyond the age of 50 years.[4]

**AETIOLOGY/ RISK FACTORS** Fractures usually arise from trauma. General risk factors include those associated with an increased risks of falling (such as ataxia, drug and alcohol intake, loose carpets), age, osteoporosis, bony metastases, and other bone disorders. Postmenopausal women are at increased risk of fracture because of hormonal bone loss. Risk factors for fractures in postmenopausal women include increasing age, low body mass index, time since menopause, alcohol consumption, smoking, some endocrine diseases, such as hyperparathyroidism or thyroid disease, and steroid use, among others.

**PROGNOSIS** Fractures may result in pain, short or long term disability, haemorrhage, thromboembolic disease (see thromboembolism, p 000), shock, and death. Vertebral fractures are associated with pain, physical impairment, muscular atrophy, changes in body shape, loss of physical function, and lower quality of life.[5] About 20% of women die in the first year after a hip fracture, representing an increase in mortality of 12–20% compared with women of similar age and no hip fracture. Half of elderly women who had been independent become partly dependent after hip fracture. A third become totally dependent.

Please refer to CD-ROM for full text and references.

# Herniated lumbar disc

## Search date December 2002

*Jo Jordan, Tamara Shawver Morgan, and James Weinstein*

Musculoskeletal disorders

---

## What are the effects of treatments?

### Microdiscectomy (as effective as standard discectomy)

We found no RCTs comparing microdiscectomy⊕ and conservative treatment. Three RCTs found no significant difference in clinical outcomes between microdiscectomy and standard discectomy. One RCT found no significant difference in satisfaction or pain between video-assisted arthroscopic microdiscectomy and standard discectomy at about 30 months, although postoperative recovery was slower with standard discectomy. We found conflicting evidence on the effects of automated percutaneous discectomy compared with microdiscectomy.

### Spinal manipulation

One RCT in people with sciatica caused by disc herniation found that after 2 weeks, spinal manipulation increased perceived improvement compared with placebo. A second RCT found no significant difference in improvement between spinal manipulation, manual traction, exercise, and corsets after 1 month. A third RCT found that spinal manipulation significantly increased the proportion of people with improved symptoms compared with traction.

### Standard discectomy

One RCT found that standard discectomy⊕ increased self reported improvement at 1 year, but not at 4 and 10 years, compared with conservative treatment (physiotherapy). Three RCTs found no significant differences in clinical outcomes between standard discectomy and microdiscectomy. Adverse effects were similar with both procedures.

### Advice to stay active

One systematic review of conservative treatments found no RCTs on giving advice to stay active.

### Automated percutaneous discectomy

We found no RCTs comparing automated percutaneous discectomy⊕ versus either conservative treatment or standard discectomy. We found conflicting evidence on the clinical effects of automated percutaneous discectomy compared with microdiscectomy.

### Bed rest

One systematic review of conservative treatment found no RCTs on bed rest for symptomatic herniated discs.

### Epidural corticosteroid injections

One systematic review found limited evidence that epidural steroid injections increased global improvement compared with placebo. One subsequent RCT found no significant difference between epidural steroid injections plus conservative treatment compared with conservative treatment alone in pain, mobility, or return to work at 6 months.

### Heat or ice

One systematic review identified no RCTs of heat or ice for sciatica caused by lumbar disc herniation.

*Clin Evid Concise* 2003;10:252–253.

◀ **Massage**

One systematic review identified no RCTs of massage in people with symptomatic lumbar disc herniation.

## Analgesics; antidepressants; laser discectomy❸; muscle relaxants

We found no systematic review or RCTs on these interventions for treatment of symptomatic herniated lumbar disc.

**UNLIKELY TO BE BENEFICIAL**

## Non-steroidal anti-inflammatory drugs

One systematic review found no significant difference in overall improvement between non-steroidal anti-inflammatory drugs and placebo in people with sciatica caused by disc herniation.

| | |
|---|---|
| **DEFINITION** | Herniated lumbar disc is a displacement of disc material (nucleus pulposus or annulus fibrosis) beyond the intervertebral disc space.[1] The diagnosis can be confirmed by radiological examination; however, magnetic resonance imaging findings of herniated disc are not always accompanied by clinical symptoms.[2,3] This review covers treatment of people who have clinical symptoms relating to confirmed or suspected disc herniation. It does not include treatment of people with spinal cord compression or people with cauda equina syndrome❸, which often requires emergency intervention. The management of non-specific acute low back pain (p 256) and chronic low back pain (p 259) are covered elsewhere. |
| **INCIDENCE/ PREVALENCE** | The prevalence of symptomatic herniated lumbar disc is around 1–3% in Finland and Italy, depending on age and sex.[4] The highest prevalence is among people aged 30–50 years,[5] with a male : female ratio of 2 : 1.[6] In people aged between 25 and 55 years, about 95% of herniated discs occur at the L4–L5 level; in people over 55 years of age, disc herniation is more common above the L4–L5 level.[7,8] |
| **AETIOLOGY/ RISK FACTORS** | Radiographical evidence of disc herniation does not reliably predict low back pain in the future or correlate with symptoms; 19–27% of people without symptoms have disc herniation on imaging.[2,9] Risk factors for disc herniation include smoking (OR 1.7, 95% CI 1.0 to 2.5), weight bearing sports, and certain work activities such as repeated lifting (lifting objects < 11.3 kg, < 25 times daily while twisting body, knees not bent, OR 7.2, 95% CI 2.0 to 25.8; lifting objects < 11.3 kg, < 25 times daily while twisting body, knees bent, OR 1.9, 95% CI 0.8 to 4.8). Driving motor vehicles is also associated with increased risk (OR 1.7, 95% CI 0.2 to 2.7, depending on the vehicle model).[6,10,11] This may be because the resonant frequency of the spine is similar to that of certain vehicles. |
| **PROGNOSIS** | The natural history of disc herniation is difficult to determine because most people take some form of treatment for their back pain, and a formal diagnosis is not always made.[6] Clinical improvement is usual in most people, and only about 10% of people still have sufficient pain after 6 weeks to consider surgery. Sequential magnetic resonance images have shown that the herniated portion of the disc tends to regress over time, with partial to complete resolution after 6 months in two thirds of people.[12] |

Please refer to CD-ROM for full text and references.

# Leg cramps

### Search date October 2002

*Gavin Young*

## What are the effects of treatments for idiopathic leg cramps?

### BENEFICIAL

#### Quinine
One systematic review has found that quinine reduces the frequency of nocturnal leg cramp attacks compared with placebo over 4 weeks.

### LIKELY TO BE BENEFICIAL

#### Quinine plus theophylline
One small RCT found limited evidence that quinine plus theophylline reduced the number of nights affected by leg cramps compared with quinine alone over 2 weeks.

### UNKNOWN EFFECTIVENESS

#### Analgesics; antiepileptic drugs; compression hosiery
We found no RCTs on the effects of these interventions on idiopathic leg cramps🜚.

### UNLIKELY TO BE BENEFICIAL

#### Vitamin E
One small RCT found no significant difference between vitamin E and placebo in the number of nights disturbed by leg cramps.

## What are the effects of treatments for leg cramps in pregnancy?

### LIKELY TO BE BENEFICIAL

#### Magnesium salts
One systematic review identified one small RCT in pregnant women, which found that magnesium tablets (primarily magnesium lactate, magnesium citrate) reduced leg cramps compared with placebo after 3 weeks.

### UNKNOWN EFFECTIVENESS

#### Calcium salts
One systematic review identified two RCTs that compared calcium versus placebo or no treatment, which found conflicting results.

#### Multivitamins and mineral supplements
One systematic review identified one small RCT in pregnant women, which found no significant difference between a multivitamin plus mineral tablet and placebo in leg cramps in the ninth month of pregnancy.

#### Sodium chloride
One systematic review found insufficient evidence about the effects of sodium chloride on leg cramps in pregnancy.

DEFINITION    Leg cramps are involuntary, localised, and usually painful skeletal muscle contractions, which commonly affect calf muscles. Leg cramps typically occur at night and usually last only seconds to minutes. Leg cramps may be idiopathic or related to a definable process or disease such as pregnancy, renal dialysis, or venous insufficiency.

**INCIDENCE/ PREVALENCE**
Leg cramps are common and their incidence increases with age. About half of the people attending a general medicine clinic have had leg cramps within 1 month of their visit, and over two thirds of people over 50 years of age have experienced leg cramps.[1]

**AETIOLOGY/ RISK FACTORS**
Very little is known about the causes of leg cramps. Risk factors include pregnancy, exercise, salt depletion, renal dialysis, electrolyte imbalances, peripheral vascular disease (both venous and arterial), peripheral nerve injury, polyneuropathies, motor neuron disease, muscle diseases, and certain drugs. Other causes of calf pain include trauma, deep venous thrombosis (see thromboembolism, p 40), and ruptured Baker's cyst**G**.

**PROGNOSIS**
Leg cramps may cause severe pain and sleep disturbance, both of which are distressing.

Please refer to CD-ROM for full text and references.

# Low back pain and sciatica (acute)

Search date February 2003

*Maurits van Tulder and Bart Koes*

## What are the effects of treatments?

**BENEFICIAL**

### Advice to stay active

Two systematic reviews and one subsequent RCT found that advice to stay active increased the rate of recovery, reduced pain, reduced disability, and reduced time spent off work compared with advice to rest in bed or bed rest.

### Non-steroidal anti-inflammatory drugs

One systematic review and one additional RCT have found that non-steroidal anti-inflammatory drugs increased overall improvement after 1 week and reduced the need for additional analgesics compared with placebo. One systematic review and additional RCTs have found no significant difference among non-steroidal anti-inflammatory drugs or between non-steroidal anti-inflammatory drugs and other treatments (paracetamol, opioids, muscle relaxants, and non-drug treatments) in pain relief.

**LIKELY TO BE BENEFICIAL**

### Behavioural therapy

One RCT found that cognitive behavioural therapy❻ reduced acute low back pain and disability compared with traditional care or electromyographic biofeedback❻.

### Multidisciplinary treatment programmes (for subacute low back pain)

We found no RCTs in people with acute low back pain. One systematic review in people with subacute low back pain found limited evidence that multidisciplinary treatment❻, including a workplace visit, reduced sick leave compared with usual care.

**TRADE OFF BETWEEN BENEFITS AND HARMS**

### Muscle relaxants

Systematic reviews have found that muscle relaxants improve symptoms (including pain and muscle tension) and increase mobility compared with placebo, but found no significant difference in outcomes among muscle relaxants. Adverse effects in people using muscle relaxants were common and included dependency, drowsiness, and dizziness.

**UNKNOWN EFFECTIVENESS**

### Acupuncture

We found no RCTs of acupuncture❻ specifically in people with acute low back pain.

### Analgesics (paracetamol, opioids)

We found no placebo controlled RCTs. Systematic reviews have found no consistent difference between analgesics and non-steroidal anti-inflammatory drugs in reducing pain.

### Back schools

One systematic review found limited evidence that back schools increased rates of recovery and reduced sick leave compared with placebo in the short term. The ▶

review found no significant difference in outcomes between back school and physiotherapy, and found that back school increased pain and sick leave compared with McKenzie exercises**G**.

## Epidural steroid injections

One RCT found that epidural steroids increased the proportion of people who were pain free compared with subcutaneous lidocaine (lignocaine) injections after 3 months. A second RCT found no significant difference in the proportion of people cured or improved between epidural steroids and epidural saline, epidural bupivacaine, or dry needling.

## Lumbar supports

We found no RCTs on the effects of lumbar supports.

## Massage

One systematic review found insufficient evidence from one RCT about the effects of massage**G** compared with spinal manipulation or electrical stimulation.

## Spinal manipulation

Systematic reviews found conflicting evidence on the effects of spinal manipulation.

## Traction

RCTs found conflicting evidence on the effects of traction.

## Colchicine; electromyographic biofeedback**G**; temperature treatments (short wave diathermy, ultrasound, ice, heat); transcutaneous electrical nerve stimulation

We found insufficient evidence on the effects of these interventions.

### UNLIKELY TO BE BENEFICIAL

## Back exercises

Systematic reviews and additional RCTs have found either no significant difference between back exercises and conservative or inactive treatments in pain or disability, or have found that back exercises increase pain or disability.

### LIKELY TO BE INEFFECTIVE OR HARMFUL

## Bed rest

Systematic reviews have found that bed rest could be worse than no treatment, advice to stay active, back exercises, physiotherapy, spinal manipulation, or non-steroidal anti-inflammatory drugs. One systematic review has found that adverse effects of bed rest include joint stiffness, muscle wasting, loss of bone mineral density, pressure sores, and venous thromboembolism.

**DEFINITION**  Low back pain is pain, muscle tension, or stiffness that is localised below the costal margin and above the inferior gluteal folds, with or without leg pain (sciatica**G**),[1] and is designated as acute when it persists for less than 12 weeks.[2] Non-specific low back pain is low back pain not attributed to a recognisable pathology (such as infection, tumour, osteoporosis, rheumatoid arthritis, fracture, or inflammation).[1] This review excludes low back pain or sciatica with symptoms or signs at presentation that suggest a specific underlying condition.

**INCIDENCE/**  Over 70% of people in developed countries will experience low back pain at
**PREVALENCE**  some time in their lives.[3] Each year, 15–45% of adults suffer low back pain, and 1/20 (5%) people present to hospital with a new episode. Low back pain is most common between the ages of 35–55 years.[3]

# Low back pain and sciatica (acute)

**AETIOLOGY/ RISK FACTORS**  Symptoms, pathology, and radiological appearances are poorly correlated. Pain is non-specific in about 85% of people. About 4% of people with low back pain in primary care have compression fractures and about 1% have a tumour. The prevalence of prolapsed intervertebral disc is about 1–3%.[3] Ankylosing spondylitis and spinal infections are less common.[4] Risk factors for the development of back pain include heavy physical work, frequent bending, twisting, lifting, and prolonged static postures. Psychosocial risk factors include anxiety, depression, and mental stress at work.[3,5]

**PROGNOSIS**  Acute low back pain is usually self limiting (90% of people recover within 6 weeks), although 2–7% develop chronic pain. One study found recurrent pain accounted for 75–85% of absenteeism from work.[6]

Please refer to CD-ROM for full text and references.

### Search date February 2003

*Maurits van Tulder and Bart Koes*

## What are the effects of treatments?

### BENEFICIAL

#### Exercise

Systematic reviews and additional RCTs have found that exercise improves pain and functional status compared with usual care. RCTs found conflicting evidence on the effects of different types of exercise, or exercise compared with inactive treatments.

#### Intensive multidisciplinary treatment programmes

One systematic review has found that intensive multidisciplinary biopsychosocial rehabilitation with functional restoration reduces pain and improves function compared with inpatient or outpatient non-multidisciplinary treatments or usual care. The review found no significant difference between less intensive multidisciplinary treatments and non-multidisciplinary treatment or usual care in pain or function.

### LIKELY TO BE BENEFICIAL

#### Analgesics

One RCT found that tramadol decreased pain and functional status compared with placebo. A second RCT found that paracetamol increased the proportion of people who rated the treatment as good or excellent compared with diflunisal.

#### Back schools in occupational settings (versus no treatment)

One systematic review has found that, in occupational settings, back schools⊕ improve pain and reduce disability compared with no treatment. Systematic reviews and one subsequent RCT found conflicting evidence on the effects of back schools compared with other treatments.

#### Behavioural therapy

Systematic reviews have found that behavioural therapy reduces pain and improves functional status and behavioural outcomes compared with no treatment, placebo, or waiting list control. Systematic reviews found no significant difference in functional status, pain, or behavioural outcomes between different types of behavioural therapy, and found conflicting results with behavioural therapy compared with other treatments.

#### Massage (versus other treatments)

One systematic review found that massage⊕ combined with exercises and education is more effective than inert treatment. The review found conflicting evidence about the effects of massage compared with other treatments.

#### Non-steroidal anti-inflammatory drugs

One RCT found that naproxen increased pain relief compared with placebo. One systematic review and additional RCTs found no significant difference with non-steroidal anti-inflammatory drugs compared with each other for symptom outcomes. Two RCTs found conflicting evidence on the effects of non-steroidal anti-inflammatory drugs compared with other analgesics.

© BMJ Publishing Group Ltd 2003

# Low back pain and sciatica (chronic)

### Trigger point and ligamentous injections

One systematic review found limited evidence that steroid plus local anaesthetic injection of trigger points increased pain relief compared with local anaesthetic injection alone, and that phenol increased pain relief compared with saline injection of the lumbar interspinal ligament.

## UNKNOWN EFFECTIVENESS

### Acupuncture

We found conflicting evidence from two systematic reviews and two subsequent RCTs about the effects of acupuncture compared with placebo or no treatment. One systematic review and one subsequent RCT have found that acupuncture reduces pain intensity and increases overall improvement compared with transcutaneous electrical nerve stimulation.

### Antidepressants

One systematic review and additional RCTs have found that antidepressants significantly increase pain relief compared with placebo. However, they found no consistent difference in functioning or depression. Additional RCTs found conflicting results on pain relief with antidepressants compared with each other or analgesics.

### Electromyographic biofeedback

One systematic review found no difference in pain relief or functional status between electromyographic biofeedback and placebo or waiting list control, but found conflicting results on the effects of electromyographic biofeedback compared with other treatments.

### Epidural steroid injections

One systematic review found no significant difference between epidural steroid injections and placebo in pain relief after 6 weeks or 6 months.

### Lumbar supports

We found insufficient evidence on the effects of lumbar supports.

### Muscle relaxants

We found insufficient evidence about the benefits of muscle relaxants. One RCT found that adverse effects in people using muscle relaxants are common and include dependency, drowsiness, and dizziness.

### Physical conditioning programmes *New*

One systematic review has found that physical conditioning programmes with a cognitive behavioural approach plus physical training for workers with back pain reduced sick days but not the risk of being off work at 12 months compared with general practitioner care.

### Spinal manipulation

We found five systematic reviews, which identified 13 RCTs. One of the reviews found that spinal manipulation improved outcomes compared with placebo; one concluded that improvements in pain and disability scores were too small to be clinically worthwhile, and the other three were conflicting.

### Transcutaneous electrical nerve stimulation

One systematic review found no significant difference in pain relief between transcutaneous electrical nerve stimulation and sham stimulation.

## Facet joint injections

One systematic review found no significant difference in pain relief between facet joint injections and placebo or facet joint nerve blocks.

## Traction

One systematic review and two additional RCTs found no significant difference between traction and placebo or between traction plus massage and interferential treatment in pain relief or functional status.

**DEFINITION**  Low back pain is pain, muscle tension, or stiffness that is localised below the costal margin and above the inferior gluteal folds, with or without leg pain (sciatica❻),[1] and is defined as chronic when it persists for 12 weeks or more (see definition of low back pain and sciatica [acute], p 257).[2] Non-specific low back pain is low back pain not attributed to a recognisable pathology (such as infection, tumour, osteoporosis, rheumatoid arthritis, fracture, or inflammation).[1] This review excludes low back pain or leg pain with symptoms or signs at presentation that suggest a specific underlying condition.

**INCIDENCE/**  Over 70% of people in developed countries will experience low back pain at
**PREVALENCE**  some time in their lives.[3] Each year, 15–45% of adults suffer low back pain, and 1/20 people present to hospital with a new episode. About 2–7% of patients with acute low back pain will go on to become chronic. Low back pain is most common between the ages of 35–55 years.[3]

**AETIOLOGY/**  Symptoms, pathology, and radiological appearances are poorly correlated. Pain
**RISK FACTORS**  is non-specific in about 85% of people. About 4% of people with low back pain in primary care have compression fractures and about 1% have a tumour. The prevalence of prolapsed intervertebral disc is about 1–3%.[3] Ankylosing spondylitis and spinal infections are less common.[4] Risk factors for the development of back pain include heavy physical work, frequent bending, twisting, lifting, and prolonged static postures. Psychosocial risk factors include anxiety, depression, and mental stress at work.[3,5] Having a previous history of low back pain and a longer duration of the present episode are significant risk factors for chronicity. A recently published systematic review of prospective cohort studies found that some psychological factors (distress, depressive mood, and somatisation) are associated with an increased risk of chronic low back pain.[6] Individual and workplace factors have also been reported to be associated with the transition to chronic low back pain.[7]

**PROGNOSIS**  Generally, the clinical course of an episode of low back pain seems to be favourable, and most pain will resolve within 2 weeks. Back pain among primary care patients typically has a recurrent course characterised by variation and change, rather than an acute, self limiting course.[8] Most back pain patients will have experienced a previous episode, and acute attacks often occur as exacerbations of chronic low back pain. In general, recurrences will occur more frequently and be more severe if patients had frequent or long lasting low back pain complaints in the past. The course of sick leave due to low back pain is similarly favourable. One study reported that 67% of patients with sick leave due to low back pain will have returned to work within a week, and 90% within 2 months. However, the longer the period of sick leave the less likely the return to work becomes. Less than half of the low back pain patients who have been off work for 6 months will return to work. After 2 years of work absenteeism, the chance to return to work is virtually zero.[9]

Please refer to CD-ROM for full text and references.

# Neck pain

**Search date January 2003**

*Allan Binder*

---

## What are the effects of treatments for uncomplicated neck pain without severe neurological deficit?

### LIKELY TO BE BENEFICIAL

**Physical treatments (active physiotherapy, pulsed electromagnetic field treatment)**

Systematic reviews and RCTs have found that active physiotherapy reduces pain compared with passive treatment, and that exercise reduces pain compared with stress management. It found limited evidence that pulsed electromagnetic field treatment reduced pain compared with sham treatment.

### UNKNOWN EFFECTIVENESS

**Drug treatments (analgesics, non-steroidal anti-inflammatory drugs, antidepressants, or muscle relaxants)**

We found insufficient evidence on the effects of analgesics, non-steroidal anti-inflammatory drugs, antidepressants, or muscle relaxants for neck pain, although they are widely used. Several drugs used to treat neck pain are associated with well documented adverse effects.

**Manual treatments (mobilisation and manipulation)**

We found insufficient evidence about the effects of manipulation or mobilisation compared with other or no treatment in people with neck pain.

**Multidisciplinary (multimodal) treatment**

We found insufficient evidence from RCTs to compare effects of multimodal cognitive behavioural therapy with other treatments in people with uncomplicated neck pain.

**Physical treatments (heat or cold, traction, biofeedback, spray and stretch, acupuncture, laser)**

Systematic reviews found insufficient evidence about the effects of these physical treatments.

**Soft collars or special pillows**

We found no reliable evidence on the effects of soft collars or special pillows in people with non-specific neck pain.

### UNLIKELY TO BE BENEFICIAL

**Patient education**

Three RCTs found no significant difference between patient education (advice or group instruction) with or without analgesics and no treatment, placebo, or usual care.

---

## What are the effects of treatments for acute whiplash injury?

### LIKELY TO BE BENEFICIAL

**Early mobilisation**

Systematic reviews and subsequent RCTs found limited evidence that early mobilisation reduced pain compared with immobilisation or rest plus a collar. ▶

◀ **Early return to normal activity**

Systematic reviews and subsequent RCTs found limited evidence that advice to "act as usual" plus anti-inflammatory drugs improved mild symptoms compared with immobilisation plus 14 days' sick leave.

**Electrotherapy**

One small RCT found limited evidence that electromagnetic field treatment reduced pain after 4 weeks but not after 3 months compared with sham treatment.

**Multimodal treatment**

One RCT found that multimodal treatment reduced pain at the end of treatment and after 6 months compared with physical treatment.

## What are the effects of treatments for chronic whiplash injury?

**LIKELY TO BE BENEFICIAL**

**Percutaneous radiofrequency neurotomy**

One RCT found limited evidence that percutaneous radiofrequency neurotomy reduced pain compared with a sham procedure after 27 weeks.

**UNKNOWN EFFECTIVENESS**

**Physiotherapy (v multimodal treatment)**

One RCT found no significant difference between physiotherapy alone and multi-modal treatment in disability, pain, or range of movement at the end of treatment or at 3 months.

## What are the effects of treatments for neck pain with radiculopathy?

**UNKNOWN EFFECTIVENESS**

**Drug treatments (epidural steroid injections, analgesics, non-steroidal anti-inflammatory drugs, or muscle relaxants)**

We found no evidence about the effects of epidural steroid injections, analgesics, non-steroidal anti-inflammatory drugs, or muscle relaxants.

**Surgery versus conservative treatment**

One RCT found no significant difference between surgery and conservative treatment in symptoms after 1 year.

**DEFINITION**  In this topic we have differentiated uncomplicated neck pain from whiplash, although many studies, particularly in people with chronic pain (duration more than 3 months), do not specify which types of participants are included. Most studies of acute pain (duration less than 3 months) are confined to whiplash. We have included under radiculopathy those studies involving people with predominantly radicular symptoms arising in the cervical spine. Neck pain often occurs in combination with limited movement and poorly defined neurological symptoms affecting the upper limbs. The pain can be severe and intractable, and can occur with radiculopathy or myelopathy.

▶

# Neck pain

| | |
|---|---|
| **INCIDENCE/ PREVALENCE** | About two thirds of people will experience neck pain at some time in their lives.[1,2] Prevalence is highest in middle age. In the UK about 15% of hospital based physiotherapy and in Canada 30% of chiropractic referrals are for neck pain.[3,4] In The Netherlands neck pain contributes up to 2% of general practitioner consultations.[5] |
| **AETIOLOGY/ RISK FACTORS** | Most uncomplicated neck pain is associated with poor posture, anxiety and depression, neck strain, occupational injuries, or sporting injuries. With chronic pain, mechanical and degenerative factors (often referred to as cervical spondylosis) are more likely. Some neck pain results from soft tissue trauma, most typically seen in whiplash injuries. Rarely disc prolapse and inflammatory, infective, or malignant conditions affect the cervical spine and present with neck pain with or without neurological features. |
| **PROGNOSIS** | Neck pain usually resolves within days or weeks but can recur or become chronic. In some industries, neck related disorders account for as much time off work as low back pain (see low back pain and sciatica [acute], p 258).[6] The percentage of people in whom neck pain becomes chronic depends on the cause but is thought to be about 10%,[1] similar to low back pain. Neck pain causes severe disability in 5% of affected people.[2] **Whiplash:** Whiplash injuries were more likely to cause disability; up to 40% of sufferers reported symptoms even after 15 years' follow up.[7] Factors associated with a poorer outcome after whiplash are not well defined.[8] The incidence of chronic disability after whiplash varies among countries, although reasons for this variation are unclear.[9] |

Please refer to CD-ROM for full text and references.

# Non-steroidal anti-inflammatory drugs

### Search date September 2002

*Peter C Gøtzsche*

## Are there any important differences between available non-steroidal anti-inflammatory drugs (NSAIDs)?

### UNKNOWN EFFECTIVENESS

**Choice between different NSAIDs**

Systematic reviews have found no important differences in benefits among different NSAIDs or doses, but found differences in harms related to choice and dose of NSAID.

### UNLIKELY TO BE BENEFICIAL

**NSAIDs in increased doses**

Systematic reviews have found that benefits of NSAIDs increase towards a maximum value at high doses. Recommended doses are close to creating the maximum benefit. In contrast, three systematic reviews found no ceiling for adverse effects, which increased in an approximately linear fashion with dose.

## What are the effects of co-treatments to reduce the risk of gastrointestinal adverse effects of NSAIDs?

### LIKELY TO BE BENEFICIAL

**$H_2$ blockers in people who cannot avoid NSAIDs**

One systematic review in people who had taken NSAIDs for 3 months has found that double doses of $H_2$ blockers versus placebo significantly reduce the development of endoscopically diagnosed gastric and duodenal ulcers. One RCT found that omeprazole versus ranitidine in double doses significantly increased remission after 6 months. One RCT with a high withdrawal and exclusion rate found weak evidence that misoprostol versus ranitidine in double doses significantly reduced the number of people with gastric ulcers.

**Omeprazole (v $H_2$ blockers) in people in people who cannot avoid NSAIDs**

One systematic review in people who had taken NSAIDs for at least 3 months has found that omeprazole versus placebo significantly reduces the incidence of endoscopically diagnosed gastric and duodenal ulcers.

### TRADE OFF BETWEEN BENEFITS AND HARMS

**Misoprostol in people who cannot avoid NSAIDs**

One systematic review in people who had taken NSAIDs for at least 3 months has found that misoprostol versus placebo significantly reduces the development of endoscopically diagnosed gastric and duodenal ulcers. One additional RCT in people with rheumatoid arthritis taking NSAIDs found that misoprostol versus placebo significantly reduced the incidence of serious upper gastrointestinal complications, such as perforation, gastric outlet obstruction, or bleeding over 6 months. Subgroup analysis found a greater absolute effect in people at high risk. RCTs have found that misoprostol versus placebo significantly increases gastrointestinal adverse events, such as diarrhoea and abdominal pain. One RCT found that more people with ulcers who had improved with either omeprazole or misoprostol, and who were then re-randomised to omeprazole or misoprostol and remained in remission with omeprazole versus misoprostol.

# Non-steroidal anti-inflammatory drugs

## What are the effects of topical NSAIDs?

**BENEFICIAL**

### Topical NSAIDs in acute and chronic pain conditions

One systematic review in people with acute and chronic pain conditions has found that topical NSAIDs versus placebo significantly reduce pain.

**UNKNOWN EFFECTIVENESS**

### Topical versus systemic NSAIDs or alternative analgesics

One systematic review found no high quality RCTs of topical NSAIDs versus oral forms of the same NSAID, or versus paracetamol.

**DEFINITION**   NSAIDs have anti-inflammatory, analgesic, and antipyretic effects, and inhibit platelet aggregation. The drugs have no documented effect on the course of musculoskeletal diseases such as rheumatoid arthritis and osteoarthritis.

**INCIDENCE/**   NSAIDs are widely used. Almost 10% of people in the Netherlands used a
**PREVALENCE**   non-aspirin NSAID in 1987, and the overall use was 11 defined daily doses**G** per 1000 population per day.[1] In Australia in 1994, overall use was 35 defined daily doses per 1000 population per day, with 36% of the people receiving NSAIDs for osteoarthritis, 42% for sprain and strain or low back pain, and 4% for rheumatoid arthritis; 35% were aged over 60 years.[2]

Please refer to CD-ROM for full text and references.

# Osteoarthritis

### Search date November 2002

*David Scott, Claire Smith, Stefan Lohmander, and Jiri Chard*

## What are the effects of treatments?

### BENEFICIAL

**Hip replacement**

One systematic review of RCTs and observational studies has found that hip replacement is effective for at least 10 years.

**Knee replacement**

Systematic reviews of observational studies have found that knee replacement is effective in relieving pain and improving function. One RCT found limited evidence that unicompartmental knee replacement is more effective than tricompartmental replacement at 5 years' follow up. One systematic review of observational studies found better outcomes with unicompartmental knee operations compared with bicompartmental operations.

**Oral non-steroidal anti-inflammatory drugs (short term pain relief)**

Systematic reviews have found that non-steroidal anti-inflammatory drugs (NSAIDs) reduce short term pain in osteoarthritis compared with placebo. NSAIDs are associated with an increased risk of gastrointestinal haemorrhage. RCTs provided insufficient evidence to compare the effects of oral versus topical NSAIDs. RCTs found no good evidence that simple analgesics, such as paracetamol (acetaminophen), are significantly different from NSAIDs in pain relief. Concerns exist relating to trial quality and commercial bias.

**Simple oral analgesics (short term pain relief)**

Systematic reviews in people with osteoarthritis of the hip or knee found limited evidence that simple analgesics, such as paracetamol, reduced pain compared with placebo. RCTs found no good evidence that simple analgesics, such as paracetamol (acetaminophen), are significantly different from NSAIDs in pain relief.

**Topical agents (short term pain relief)**

One systematic review and RCTs have found that topical agents containing NSAIDs reduce pain compared with placebo. One systematic review found that systemic adverse events were no more common than with placebo. RCTs provided insufficient evidence to compare the effects of oral versus topical NSAIDs. We found no RCTs comparing topical agents versus other local treatments such as heat or cold packs. RCTs found limited evidence that capsaicin improved pain compared with placebo.

### LIKELY TO BE BENEFICIAL

**Exercise (pain relief and improved function)**

Systematic reviews and subsequent RCTs have found that exercise and physical therapy reduce pain and disability in people with hip or knee osteoarthritis, although many of the RCTs were limited by poor methods and reporting.

**Intra-articular glucocorticoid injections of the knee (short term pain relief)**

One systematic review and one subsequent RCT found limited evidence that intra-articular glucocorticoids reduced pain for 1–4 weeks compared with placebo.

# Osteoarthritis

### Intra-articular hyaluronan injections of the knee

One systematic review and RCTs found limited evidence that hyaluronan reduced pain for 1–6 months compared with placebo.

### Osteotomy

We found no RCTs comparing osteotomy versus conservative treatment. Two RCTs found similar functional outcomes with osteotomy compared with knee replacement. Two RCTs provided insufficient evidence on the effects of different types of osteotomy

### Physical aids

RCTs in people with knee osteoarthritis found limited evidence that joint bracing or taping may improve disease specific quality of life and symptoms compared with control treatment. RCTs provided insufficient evidence to compare the effects of different insoles.

## UNKNOWN EFFECTIVENESS

### Chondroitin

One systematic review and RCTs provided insufficient evidence on the effects of chondroitin in people with osteoarthritis.

### Education

RCTs provided insufficient evidence to assess the effects of education and behavioural change in people with hip or knee osteoarthritis.

### Glucosamine

Systematic reviews and subsequent RCTs found limited evidence that glucosamine improved symptoms compared with placebo, but publication bias and poor trial quality makes the results difficult to interpret.

### Glucosamine plus chondroitin

We found no RCTs of glucosamine plus chondroitin alone. RCTs found limited evidence that glucosamine plus chondroitin plus manganese ascorbate improved disease severity scores compared with placebo.

### Hip replacement (who is most likely to benefit)

We found no RCTs. One systematic review of observational studies has suggested younger age (< 45 years), older age (> 75 years), and weight over 70 kg may be associated with worse outcomes in terms of pain relief and function after hip replacement. One cohort study found that younger people were at greater risk of revision, whereas another study found lower rates of implant survival in obese people.

### Intra-articular injection of the knee other than glucocorticoid or hyaluronan

We found insufficient evidence on the effects of other intra-articular treatments, such as radioactive isotopes, glycosaminoglycan polysulphuric acid, orgotein, and morphine.

### Knee replacement (who is most likely to benefit)

We found no RCTs. We found insufficient evidence from observational studies on the effects of obesity on knee replacement outcomes. We found limited evidence from observational studies that knee replacement is effective in elderly people. ▶

◄ **LIKELY TO BE INEFFECTIVE OR HARMFUL**

### Oral NSAIDs in older people and people at risk of renal disease or peptic ulceration

Studies have found that NSAIDs increased the risk of renal or gastrointestinal damage in older people with osteoarthritis, particularly those with intercurrent disease.

### Simple oral analgesics in people with existing liver damage

Observational evidence suggests that lower doses of paracetamol may cause liver damage in people with liver disease.

**DEFINITION**  Osteoarthritis is a heterogeneous condition for which the prevalence, risk factors, clinical manifestations, and prognosis vary according to the joints affected. It most commonly affects hands, knees, hips, and spinal apophyseal joints. It is usually defined by pathological or radiological criteria rather than clinical features, and is characterised by focal areas of damage to the cartilage surfaces of synovial joints, associated with remodelling of the underlying bone and mild synovitis. When severe, there is characteristic joint space narrowing and osteophyte formation, with visible subchondral bone changes on radiography.

**INCIDENCE/ PREVALENCE**  Osteoarthritis is common and an important cause of pain and disability in older adults.[1,2] Radiographic features are practically universal in at least some joints in people aged over 60 years, but significant clinical disease probably affects 10–20% of people. Knee disease is about twice as prevalent as hip disease in people aged over 60 years (about 10% v 5%).[3,4]

**AETIOLOGY/ RISK FACTORS**  The main initiating factors are abnormalities in joint shape or injury. Genetic factors are probably implicated.

**PROGNOSIS**  The natural history of osteoarthritis is poorly understood. Only a minority of people with clinical disease of the hip or knee joint progress to requiring surgery.

Please refer to CD-ROM for full text and references.

# Plantar heel pain and fasciitis

Search date January 2003

*Fay Crawford*

---

## What are the effects of treatments?

### TRADE OFF BETWEEN BENEFITS AND HARMS

**Corticosteroid injection plus local anaesthesia versus local anaesthetic injection alone (short term)**

One RCT found that prednisolone plus lidocaine injection reduced pain compared with lidocaine alone after 1 month. Observational studies have found a high rate of plantar fascia rupture and other complications associated with corticosteroid injections, which may lead to chronic disability in some people.

### UNKNOWN EFFECTIVENESS

**Casted orthoses☉ (custom made insoles)**

We found no RCTs on the effects of orthoses compared with placebo or no treatment. One systematic review and three RCTs found limited and conflicting evidence about the effects of orthoses compared with corticosteroids, corticosteroids plus local anaesthesia, or other physical supports.

**Corticosteroid injection plus local anaesthesia versus heel pads (short term)**

One RCT found that triamcinolone plus lidocaine injection improved pain compared with heel pad after 1 month. One small RCT found no significant difference in pain between triamcinolone plus lidocaine injection and heel pad at 1, 2, or 12 weeks. One RCT found no significant difference in pain between dexamethasone plus local anaesthetic injection plus oral etodolac and heel pads plus paracetamol at 3 months. Observational studies have found a high rate of plantar fascia rupture and other complications associated with corticosteroid injections, which may lead to chronic disability in some people.

**Corticosteroid injections plus local anaesthetic injection versus placebo (short term)**

One systematic review identified no RCTs comparing corticosteroid injection plus local anaesthesia versus placebo.

**Corticosteroid injections versus placebo (short term)**

We found no RCTs comparing short term effects of corticosteroid injection alone and placebo.

**Extracorporeal shock wave therapy**

We found insufficient evidence from four small RCTs about effects of extracorporeal shock wave therapy☉ compared with placebo. Two RCTs found limited evidence that high dose extracorporeal shock wave therapy reduced pain and walking scores compared with low dose therapy. However, the clinical importance of these effects is not clear.

**Heel pads and heel cups**

We found no RCTs on the effects of heel pads☉ and heel cups☉ compared with placebo or no treatment. One systematic review and subsequent RCTs found limited and conflicting evidence on the effects of heel pads and heel cups compared with other treatment modalities. ▶

### Lasers
One small RCT identified by a systematic review found no significant difference between laser treatment and placebo.

### Local anaesthetic injection
We found no RCTs on the effects of local anaesthesia compared with placebo or no treatment. One RCT found that prednisolone plus lidocaine injection reduced pain compared with lidocaine alone after 1 month, although the difference was not significant after 3 or 6 months.

### Night splints
One RCT found no significant difference in pain between a night splint and no splint after 3 months.

### Stretching *New*
We found no RCTs comparing stretching versus no treatment in people with heel pain. We found insufficient evidence from two RCTs to compare stretching versus stretching plus custom made orthoses, or to compare different types of stretching in people with heel pain.

### Surgery
One systematic review found no RCTs of surgery for heel pain.

### Ultrasound
One systematic review of one small RCT found no significant difference in pain between ultrasound and sham ultrasound.

## LIKELY TO BE INEFFECTIVE OR HARMFUL

### Corticosteroid injection plus local anaesthesia versus heel pads (medium to long term)
One RCT found no significant difference in pain between triamcinolone plus lidocaine injection and heel pad after 24 weeks. One RCT found no significant difference in pain between dexamethasone plus local anaesthetic injection plus oral etodolac and heel pads plus paracetamol at 3 months. Observational studies have found a high rate of plantar fascia rupture and other complications associated with corticosteroid injections, which may lead to chronic disability in some people.

### Corticosteroid injections plus local anaesthesia versus local anaesthetic injection alone (medium to long term)
One RCT found no significant difference in pain between prednisolone plus lidocaine injection and lidocaine alone after 3 or 6 months. Observational studies have found a high rate of plantar fascia rupture and other complications associated with corticosteroid injections, which may lead to chronic disability in some people.

### Corticosteroid injections plus local anaesthetic injection versus placebo (medium to long term)
One systematic review identified no RCTs comparing corticosteroid plus local anaesthetic injection versus placebo. Observational studies have found a high rate of plantar fascia rupture and other complications associated with corticosteroid injections, which may lead to chronic disability in some people.

### Corticosteroid injections versus placebo (medium to long term)
We found insufficient evidence from one RCT about clinical effects of corticosteroid injection versus placebo. Observational studies have found a high rate of plantar fascia rupture and other complications associated with corticosteroid injections, which may lead to chronic disability in some people.

# Plantar heel pain and fasciitis

**DEFINITION**    Plantar heel pain is soreness or tenderness of the heel. It often radiates from the central part of the heel pad or the medial tubercle of the calcaneum, but may extend along the plantar fascia into the medial longitudinal arch of the foot. Severity may range from an irritation at the origin of the plantar fascia, which is noticeable on rising after rest, to an incapacitating pain. This review excludes clinically evident underlying disorders, for example, infection, calcaneal fracture, and calcaneal nerve entrapment, which may be distinguished clinically — a calcaneal fracture may present after trauma, and calcaneal nerve entrapment gives rise to shooting pains and feelings of "pins and needles" on the medial aspect of the heel.

**INCIDENCE/**    The incidence and prevalence of plantar heel pain is uncertain. Plantar heel
**PREVALENCE**    pain primarily affects those in mid to late life.[1]

**AETIOLOGY/**    Unknown.
**RISK FACTORS**

**PROGNOSIS**    One systematic review (search date 1997) found that almost all of the included trials reported an improvement in discomfort regardless of the intervention received (including placebo), suggesting that the condition is at least partially self limiting.[1] A telephone survey of 100 people treated conservatively (average follow up 47 months) found that 82 people had resolution of symptoms, 15 had continued symptoms but no limitations of activity or work, and three had continued symptoms that limited activity or changed work status.[2] Thirty one people said that they would have seriously considered surgical treatment at the time medical attention was sought. The three people still affected had bilateral symptoms but no other clear risk factors.

Please refer to CD-ROM for full text and references.

### Search date February 2003

*Janet Pope*

## What are the effects of treatments?

### TRADE OFF BETWEEN BENEFITS AND HARMS

**Nifedipine**

Six RCTs found that nifedipine reduced the frequency and severity of attacks over 4–12 weeks compared with placebo, and was rated by participants as more effective than placebo in improving overall symptoms. The RCTs found that nifedipine was associated with higher rates of adverse effects compared with placebo, including flushing, headache, oedema, and tachycardia.

### UNKNOWN EFFECTIVENESS

**Amlodopine; diltiazem; moxisylyte (thymoxamine)**

We found no good RCTs of these interventions.

**Inositol nicotinate; naftidrofuryl oxalate; nicardipine; prazosin**

RCTs provided insufficient evidence to assess these interventions.

**DEFINITION**
Raynaud's phenomenon is episodic vasospasm of the peripheral arteries, causing pallor followed by cyanosis and redness with pain and sometimes paraesthesia, and, rarely, ulceration of the fingers and toes (and in some cases of the ears or nose). Primary or idiopathic Raynaud's phenomenon (Raynaud's disease) occurs without an underlying disease. Secondary Raynaud's phenomenon (Raynaud's syndrome) occurs in association with an underlying disease — usually connective tissue disorders such as scleroderma, systemic lupus erythematosus, rheumatoid arthritis, or polymyositis. This review excludes secondary Raynaud's phenomenon.

**INCIDENCE/ PREVALENCE**
The prevalence of primary Raynaud's phenomenon varies by gender, country, and exposure to workplace vibration. One large US cohort study (4182 people) found symptoms in 9.6% of women and 8.1% of men, of whom 81% had primary Raynaud's phenomenon.[1] Smaller cohort studies in Spain have estimated the prevalence of Raynaud's phenomenon to be 3.7–4.0%, of which 90% is primary Raynaud's phenomenon.[2,3] One cohort study in Japan (332 men, 731 women) found symptoms of primary Raynaud's phenomenon in 3.4% of women and 3.0% of men.[4]

**AETIOLOGY/ RISK FACTORS**
The aetiology of primary Raynaud's phenomenon is unknown.[5] There is evidence for genetic predisposition,[6,7] most likely in those people with early onset Raynaud's phenomenon (aged < 40 years).[8] One prospective observational study (424 people with Raynaud's phenomenon) found that 73% of sufferers first developed symptoms before age 40 years.[8] Women are more at risk than men (OR 3.0, 95% CI 1.2 to 7.8, in 1 US case control study [235 people]).[9] The other known risk factor is occupational exposure to vibration from tools (symptoms developed in about 8% with exposure *v* 2.7% with no exposure in 2 cohorts from Japan).[10,11] People who are obese may be less at risk.[9] Symptoms are often worsened by cold or emotion.

**PROGNOSIS**
Attacks may last from several minutes to a few hours. One systematic review (search date 1996, 10 prospective observational studies, 639 people with primary Raynaud's phenomenon) found that only 13% of long term sufferers later manifested an underlying disorder such as scleroderma.[12]

Please refer to CD-ROM for full text and references.

Musculoskeletal disorders

# Rheumatoid arthritis

## Search date July 2002

*Paul Emery and Maria Suarez-Almazor*

## What are the effects of treatments?

### BENEFICIAL

#### Antimalarials

One systematic review has found that hydroxychloroquine reduces disease activity and joint inflammation compared with placebo in people with rheumatoid arthritis. We found insufficient evidence about effects on functional status. One systematic review found no consistent difference in effectiveness between antimalarials and other disease modifying antirheumatic drugs (DMARDs).

#### Early intervention with DMARDs

One systematic review and one additional RCT found that early DMARDs (oral gold, im gold, hydroxychloroquine, methotrexate, minocycline) significantly improved radiological progression, swollen joint counts, and quality of life scores at 12–60 months compared with delayed treatment.

#### Methotrexate

One systematic review has found that methotrexate reduces joint inflammation and radiological progression and improves functional status compared with placebo in people with rheumatoid arthritis. One systematic review and subsequent RCTs have found no consistent differences in efficacy between methotrexate versus leflunomide, parenteral gold, or etanercept.

#### Minocycline

RCTs have found that minocycline improves control of disease activity compared with placebo. We found no RCTs comparing minocycline versus other DMARDs.

#### Short term low dose oral corticosteroids

One systematic review has found that low dose oral corticosteroids for several weeks significantly reduces disease activity and joint inflammation compared with placebo.

#### Sulfasalazine

Systematic reviews have found that sulfasalazine versus placebo for 6 months significantly reduces disease activity and joint inflammation. We found inadequate evidence on radiological progression and functional status. One systematic review found no consistent differences between sulfasalazine and other DMARDs. Another systematic review of observational studies and RCTs found that over 5 years people were less likely to continue sulfasalazine than methotrexate.

### LIKELY TO BE BENEFICIAL

#### Auranofin (less effective than other DMARDs)

One systematic review has found that auranofin (oral gold) versus placebo reduces disease activity and joint inflammation, but found no evidence on radiological progression or long term functional status. Limited evidence from RCTs suggests that auranofin is less effective than DMARDs.

#### Leflunomide (long term safety unclear)

One systematic review has found that leflunomide versus placebo reduces disease activity and joint inflammation, improves functional status and health related quality of life, and decreases radiological progression. We found no good evidence ▶

on long term adverse effects. We found no consistent evidence of a difference in clinical efficacy between leflunomide and methotrexate or sulfasalazine.

### Treatment with several DMARDs combined

One systematic review and subsequent RCTs have found that combining certain DMARDs is more effective than using individual drugs alone. However, the balance between benefit and harm varies among combinations.

### Tumour necrosis factor antagonists (long term safety unclear)

RCTs have found that tumour necrosis factor antibodies (etanercept and infliximab) significantly improve symptoms, and reduce long term disease activity and joint inflammation compared with placebo. One RCT found no significant difference between etanercept and methotrexate for quality of life at 1 year. Short term toxicity is relatively low, but long term safety is less clear.

## TRADE OFF BETWEEN BENEFITS AND HARMS

### Azathioprine

One systematic review has found that azathioprine versus placebo reduces disease activity in the short term (16 wks to 6 months). We found no evidence on radiological progression or long term functional status. A high level of toxicity limits the usefulness of azathioprine.

### Ciclosporin

One systematic review has found that ciclosporin for a minimum of 4 months significantly reduces disease activity and joint inflammation, improves functional status, and may decrease the rate of radiological progression compared with methotrexate. One RCT found no significant difference between parenteral gold versus ciclosporin for radiological joint damage or self assessment of change in disease activity at 36 months. A very high frequency of toxicity limits the usefulness of ciclosporin.

### Cyclophosphamide

One systematic review has found that cyclophosphamide significantly reduces disease activity and joint inflammation compared with placebo at 6 months. It may also reduce the rate of radiological progression, but evidence was limited. We found no evidence of its effect on long term functional status. Severe toxicity limits its usefulness.

### Long term low dose oral corticosteroids

One systematic review and one subsequent RCT have found that low dose oral corticosteroids for at least 3 months significantly reduce pain, joint inflammation, and functional status compared with placebo. However, long term use is associated with considerable adverse effects.

### Parenteral gold

One systematic review has found that parenteral gold reduces disease activity and joint inflammation, and slows radiological progression compared with placebo in people with rheumatoid arthritis. We found no evidence on long term functional status. One systematic review and one RCT both indicate increased withdrawals because of toxicity. RCTs found no significant differences in clinical efficacy between parenteral gold versus methotrexate or ciclosporin at 1–3 years.

### Penicillamine

One systematic review has found that penicillamine reduces disease activity and joint inflammation compared with placebo at 4–6 months. We found no evidence about effects of penicillamine on radiological progression or long term functional

# Rheumatoid arthritis

status. One systematic review has found no consistent difference between penicillamine versus other DMARDs. Common and potentially serious adverse effects limit the usefulness of penicillamine.

**DEFINITION**   Rheumatoid arthritis is a chronic inflammatory disorder. It is characterised by a chronic polyarthritis that primarily affects the peripheral joints and related periarticular tissues. It usually starts as an insidious symmetric polyarthritis, often with non-specific systemic symptoms. Diagnostic criteria include arthritis lasting longer than 6 weeks (although evidence suggests that 12 wks is more specific), positive rheumatoid factor, and radiological damage.[1]

**INCIDENCE/**
**PREVALENCE**   Prevalence ranges from 0.5–1.5% of the population in industrialised countries.[2,3] Rheumatoid arthritis occurs more frequently in women than men (ratio 2.5 : 1).[2,3] The annual incidence in women was recently estimated at 36/100 000 and in men at 14/100 000.[3]

**AETIOLOGY/**
**RISK FACTORS**   The evidence suggests that the cause is multifactorial in people with genetic susceptibility.[4]

**PROGNOSIS**   The course of rheumatoid arthritis is variable and unpredictable. Some people experience flares and remissions, and others a progressive course. Over years, structural damage occurs, leading to articular deformities and functional impairment. About half of people will be unable to work within 10 years.[5] Rheumatoid arthritis shortens life expectancy.[6]

Please refer to CD-ROM for full text and references.

### Search date October 2002

*Cathy Speed and Brian Hazleman*

## What are the effects of treatments?

Shoulder pain is not a specific diagnosis. Well designed, double blind RCTs of specific interventions in specific shoulder disorders are needed. Systematic reviews have found RCTs mostly with poor methods, and pronounced heterogeneity of study populations and outcome measures. We found insufficient evidence on the effects of most interventions in people with non-specific shoulder pain.

### UNKNOWN EFFECTIVENESS

**Arthroscopic laser subacromial decompression**

One systematic review found no RCTs on arthroscopic laser subacromial decompression.

**Electrical stimulation**

One RCT found no significant difference in pain between electrical stimulation versus control. However, the study may have lacked power to detect clinically important differences.

**Extracorporeal shock wave therapy**

We found mixed results from three RCTs. The first RCT found that one or two sessions of high energy extracorporeal shock wave therapy versus placebo improved pain and function in people with calcific tendinitis. However, two further RCTs in people with rotator cuff tendinosis found no significant difference for extracorporeal shock wave therapy versus sham treatment for pain or function at 3–6 months.

**Intra-articular corticosteroid injection**

One small RCT found no significant difference for intra-articular triamcinolone versus saline in pain score, change in mobility, or function at 3 weeks. One small RCT found no significant difference for intra-articular methylprednisolone plus lidocaine (lignocaine) versus lidocaine alone in pain or shoulder motion at 24 weeks. The RCTs were small and may have lacked power to detect clinically important differences.

**Intra-articular guanethidine**

We found no systematic review or RCTs of intra-articular guanethidine in people with non-arthritic shoulder pain.

**Laser treatment**

We found mixed results from four small RCTs that compared laser treatment versus placebo in shoulder pain. Two short term RCTs found that laser improved recovery rate and pain compared with placebo at 2–4 weeks. However, two longer term RCTs found no significant difference in pain or recovery rate at 8–12 weeks.

**Multidisciplinary biopsychosocial rehabilitation**

One systematic review found no good quality RCTs of multidisciplinary biopsychosocial rehabilitation⊕ in people with shoulder pain.

**Oral non-steroidal anti-inflammatory drugs**

We found insufficient evidence from one systematic review and one additional RCT to draw firm conclusions about effects of oral non-steroidal anti-inflammatory drugs versus placebo in people with non-specific shoulder pain.

# Shoulder pain

### Phonophoresis©

We found no RCTs solely in people with shoulder pain.

### Physiotherapy (exercises and manual treatments)

One systematic review has found insufficient evidence about effects of physiotherapy alone versus no treatment or advice to exercise in people with shoulder pain.

### Subacromial corticosteroid injection

We found no RCTs comparing subacromial injection of steroids versus placebo. We found insufficient evidence from two small RCTs to compare clinical effects of corticosteroid plus lidocaine versus lidocaine alone in people with rotator cuff tendinitis. One small RCT found limited evidence that intra-articular plus subacromial corticosteroid injections versus intra-articular and subacromial lidocaine alone increased remission rates at 4 weeks.

### Surgery/forced manipulation

We found no placebo-controlled RCTs. One small RCT found that forced manipulation plus intra-articular hydrocortisone injection versus intra-articular hydrocortisone injection alone increased recovery rate at 3 months.

### Transdermal glyceryl trinitrate

We found no reliable RCTs.

### Ice; paracetamol or opiates; topical or intra-articular non-steroidal anti-inflammatory drugs

We found no RCTs about these interventions.

## UNLIKELY TO BE BENEFICIAL

### Oral corticosteroids

Two small RCTs found no evidence of reduced pain or improved abduction with oral corticosteroids versus placebo or versus no treatment at 4–8 months. Adverse effect of corticosteroids are well documented (see rheumatoid arthritis, p 274 and asthma, p 328).

### Ultrasound

One systematic review and two subsequent RCTs found no clinically important difference in pain, abduction or quality of life with ultrasound versus sham treatment or no treatment.

**DEFINITION**     Shoulder pain arises in or around the shoulder from the glenohumeral, acromioclavicular, sternoclavicular, "subacromial", and scapulothoracic articulations, and surrounding soft tissues. Regardless of the disorder, pain is the most common reason for consulting a practitioner. In adhesive capsulitis (frozen shoulder), pain is associated with pronounced restriction of movement. For most shoulder disorders, diagnosis is based on clinical features, with imaging studies playing a role in some people. Post-stroke shoulder pain is not addressed in this topic.

**INCIDENCE/**     Each year in primary care in the UK, about 1% of adults aged over 45 years
**PREVALENCE**     present with a new episode of shoulder pain.[1] Prevalence is uncertain, with estimates from 4–20%.[2–6] One community survey (392 people) found a 1 month prevalence of shoulder pain of 34%.[7] A second community survey (644 people aged ≥ 70 years) reported a point prevalence of 21%, with a higher frequency in women than men (25% v 17%).[8] Seventy per cent of cases involved the rotator cuff. One survey of 134 people in a community based rheumatology clinic found that 65% of cases were rotator cuff lesions; 11% were caused by localised tenderness in the pericapsular musculature; 10% acromioclavicular joint pain; 3% glenohumeral joint arthritis; and 5%

were referred pain from the neck.[9] One survey found that in adults, the annual incidence of frozen shoulder was about 2%, with those aged 40–70 years most commonly affected.[10] The age distribution of specific shoulder disorders in the community is unknown.

**AETIOLOGY/ RISK FACTORS** Rotator cuff disorders are associated with excessive overloading, instability of the glenohumeral and acromioclavicular joints, muscle imbalance, adverse anatomical features (narrow coracoacromial arch and a hooked acromion), cuff degeneration with aging, ischaemia, and musculoskeletal diseases that result in wasting of the cuff muscles.[11–14] Risk factors for frozen shoulder include female sex, older age, shoulder trauma, surgery, diabetes, cardiorespiratory disorders, cerebrovascular events, thyroid disease, and hemiplegia.[10,15,16] Arthritis of the glenohumeral joint can occur in numerous forms, including primary and secondary osteoarthritis, rheumatoid arthritis, and crystal arthritides.[11]

**PROGNOSIS** One survey in an elderly community found that most people with shoulder pain were still affected 3 years after the initial survey.[17] One prospective cohort study of 122 people in primary care found that 25% of people with shoulder pain reported previous episodes and 49% reported full recovery at 18 months' follow up.[18]

Please refer to CD-ROM for full text and references.

# Tennis elbow

**Search date August 2002**

*Willem Assendelft, Sally Green, Rachelle Buchbinder, Peter Struijs, and Nynke Smidt*

## What are the effects of treatments for tennis elbow (lateral epicondylitis)?

### BENEFICIAL

**Topical non-steroidal anti-inflammatory drugs for short term pain relief**

One systematic review has found that topical non-steroidal anti-inflammatory drugs versus placebo significantly improve pain in the short term. Minor adverse effects have been reported. We found no RCTs comparing oral versus topical non-steroidal anti-inflammatory drugs.

### LIKELY TO BE BENEFICIAL

**Oral non-steroidal anti-inflammatory drugs**

One systematic review found limited evidence of a short term improvement in pain and function with an oral non-steroidal inflammatory drug versus placebo. The review found limited evidence that fewer people receiving an oral non-steroidal anti-inflammatory drug versus a corticosteroid injection had self perceived improvement at 4 weeks, but found that an oral non-steroidal anti-inflammatory drug significantly reduced pain at 26 weeks.

### TRADE OFF BETWEEN BENEFITS AND HARMS

**Corticosteroid injections**

We found one systematic review and two subsequent RCTs of corticosteroid injections, which found limited evidence of a short term improvement in symptoms with steroid injections versus placebo, a local anaesthetic, elbow strapping, or physiotherapy. It found no good evidence on long term effects of corticosteroids versus placebo or local anaesthetic. It found no evidence of a difference with corticosteroid injection versus mobilisation plus massage or elbow strapping in overall improvement at 1 year. However, one RCT identified by the review found significantly greater improvement in symptoms with physiotherapy versus an injection at 26 and 52 weeks. The review found limited evidence of greater self perceived improvement at 4 weeks with a corticosteroid injection versus an oral non-steroidal anti-inflammatory drug (NSAID), but found greater improvement in pain at 26 weeks with an oral non-steroidal anti-inflammatory drug.

### UNKNOWN EFFECTIVENESS

**Acupuncture**

One systematic review and one subsequent RCT found insufficient evidence to assess the effects of acupuncture (either needle or laser).

**Exercise and mobilisation**

One systematic review found limited evidence of a better outcome with exercise versus ultrasound plus friction massage at 8 weeks.

**Extra-corporeal shock wave therapy**

One systematic review found conflicting evidence from two RCTs of the effects on symptoms of extra-corporeal shock wave therapy versus sham treatment.

◀ **Non-steroidal anti-inflammatory drugs for longer term pain relief**

We found insufficient evidence to assess the longer term effects of oral or topical non-steroidal anti-inflammatory drugs.

## Orthoses

One systematic review found insufficient evidence about the effects of orthoses (braces).

## Surgery

One systematic review found no RCTs of surgical treatment for tennis elbow.

**DEFINITION**     Tennis elbow has many analogous terms, including lateral elbow pain, lateral epicondylitis, rowing elbow, tendonitis of the common extensor origin, and peritendonitis of the elbow. Tennis elbow is characterised by pain and tenderness over the lateral epicondyle of the humerus and pain on resisted dorsi-flexion of the wrist, middle finger or both. For the purposes of this review, tennis elbow was restricted to lateral elbow pain, or lateral epicondylitis.

**INCIDENCE/**     Lateral elbow pain is common (population prevalence 1–3%).[1] Peak inci-
**PREVALENCE**   dence is 40–50 years and for women of 42–46 years of age the incidence increases to 10%.[2,3] The incidence of lateral elbow pain in general practice is 4–7/1000 people a year.[3–5]

**AETIOLOGY/**     Tennis elbow is considered to be an overload injury, typically after minor and
**RISK FACTORS** often unrecognised trauma of the extensor muscles of the forearm. Despite the title tennis elbow, tennis is a direct cause in only 5% of those with epicondylitis.[6]

**PROGNOSIS**     Although lateral elbow pain is generally self limiting, in a minority of people symptoms persist for 18 months to 2 years and in some cases for much longer.[7] The cost is therefore high, both in terms of lost productivity, and healthcare use. In a general practice trial of an expectant waiting policy 80% of the people with elbow pain of already greater than 4 weeks' duration were recovered after 1 year.[8]

---

Please refer to CD-ROM for full text and references.

# Bell's palsy

**Search date November 2002**

*Rodrigo Salinas*

---

## *What are the effects of treatments in adults and children?*

### UNKNOWN EFFECTIVENESS

#### Antiviral treatment

Two systematic reviews found no RCTs of aciclovir versus placebo. One RCT found limited evidence that aciclovir plus prednisone improved facial function compared with prednisone alone after 4 months.

#### Corticosteroids

One systematic review found no clear evidence that corticosteroid improved the recovery of facial motor function or cosmetically disabling sequelae compared with placebo after 6 months.

#### Facial nerve decompression surgery

One systematic review identified no RCTs of facial nerve decompression.

| | |
|---|---|
| **DEFINITION** | Bell's palsy is an acute, unilateral paresis or paralysis of the face in a pattern consistent with peripheral nerve dysfunction, without detectable causes.[1] Additional symptoms may include pain in or behind the ear, numbness in the affected side of the face, hyperacusis, and disturbed taste on the ipsilateral anterior part of the tongue.[2–5] |
| **INCIDENCE/ PREVALENCE** | The incidence is about 23/100 000 people a year, or about 1/60–70 people in a lifetime.[6] Bell's palsy affects men and women more or less equally, with a peak incidence between the ages of 10 and 40 years. It occurs with equal frequency on the right and left sides of the face.[7] |
| **AETIOLOGY/ RISK FACTORS** | The cause is unclear. Viral infection, vascular ischaemia, autoimmune inflammatory disorders, and heredity have been proposed as underlying causes.[2,8,9] A viral cause has gained popularity since the isolation of the herpes simplex virus-1 genome from facial nerve endoneurial fluid in people with Bell's palsy.[10] |
| **PROGNOSIS** | More than two thirds of people with Bell's palsy achieve full spontaneous recovery. The largest series of people with Bell's palsy who received no specific treatment (1011 people) found the first signs of improvement within 3 weeks of onset in 85% of people.[11] For the other 15%, some improvement occurred 3–6 months later. The same series found that 71% of people recovered normal function of the face, 13% had insignificant sequelae, and the remaining 16% had permanently diminished function, with contracture and synkinesis**G**. These figures are roughly similar to those of other series of people receiving no specific treatment for Bell's palsy.[7,8,12] |

---

Please refer to CD-ROM for full text and references.

Neurological disorders

---

## What are the effects of treatments?

### BENEFICIAL

**Addition of second line drugs for drug resistant partial epilepsy**

Systematic reviews in people with drug resistant partial epilepsy have found that adding gabapentin, levetiracetam, lamotrigine, oxcarbazepine, tiagabine, topiramate, vigabatrin, or zonisamide to usual treatment reduces seizure frequency compared with adding placebo. The reviews have found that adding any of the drugs increases the frequency of adverse effects compared with adding placebo. We found no good evidence from RCTs on which to base a choice among drugs.

**Antiepileptic monotherapy in generalised epilepsy***

We found no placebo controlled trials of the main antiepileptic drugs (carbamazepine, phenobarbital, phenytoin, sodium valproate), but widespread consensus holds that these drugs are effective. Systematic reviews found no good evidence on which to base a choice among these drugs in terms of seizure control.

**Antiepileptic monotherapy in partial epilepsy***

We found no placebo controlled RCTs of the main antiepileptic drugs (carbamazepine, phenobarbital, phenytoin, sodium valproate) used as monotherapy in people with partial epilepsy, but widespread consensus holds that these drugs are effective. Systematic reviews found no reliable evidence on which to base a choice among drugs in terms of seizure control. Systematic reviews have found that phenobarbital is more likely to be withdrawn than phenytoin or carbamazepine and that phenytoin is more likely to be withdrawn than carbamazepine.

*We found no placebo controlled RCTs. However, widespread consensus holds that these drugs are effective.

### LIKELY TO BE BENEFICIAL

**Educational programmes**

One RCT found that a 2 day education programme reduced seizure frequency at 6 months compared with waiting list control, although it found no significant difference in health related quality of life. Two RCTs found that an educational package improved knowledge and understanding of epilepsy, adjustment to epilepsy, and psychosocial functioning compared with control.

### TRADE OFF BETWEEN BENEFITS AND HARMS

**Antiepileptic drug withdrawal for people in remission**

One systematic review of observational studies and one RCT have found that antiepileptic drug withdrawal for people in remission is associated with a higher risk of seizure recurrence than is continued treatment. Clinical predictors of relapse after drug withdrawal include age, seizure type, number of antiepileptic drugs being taken, whether seizures have occurred since antiepileptic drugs were started, and the period of remission before drug withdrawal.

**Antiepileptic drugs after a single seizure**

RCTs have found that immediate treatment of a single seizure with antiepileptic drugs reduces seizure recurrence at 2 years compared with no treatment. However, we found no evidence that treatment alters long term prognosis. Long term antiepileptic drug treatment is potentially harmful.

Neurological disorders

## Cognitive behavioural therapy
We found insufficient evidence about the effects of cognitive behavioural therapy🇬 in people with epilepsy from two small RCTs.

## Family counselling
We found insufficient evidence on family counselling from one small RCT that employed weak methods.

## Relaxation plus behavioural modification therapy
RCTs found insufficient evidence about the effects of combined relaxation and behavioural modification on seizures.

## Biofeedback; relaxation therapy🇬; yoga
Systematic reviews found insufficient evidence on the effects of these interventions.

**DEFINITION**  Epilepsy is a group of disorders rather than a single disease. Seizures can be classified by type as partial (categorised as simple partial🇬, complex partial🇬, and secondary generalised tonic clonic seizures), or generalised (categorised as generalised tonic clonic, absence, myoclonic, tonic, and atonic seizures🇬).[1]

**INCIDENCE/ PREVALENCE**  Epilepsy is common, with an estimated prevalence in the developed world of 5–10/1000, and an annual incidence of 50/100 000 people.[2] About 3% of people will be given a diagnosis of epilepsy at some time in their lives.[3]

**AETIOLOGY/ RISK FACTORS**  Epilepsy can also be classified by cause.[1] Idiopathic generalised epilepsies (such as juvenile myoclonic epilepsy or childhood absence epilepsy) are largely genetic. Symptomatic epilepsies result from a known cerebral abnormality; for example, temporal lobe epilepsy may result from a congenital defect, mesial temporal sclerosis, or a tumour. Cryptogenic epilepsies are those that cannot be classified as idiopathic or symptomatic and in which no causative factor has been identified, but is suspected.

**PROGNOSIS**  For most people with epilepsy the prognosis is good. About 70% go into remission, defined as being seizure free for 5 years on or off treatment. This leaves 20–30% who develop chronic epilepsy, which is often treated with multiple antiepileptic drugs.[4] About 60% of untreated people have no further seizures in the 2 years after their first seizure.[5]

Please refer to CD-ROM for full text and references.

Search date September 2002

*Joaquim Ferreira and Cristina Sampaio*

Neurological disorders

## What are the effects of drug treatments in people with essential tremor of the hand?

### LIKELY TO BE BENEFICIAL

#### Propranolol (evidence for short term only)
Small RCTs have found that propranolol versus placebo significantly improves short term clinical scores, tremor amplitude, and symptom severity for up to 6 weeks.

### TRADE OFF BETWEEN BENEFITS AND HARMS

#### Botulinum A toxin–haemagglutinin complex (evidence for short term only)
RCTs comparing botulinum A toxin–haemagglutinin complex versus placebo found short term improvement of clinical rating scales, but no consistent improvement of motor task performance or functional disability. Hand weakness, which is dose dependent and transient, is a frequent adverse effect.

#### Phenobarbital (evidence for short term only)
One small RCT found limited evidence that phenobarbital (phenobarbitone) versus placebo significantly improved tremor scores at 5 weeks. However, two further RCTs found no significant difference between phenobarbital and placebo. Phenobarbital is associated with depression and cognitive and behavioural effects.

#### Primidone (evidence for short term only)
Three small, short term RCTs found limited evidence that primidone versus placebo improved tremor and functional ability. We found no long term RCTs. Primidone is associated with depression and cognitive and behavioural adverse effects.

#### Topiramate (evidence for short term only)
One RCT found that topiramate improved observer rated tremor score but was associated with more adverse effects compared with placebo. The clinical importance of the difference in tremor score is uncertain.

### UNKNOWN EFFECTIVENESS

#### All treatment options (long term)
We found no RCTs that reported the long term effects of drug treatments for essential tremor.

#### β Blockers other than propranolol (atenolol, sotalol)
Small RCTs found weak evidence that sotalol or atenolol versus placebo significantly improved symptoms and self evaluated measures of tremor at 5 days to 4 weeks. However, we were unable to draw reliable conclusions about effects.

#### Benzodiazepines
Two small short term RCTs found weak evidence that alprazolam may improve tremor and function compared with placebo. However, we were unable to draw reliable conclusions about effects. We found insufficient evidence to compare effects of clonazepam versus placebo. Adverse effects with benzodiazepines, including sedation and cognitive and behavioural effects, have been well described for other conditions (see panic disorder, p 231).

#### Calcium channel blockers (nicardipine, nimodipine)
Poor quality RCTs found insufficient evidence about the effects of dihydropyridine calcium channel blockers versus placebo.

# Essential tremor

### Carbonic anhydrase inhibitors
Two RCTs found no evidence of benefit with carbonic anhydrase inhibitors compared with placebo.

### Clonidine
One RCT found no significant difference between clonidine and placebo for clinical improvement. However, the study may have lacked power to detect clinically important differences.

### Flunarizine
One small RCT found weak evidence that flunarizine versus placebo may improve symptoms after 1 month of treatment.

### Gabapentin
Small crossover RCTs found insufficient evidence about the effects of gabapentin versus placebo.

### Isoniazid
One RCT found no significant difference with isoniazid versus placebo in clinical score. However, the study may have lacked power to detect clinically important differences.

**DEFINITION**  Tremor is a rhythmic, mechanical oscillation of at least one body region. The term essential tremor is used when there is either a persistent bilateral tremor of hands and forearms, or an isolated tremor of the head without abnormal posturing, and when there is no evidence that the tremor arises from another identifiable or separately named cause. The diagnosis is not made if there are abnormal neurological signs, known causes of enhanced physiological tremor, a history or signs of psychogenic tremor, sudden change in severity, primary orthostatic tremor, isolated voice tremor, isolated position specific or task specific tremors, and isolated tongue, chin, or leg tremor.[1]

**INCIDENCE/**  Essential tremor is one of the most common movement disorders throughout
**PREVALENCE**  the world, with a prevalence of 0.4–3.9% in the general population.[2]

**AETIOLOGY/**  Essential tremor is sometimes inherited with an autosomal dominant pattern.
**RISK FACTORS**  About 40% of people with essential tremor have no family history. Alcohol ingestion provides symptomatic benefit in 50–70% of people.[3]

**PROGNOSIS**  Essential tremor is a persistent and progressive condition. It usually begins during young adulthood and the severity of the tremor increases slowly. Only a small proportion of people with essential tremor seek medical advice, but the proportion in different surveys varies from 0.5–11%.[2] Most people with essential tremor are only mildly affected. However, most of the people who seek medical care are disabled to some extent, and most are socially handicapped by the tremor.[4] A quarter of people receiving medical care for the tremor change jobs or retire because of essential tremor induced disability.[3,5]

---

Please refer to CD-ROM for full text and references.

**Search date February 2003**

*Peter J Goadsby*

## What are the effects of treatments?

We found only limited evidence about the treatment of chronic tension-type headache.

### BENEFICIAL

**Amitriptyline (only short term evidence)**
One systematic review and three small, short duration RCTs have found that amitriptyline reduces duration and frequency of chronic tension-type headache compared with placebo.

### LIKELY TO BE BENEFICIAL

**Cognitive behavioural therapy**
One systematic review of three small RCTs and one subsequent RCT found limited evidence that cognitive behavioural therapy reduced symptoms at 6 months compared with no treatment.

### UNKNOWN EFFECTIVENESS

**Acupuncture**
We found insufficient evidence from heterogeneous RCTs about effects of acupuncture compared with placebo in people with episodic or chronic tension-type headache. Many of the RCTs were of poor quality. Some of the RCTs may have lacked power to exclude a clinically important effect.

**Botulinum toxin; relaxation☺ and electromyographic biofeedback therapy☺; serotonin reuptake inhibitors; tricyclic antidepressants other than amitriptyline**
We found insufficient evidence about the effects of these interventions.

### LIKELY TO BE INEFFECTIVE OR HARMFUL

**Benzodiazepines**
Two RCTs found insufficient evidence about the effects of benzodiazepines compared with placebo or other treatments. Benzodiazepines are commonly associated with adverse effects if taken regularly.

**Regular acute pain relief medication**
We found no RCTs. We found insufficient evidence from one non-systematic review of observational studies about benefits of common analgesics in people with chronic tension-type headache. It found that sustained and frequent use of some analgesics was associated with chronic headache and reduced the effectiveness of prophylactic treatment.

**DEFINITION**    The 1988 International Headache Society criteria for chronic tension-type headache (CTTH) are headaches on 15 or more days a month (180 days/ year) for at least 6 months; pain that is bilateral, pressing, or tightening in quality, of mild or moderate intensity, which does not prohibit activities and is not aggravated by routine physical activity; presence of no more than one additional clinical feature (nausea, photophobia, or phonophobia) and no vomiting.[1] CTTH is distinguished from chronic daily headache, which is simply a descriptive term for any headache type that occurs for 15 days or more a month that may be due to CTTH as well as migraine or analgesic associated headache.[2] In contrast to CTTH, episodic tension-type headache can last for ▶

# Headache (chronic tension-type)

30 minutes to 7 days and occurs for fewer than 180 days a year. Terms based on assumed mechanisms (muscle contraction headache, tension headache) are not operationally defined. Old studies that used these terms may have included people with many different types of headache. The greatest obstacle to studying tension-type headache is the lack of any single proved specific or reliable, clinical, or biological defining characteristic of the disorder.

**INCIDENCE/ PREVALENCE**
The prevalence of chronic daily headache from a survey of the general population in the USA was 4.1%. Half of sufferers met the International Headache Society criteria for CTTH.[3] In a survey of 2500 undergraduate students in the USA, the prevalence of CTTH was 2%.[4] The prevalence of CTTH was 2.5% in a Danish population based survey of 975 individuals.[5] One community based survey in Singapore (2096 people from the general population) found that prevalence was 1.8% in females and 0.9% males.[6]

**AETIOLOGY/ RISK FACTORS**
Tension type headache is more prevalent in women (65% of cases in one survey).[7] Symptoms begin before the age of 10 years in 15% of people with CTTH. Prevalence declines with age.[8] There is a family history of some form of headache in 40% of people with CTTH,[9] although a twin study found that risk of CTTH was similar for identical and non-identical twins.[10]

**PROGNOSIS**
The prevalence of CTTH declines with age.[8]

---

Please refer to CD-ROM for full text and references.

## What are the effects of drug treatment?

### BENEFICIAL

#### Eletriptan
One systematic review and subsequent RCTs have found that eletriptan increases headache relief❻ compared with placebo. Two RCTs found that eletriptan increased headache relief compared with sumatriptan.

#### Naratriptan
Four RCTs have found that naratriptan increases headache relief at 4 hours compared with placebo. One RCT comparing naratriptan versus sumatriptan found no significant difference in headache recurrence❻.

#### Rizatriptan
One systematic review and subsequent RCTs have found that rizatriptan improves headache relief compared with placebo.

#### Salicylates
RCTs have found that oral or intravenous lysine acetylsalicylic acid (alone or in combination with metoclopramide) and oral aspirin (alone or in combination with metoclopramide, paracetamol, or caffeine) increase headache relief compared with placebo. One RCT found no significant difference between aspirin and paracetamol plus codeine in headache relief, although both were more effective than placebo. One RCT found no significant difference between aspirin plus metoclopramide and sumatriptan in headache relief.

#### Sumatriptan
RCTs have found that subcutaneous, oral, or intranasal sumatriptan increases headache relief compared with placebo. RCTs found no significant difference in headache relief between sumatriptan and aspirin plus metoclopramide, tolfenamic acid, or zolmitriptan. RCTs found that oral or nasal sumatriptan increased headache relief compared with oral or nasal ergotamine. One RCT found no significant difference between sumatriptan and naratriptan in headache recurrence.

#### Zolmitriptan
Three large RCTs have found that oral zolmitriptan increases headache relief compared with placebo. Two RCTs found no significant difference between zolmitriptan and sumatriptan in headache relief.

### LIKELY TO BE BENEFICIAL

#### Diclofenac
RCTs found that oral or intramuscular diclofenac improved headache symptoms compared with placebo. One RCT found that intramuscular diclofenac improved migraine symptoms compared with intramuscular paracetamol.

#### Ergotamine
One systematic review found limited evidence from four RCTs that ergotamine or ergotamine plus caffeine improved headache relief compared with placebo. RCTs found that ergotamine (or its derivatives, with or without caffeine and cyclizine) was ▶

# Migraine headache

less effective for migraine symptoms than sumatriptan, and limited evidence that it was less effective than naproxen. One overview of harms suggested that ergotamine increased nausea and vomiting compared with placebo.

## Ibuprofen

Five RCTs found that ibuprofen improved migraine symptoms compared with placebo.

## Naproxen

Three small RCTs found that naproxen reduced migraine symptoms compared with placebo. Two RCTs found that naproxen reduced symptoms compared with ergotamine (with or without caffeine plus cyclizine). However, one further RCT found no significant difference between naproxen and ergotamine in pain relief after 1 hour.

## Tolfenamic acid

RCTs found limited evidence that tolfenamic acid improved duration and severity of headache compared with placebo. RCTs found no significant difference in symptoms between tolfenamic acid and sumatriptan or paracetamol.

**DEFINITION**    Migraine is a primary headache disorder manifesting as recurring attacks usually lasting for 4–72 hours and involving pain of moderate to severe intensity, often with nausea, sometimes vomiting, and/or sensitivity to light, sound, and other sensory stimuli. The 1988 International Headache Society criteria⊙ include separate criteria for migraine with and migraine without associated aura.[1] Unless stated otherwise, RCTs used International Headache Society criteria for migraine with or without aura

**INCIDENCE/**    Migraine is common worldwide. Prevalence has been reported to be 5–25%
**PREVALENCE** in women and 2–10% in men. Overall, the highest incidence for migraine without aura has been reported between the ages of 10 and 11 years (10/1000 person years). The peak incidence of migraine without aura in males is between ages 10 and 11 years (10/1000 person years) and in females between ages 14 and 17 years (19/1000 person years).[2] The incidence of migraine with aura peaks in males at around age 5 years (7/1000 person years) and in females at around age 12–13 years (14/1000 person years).[2] Female prevalence of migraine with or without aura has a declining trend after age 45–50 years

**AETIOLOGY/**    Data from independent representative samples from Canada,[3,4] the USA,[5,6]
**RISK FACTORS** several countries in Latin America,[7] several countries in Europe,[8–11] Hong Kong,[12] and Japan[13] demonstrate a female to male predominance and a peak in middle aged women. Migraine has been reported to be 50% more likely in people with a family history of migraine.[14]

**PROGNOSIS**    Acute migraine is self limiting and only rarely results in permanent neurological complications. Chronic recurrent migraine may cause disability through pain, and may affect daily functioning and quality of life.

Please refer to CD-ROM for full text and references.

## What are the effects of interventions aimed at reducing relapse rates and disability?

We found no evidence from RCTs that any treatment alters long term outcome in multiple sclerosis.

### LIKELY TO BE BENEFICIAL

**Glatiramer acetate**

One RCT in people with relapsing and remitting multiple sclerosis found that, compared with placebo, glatiramer acetate reduced relapse rates over 2 years, but had no effect on disability. We found no good quality RCTs in people with secondary progressive multiple sclerosis.

**Interferon beta**

Two RCTs in people experiencing a first demyelinating event found that interferon beta-1a decreased the risk of conversion to clinically definite multiple sclerosis over 2–3 years compared with placebo. One systematic review in people with active relapsing remitting multiple sclerosis found limited evidence that, compared with placebo, interferon beta-1a/b reduced exacerbations and disease progression over 2 years. One subsequent RCT in people with relapsing remitting multiple sclerosis found that interferon beta-1b reduced the proportion of people with relapse over 2 years compared with interferon beta-1a. We found conflicting evidence from three RCTs about the effects of interferon beta on disease progression in people with secondary progressive multiple sclerosis.

### UNKNOWN EFFECTIVENESS

**Azathioprine**

One systematic review in people with relapsing and remitting or progressive multiple sclerosis comparing azathioprine versus placebo or no treatment found a modest reduction in relapse rates over 2 years, but no evidence of a difference in disability. However, we were unable to draw reliable conclusions because of clinical heterogeneity among included RCTs.

**Intravenous immunoglobulin**

One RCT in people with relapsing and remitting multiple sclerosis found limited evidence from baseline comparisons that intravenous immunoglobulin may reduce disability over 2 years compared with placebo. However, the clinical importance of this difference is unclear. We found no good quality RCTs in people with secondary progressive multiple sclerosis.

**Methotrexate**

We found insufficient evidence from one small RCT about the effects of methotrexate in people with multiple sclerosis.

### TRADE OFF BETWEEN BENEFITS AND HARMS

**Mitoxantrone**

One RCT in people with worsening, relapsing, remitting, or progressive multiple sclerosis found that mitoxantrone reduced progression of disability compared with placebo. One small RCT in people with active multiple sclerosis found limited ▶

# Multiple sclerosis

evidence that mitoxantrone plus methylprednisolone reduced relapse compared with methylprednisolone alone. However, mitoxantrone is associated with leukopenia, menstrual disorders, and arrhythmia.

---

## What are the effects of treatments for acute relapse?

### LIKELY TO BE BENEFICIAL

#### Corticosteroids (methylprednisolone or corticotrophin)

One systematic review in people with multiple sclerosis requiring treatment for acute exacerbations has found that corticosteroids (methylprednisolone or corticotrophin) improves symptoms compared with placebo within the first 5 weeks of treatment. The optimal dose, route, and duration of treatment are unclear.

### UNKNOWN EFFECTIVENESS

#### Plasma exchange

One small RCT provided insufficient evidence to assess plasma exchange in people with acute relapses of multiple sclerosis.

---

## What are the effects of treatments for fatigue?

### UNKNOWN EFFECTIVENESS

#### Amantadine

We found insufficient evidence from one systematic review of poor quality RCTs about the effects of amantadine on fatigue in people with multiple sclerosis.

#### Behaviour modification

We found no RCTs on the effects of behavioural modification treatment in people with multiple sclerosis related fatigue.

#### Exercise

We found insufficient evidence from two RCTs about the effects of exercise in people with multiple sclerosis related fatigue.

### UNLIKELY TO BE BENEFICIAL

#### Pemoline

One systematic review found no significant difference in the self reporting of fatigue with pemoline compared with placebo.

---

## What are the effects of treatments for spasticity?

### UNKNOWN EFFECTIVENESS

#### Botulinum toxin

We found insufficient evidence from one small RCT about the effects of botulinum toxin on functional outcomes in people with spasticity due to multiple sclerosis.

#### Intrathecal baclofen

One small crossover RCT provided insufficient evidence to assess functional effects of intrathecal baclofen.

#### Oral drug treatments

One systematic review found insufficient evidence about the effects of oral drugs on functional outcomes in people with spasticity due to multiple sclerosis. RCTs provided insufficient evidence to assess other oral drug treatments.

### Physiotherapy

We found insufficient evidence from two small RCTs about the effects of physiotherapy. One of the RCTs found limited evidence that twice weekly hospital or home based physiotherapy for 8 weeks briefly improved mobility compared with no physiotherapy. The other, in people with progressive multiple sclerosis, found no significant difference between early versus delayed physiotherapy in mobility or activities of daily living.

## What are the effects of multidisciplinary care?

### UNKNOWN EFFECTIVENESS

### Inpatient rehabilitation

Two small RCTs provided insufficient evidence to assess the effectiveness of inpatient rehabilitation. Both RCTs found short term benefit, but no reduction in neurological impairment. Longer term effects are uncertain.

### Outpatient rehabilitation

One small RCT provided insufficient evidence to assess the effectiveness of outpatient rehabilitation.

| | |
|---|---|
| **DEFINITION** | Multiple sclerosis is a chronic inflammatory disease of the central nervous system. Diagnosis requires evidence of lesions that are separated in both time and space, and the exclusion of other inflammatory, structural, or hereditary conditions that might give a similar clinical picture. The disease takes three main forms: relapsing and remitting multiple sclerosis, characterised by episodes of neurological dysfunction interspersed with periods of stability; primary progressive multiple sclerosis, where progressive neurological disability occurs from the outset; and secondary progressive multiple sclerosis, where progressive neurological disability occurs later in the course of the disease. |
| **INCIDENCE/ PREVALENCE** | Prevalence varies with geography and racial group; it is highest in white populations in temperate regions.[1] In Europe and North America, prevalence is 1/800 people, with an annual incidence of 2–10/100 000, making multiple sclerosis the most common cause of neurological disability in young adults. Age of onset is broad, peaking between 20 and 40 years.[2] |
| **AETIOLOGY/ RISK FACTORS** | The cause remains unclear, although current evidence suggests that multiple sclerosis is an autoimmune disorder of the central nervous system resulting from an environmental stimulus in genetically susceptible individuals. Multiple sclerosis is currently regarded as a single disorder with clinical variants, but there is some evidence that it may consist of several related disorders with distinct immunological, pathological, and genetic features.[1,3] |
| **PROGNOSIS** | In 90% of people, early disease is relapsing and remitting. Although some people follow a relatively benign course over many years, most develop secondary progressive disease, usually 6–10 years after onset. In 10% of people, initial disease is primary progressive. Apart from a minority of people with "aggressive" multiple sclerosis, life expectancy is not greatly affected and the disease course is often of more than 30 years' duration. |

Please refer to CD-ROM for full text and references.

# Parkinson's disease

**Search date December 2002**

*Carl Clarke and A Peter Moore*

## What are the effects of treatments?

### LIKELY TO BE BENEFICIAL

**Selegiline in people with early disease**

RCTs have found that selegiline improves the symptoms of Parkinson's disease and delays the need for levodopa compared with placebo. One of these RCTs found weak evidence of increased mortality in people treated with selegiline.

### TRADE OFF BETWEEN BENEFITS AND HARMS

**Dopamine agonists plus levodopa in people with a fluctuating response to levodopa***

Systematic reviews in people with later stage disease taking levodopa have found that adjuvant dopamine agonists reduce "off" time⊕, improve motor impairments and activities of daily living, and reduce levodopa dose, but increase dopaminergic adverse effects⊕ and dyskinesias.

**Dopamine agonists plus levodopa* versus levodopa alone in people with early disease**

One systematic review and subsequent RCTs have found that dopamine agonist treatment plus levodopa reduces dyskinesia compared with levodopa alone. However, some of the RCTs found that dopamine agonist plus levodopa worsened motor impairments and disability compared with levodopa alone.

**Dopamine agonists versus levodopa* in people with early disease**

One systematic review and one subsequent RCT have found that dopamine agonist monotherapy reduces the incidence of dyskinesias and fluctuations in motor response compared with levodopa monotherapy.

**Levodopa* in people with early disease**

We found no placebo controlled RCTs, although experience suggests that levodopa improves motor function, but that dyskinesias⊕ and fluctuations in motor response⊕ are related to long term levodopa treatment and are irreversible.

**Pallidal surgery in people with later disease**

One systematic review found limited evidence that unilateral pallidotomy⊕ improved motor examination and activities of daily living compared with medical treatment. One RCT found insufficient evidence to assess the effects of pallidotomy versus deep brain stimulation⊕. We found no systematic review or RCTs comparing pallidal deep brain stimulation versus medical treatment. One small RCT found insufficient evidence to assess the effects of pallidal deep brain stimulation versus subthalamic deep brain stimulation. There is a high incidence of adverse effects with pallidotomy.

### UNKNOWN EFFECTIVENESS

**Subthalamic surgery in people with later disease**

One systematic review found no RCTs comparing subthalamic surgery versus medical treatment. One small RCT comparing subthalamic deep brain stimulation versus pallidal deep brain stimulation found no significant difference in motor scores.

◀ **Thalamic surgery in people with later disease**

One systematic review identified no RCTs comparing thalamic surgery versus medical treatment. One RCT found that thalamic deep brain stimulation versus thalamotomy improved functional status and caused fewer adverse effects. Case series found that thalamotomy was associated with permanent complications, including speech disturbance, apraxia, and death in 14–23% of people.

**Occupational therapy in people with later disease; physiotherapy in people with later disease; speech and language therapy for speech disturbance in people with later disease; swallowing therapy for dysphagia in people with later disease**

Systematic reviews of poor quality RCTs found insufficient evidence about the effects of these interventions.

**UNLIKELY TO BE BENEFICIAL**

**Modified release levodopa (v immediate release levodopa*) in people with early disease**

RCTs found no significant difference with modified versus immediate release levodopa in motor complications or disease control after 5 years.

*We have used the term "levodopa" to refer to a combination of levodopa and a peripheral decarboxylase inhibitor.

**DEFINITION** Idiopathic Parkinson's disease is an age related neurodegenerative disorder, associated with a combination of asymmetric bradykinesia, hypokinesia, and rigidity, sometimes combined with rest tremor and postural changes. Clinical diagnostic criteria have a sensitivity of 80% and specificity of 30% compared with the gold standard of diagnosis at autopsy.[1] The primary pathology is progressive loss of cells producing the neurotransmitter dopamine from the substantia nigra in the brainstem. Treatment aims to replace or compensate for the lost dopamine. A good response to treatment supports, but does not confirm, the diagnosis. Several other catecholaminergic neurotransmitter systems are also affected in Parkinson's disease. There is no consistent definition of early and late stage Parkinson's disease. In this review, we consider people with early stage disease to be those who have not yet developed motor complications associated with long term levodopa treatment (such as dyskinesias and "on/off" fluctuations). Late stage Parkinson's disease is taken to mean that motor complications of long term levodopa treatment are present.

**INCIDENCE/** Parkinson's disease occurs worldwide with equal incidence in both sexes. In
**PREVALENCE** 5–10% of people who develop Parkinson's disease it appears before the age of 40 years (young onset), with a mean age of onset of about 65 years. Overall age adjusted prevalence is 1% worldwide and 1.6% in Europe, rising from 0.6% at age 60–64 years to 3.5% at age 85–89 years.[2,3]

**AETIOLOGY/** The cause is unknown. Parkinson's disease may represent different conditions
**RISK FACTORS** with a final common pathway. People may be affected differently by a combination of genetic and environmental factors (viruses, toxins, 1-methyl-4-phenyl-1,2,3,6-tetrahydropyridine, well water, vitamin E, and smoking).[4–7] First degree relatives of affected people may have twice the risk of developing Parkinson's disease (17% chance of developing the condition in their lifetime) compared with people in the general population.[8–10] However, purely genetic varieties probably affect a small minority of people with Parkinson's disease.[11,12] The parkin gene on chromosome 6 may be associated with Parkinson's disease in families with at least one member with young onset Parkinson's disease, and multiple genetic factors, including the tau gene on chromosome 17q21, may be involved in idiopathic late onset disease.[13,14]

# Parkinson's disease

**PROGNOSIS**   Parkinson's disease is currently incurable. Disability is progressive and associated with increased mortality (RR of death compared with matched control populations ranges from 1.6 to 3.0).[15] Treatment can reduce symptoms and slow progression but rarely achieves complete control. The question of whether treatment reduces mortality remains controversial.[16] Levodopa seemed to reduce mortality in the UK for 5 years after its introduction, before a "catch up" effect was noted and overall mortality rose toward previous levels. This suggested a limited prolongation of life.[17] An Australian cohort study followed 130 people treated for 10 years.[18] The standardised mortality ratio was 1.58 ($P < 0.001$). At 10 years, 25% had been admitted to a nursing home and only four were still employed. The mean duration of disease until death was 9.1 years. In a similar Italian cohort study conducted over 8 years, the relative risk of death for affected people versus healthy controls was 2.3 (95% CI 1.60 to 3.39).[19] Age at initial census date was the main predictor of outcome (for people aged < 75 years: RR of death 1.80, 95% CI 1.04 to 3.11; for people aged > 75 years: RR of death 5.61, 95% CI 2.13 to 14.80).

Please refer to CD-ROM for full text and references.

Neurological disorders

## What are the effects of treatments?

### LIKELY TO BE BENEFICIAL

**Carbamazepine**

One systematic review of three crossover RCTs found that carbamazepine increased pain relief compared with placebo. The review found that carbamazepine increased adverse effects (drowsiness, dizziness, constipation, and ataxia) compared with placebo. One small RCT provided insufficient evidence to compare tizanidine versus carbamazepine. One RCT found that pimozide reduced pain over 8 weeks compared with carbamazepine, but increased adverse effects (including hand tremors, memory impairment, and involuntary movements). One systematic review found one RCT of tocainide versus carbamazepine that was of insufficient quality.

### TRADE OFF BETWEEN BENEFITS AND HARMS

**Pimozide**

One RCT found that pimozide reduced pain over 8 weeks compared with carbamazepine, but increased adverse effects (including hand tremors, memory impairment, and involuntary movements). Cardiac toxicity and sudden death have been reported with pimozide.

### UNKNOWN EFFECTIVENESS

**Baclofen**

We found insufficient evidence on the effects of baclofen versus placebo or versus other active drugs.

**Combined streptomycin and lidocaine nerve block**

Small RCTs provided insufficient evidence about the effects of nerve block with streptomycin plus lidocaine compared with nerve block with lidocaine alone.

**Lamotrigine**

One systematic review provided insufficient evidence to compare lamotrigine versus placebo in people with trigeminal neuralgia.

**Other drugs (phenytoin, clonazepam, sodium valproate, gabapentin, mexiletine, oxcarbazepine, topiramate)**

We found insufficient evidence about the effects of these drugs in people with trigeminal neuralgia.

**Peripheral laser treatment**

We found insufficient evidence on the effects of peripheral laser treatment❺ in people with trigeminal neuralgia.

**Stereotactic radiosurgery** *New*

We found insufficient evidence about the effects of stereotactic radiosurgery in people with trigeminal neuralgia.

**Tizanidine**

One small RCT provided insufficient evidence to compare tizanidine versus carbamazepine.

▶

© BMJ Publishing Group Ltd 2003

# Trigeminal neuralgia

◄ **Cryotherapy⊖ of peripheral nerves; peripheral acupuncture; peripheral alcohol injection; peripheral injection of phenol; peripheral neurectomy; peripheral radiofrequency thermocoagulation⊖**

We found no RCTs about the effects of these interventions.

## UNLIKELY TO BE BENEFICIAL

### Proparacaine eye drops

One RCT found no significant difference in pain at 30 days between placebo and a single application of proparacaine hydrochloride eye drops to the eye on the same side as the pain.

## LIKELY TO BE INEFFECTIVE OR HARMFUL

### Tocainide

One systematic review found one RCT of tocainide versus carbamazepine which was of insufficient quality. The use of tocainide is limited by considerable harms (including serious haematological effects).

**DEFINITION**  Trigeminal neuralgia is a characteristic pain in the distribution of one or more branches of the fifth cranial nerve. The diagnosis is made on the history alone, based on characteristic features of the pain. It occurs in paroxysms that last a few seconds to 2 minutes. The frequency of paroxysms is highly variable: from hundreds of attacks a day to long periods of remission that can last years. The pain is severe and described as intense, sharp, superficial, stabbing, burning, or like an electric shock. In any individual, the pain has the same character in different attacks. It is often triggered by touch in a specific area or by eating, talking, washing the face, or cleaning the teeth. Between paroxysms the person is asymptomatic. Other causes of facial pain may need to be excluded.[1] In trigeminal neuralgia the neurological examination is usually normal.[2,3]

**INCIDENCE/**  Most evidence about the incidence and prevalence of trigeminal neuralgia is
**PREVALENCE**  from the USA.[4] The annual incidence (when age adjusted to 1980 age distribution of the USA) is 5.9/100 000 women and 3.4/100 000 men. The incidence tends to be slightly higher in women at all ages. The incidence increases with age. In men aged over 80 years the incidence is 45.2/100 000.[5] Other published surveys are small. One questionnaire survey of neurological disease in a single French village found one person with trigeminal neuralgia among 993 people.[6]

**AETIOLOGY/**  The cause of trigeminal neuralgia remains unclear.[7] It is more common in
**RISK FACTORS**  people with multiple sclerosis (RR 20.0, 95% CI 4.1 to 59.0).[5] Hypertension is a risk factor in women (RR 2.1, 95% CI 1.2 to 3.4) but the evidence is less clear for men (RR 1.53, 95% CI 0.30 to 4.50).[5] A study in the USA found that people with trigeminal neuralgia smoked less, consumed less alcohol, had fewer tonsillectomies, and were less likely than matched controls to be Jewish or an immigrant.[8]

**PROGNOSIS**  One study found no reduction of 10 year survival with trigeminal neuralgia.[9] We found no evidence about the natural history of trigeminal neuralgia. The illness is characterised by recurrences and remissions. Many people have periods of remission with no pain for months or years.[3] Anecdotal reports suggest that in many people it becomes more severe and less responsive to treatment with time.[10] Most people with trigeminal neuralgia are initially managed medically, and a proportion eventually have a surgical procedure.[5] We found no good evidence about the proportion of people who require surgical treatment for pain control.

Please refer to CD-ROM for full text and references.

### Search date December 2002

*Stephen Porter and Crispian Scully CBE*

## What are the effects of treatments?

### LIKELY TO BE BENEFICIAL

**Chlorhexidine (but no effect on recurrence rates)**

RCTs found that chlorhexidine gluconate mouth rinses increased the number of ulcer free days and reduced the severity of each episode of ulceration compared with control preparations but did not affect the incidence of recurrent ulceration.

### UNKNOWN EFFECTIVENESS

**Topical corticosteroids**

Nine small RCTs found no consistent difference in the incidence of new ulcers between topical corticosteroids and control preparations. They found weak evidence that topical corticosteroids may reduce the duration of ulcers and hasten pain relief.

### UNLIKELY TO BE BENEFICIAL

**Hexitidine**

One RCT found no significant difference in the incidence or duration of ulceration between hexitidine mouthwash and a control mouthwash.

**DEFINITION**  Recurrent aphthous ulcers are superficial and rounded, with painful mouth ulcers usually occurring in recurrent bouts at intervals of a few days to a few months.[1]

**INCIDENCE/ PREVALENCE**  The point prevalence of recurrent aphthous ulcers in Swedish adults has been reported as 2%.[1] Prevalence may be 5–10% in some groups of children. Up to 66% of young adults give a history consistent with recurrent aphthous ulceration.[1]

**AETIOLOGY/ RISK FACTORS**  The causes of aphthous ulcers remain unknown. Associations with haematinic deficiency, infections, gluten sensitive enteropathy, food sensitivities, and psychological stress have rarely been confirmed. Similar ulcers are seen in Behçet's syndrome.

**PROGNOSIS**  About 80% of people with recurrent aphthous ulcers develop a few ulcers smaller than 1 cm in diameter that heal within 5–14 days without scarring (the pattern known as minor aphthous ulceration). The episodes recur typically after an interval of 1–4 months. One in 10 sufferers has a more severe form (major aphthous ulceration) with lesions larger than 1 cm that may recur after a shorter interval and can cause scarring. Likewise, 1/10 people with such recurrent ulceration may have multiple minute ulcers (herpetiform ulceration).

Please refer to CD-ROM for full text and references.

**Oral health**

# Burning mouth syndrome

**Search date October 2002**

*John Buchanan and Joanna Zakrzewska*

## What are the effects of treatments?

**LIKELY TO BE BENEFICIAL**

**Cognitive behavioural therapy**
One small RCT found that cognitive behavioural therapy in people with resistant burning mouth syndrome versus no cognitive behavioural therapy significantly reduced symptom intensity after 6 months.

**UNKNOWN EFFECTIVENESS**

**Antidepressants; benzydamine hydrochloride; dietary supplementation; hormone replacement therapy in postmenopausal women**
We found insufficient evidence on the effects of these interventions.

| | |
|---|---|
| **DEFINITION** | Burning mouth syndrome is a psychogenic or idiopathic burning discomfort or pain affecting people with clinically normal oral mucosa in whom a medical or dental cause has been excluded.[1–3] Terms previously used to describe what is now called burning mouth syndrome include glossodynia, glossopyrosis, stomatodynia, stomatopyrosis, sore tongue, and oral dysaesthesia.[4] A survey of 669 men and 758 women randomly selected from 48 500 people aged between 20 and 69 years found that people with burning mouth also have subjective dryness (66%), take some form of medication (64%), report other systemic illnesses (57%), and have altered taste (11%).[5] Many studies of people with symptoms of burning mouth do not distinguish those with burning mouth syndrome (i.e. idiopathic disease) from those with other conditions (such as vitamin B deficiency), making results unreliable. |
| **INCIDENCE/ PREVALENCE** | Burning mouth syndrome mainly affects women,[6–8] particularly after the menopause when its prevalence may be 18–33%.[9] One recent study in Sweden found a prevalence of 4% for the symptom of burning mouth without clinical abnormality of the oral mucosa (11/669 [2%] men, mean age 59 years; 42/758 [6%] women, mean age 57 years), with the highest prevalence (12%) in women aged 60–69 years.[5] Reported prevalence in general populations varies from 1%[10] to 15%.[6] Incidence and prevalence vary according to diagnostic criteria,[4] and many studies included people with the symptom of burning mouth rather than with burning mouth syndrome as defined above. |
| **AETIOLOGY/ RISK FACTORS** | The cause is unknown, and we found no good aetiological studies. Hormonal disturbances associated with the menopause[7–9] and psychogenic factors (including anxiety, depression, stress, life events, personality disorders, and phobia of cancer) are possible causal factors.[11–13] Local and systemic factors (such as infections, allergies, ill fitting dentures,[12] hypersensitivity reactions,[14] and hormone and vitamin deficiencies[15–17]) may cause the symptom of burning mouth and should be excluded before diagnosing burning mouth syndrome. |
| **PROGNOSIS** | We found no prospective cohort studies or other reliable evidence describing the natural history of burning mouth syndrome.[18] We found anecdotal reports of at least partial spontaneous remission in about half of people with burning mouth syndrome within 6–7 years.[12] |

Please refer to CD-ROM for full text and references.

### Search date February 2003

*Caroline Pankhurst*

---

## What are the effects of preventive interventions?

**BENEFICIAL**

### Antifungal prophylaxis in people undergoing cancer treatments

One systematic review in people undergoing treatment for cancer found that antifungal drugs reduced the risk of oropharyngeal candidiasis compared with placebo or no treatment. One review found that drugs that were absorbed or partially absorbed via the gastrointestinal tract were more effective than non-absorbed drugs in preventing oral candidiasis.

### Antifungal prophylaxis in people with advanced HIV disease

RCTs in people with HIV infection have found that daily or weekly antifungal prophylaxis with fluconazole, itraconazole, or nystatin reduces incidence and relapse of oropharyngeal candidiasis compared with placebo.

**LIKELY TO BE BENEFICIAL**

### Antifungal prophylaxis in immunocompromised infants and children

One large RCT in immunocompromised infants and children found that fluconazole reduced the incidence of oropharyngeal candidiasis compared with oral nystatin or amphotenicin B.

**UNKNOWN EFFECTIVENESS**

### Antifungal prophylaxis in people receiving tissue transplants

Two small RCTs in people with liver transplant found no significant difference in the risk of oropharyngeal candidiasis between nystatin and fluconazole or clotrimazole. However, the trials may have lacked power to exclude clinically important differences. We found insufficient evidence from two RCTs about the effects of prophylactic chlorhexidine mouth rinse with or without nystatin compared with placebo in people receiving bone marrow transplant.

### Continuous prophylaxis versus intermittent treatment in people with HIV infection and acute episodes of oropharyngeal candidiasis (in preventing antifungal resistance)

One RCT in people with HIV infection and acute episodes of oropharyngeal candidiasis found no significant difference in emergence of antifungal resistance between continuous antifungal prophylaxis with fluconazole and intermittent antifungal treatment with fluconazole.

### Preventive interventions in people with diabetes

We found no systematic review or RCTs.

---

## What are the effects of treatments?

**BENEFICIAL**

### Antifungal treatment in immunocompetent and immunocompromised infants and children

RCTs found that miconazole and fluconazole increased clinical cure of oropharyngeal candidiasis compared with nystatin in immunocompetent and immunocompromised infants and children.

*Clin Evid Concise* 2003;10:301–303.

# Candidiasis (oropharyngeal)

## Oral suspension of systemically absorbed azoles in people with HIV infection

RCTs have found that topical preparations of itraconazole, fluconazole, and clotrimazole effectively treat oropharyngeal candidiasis in people with HIV infection. One RCT found that fluconazole significantly reduced symptoms and signs of oropharyngeal candidiasis compared with topical nystatin.

**UNKNOWN EFFECTIVENESS**

### Antifungal treatment for denture stomatitis

We found insufficient evidence from small RCTs to compare effects of antifungals versus placebo or versus each other for treating oropharyngeal candidiasis in people who wear dentures.

### Antifungal treatment in people undergoing chemotherapy, radiotherapy, or both treatments for cancer

One systematic review found insufficient evidence from RCTs about the clinical effects of antifungals compared with placebo for treating oropharyngeal candidiasis in people undergoing chemotherapy or radiotherapy. It also found insufficient evidence about the effects of different antifungal agents or doses in people with oropharyngeal candidiasis who are receiving radiotherapy or chemotherapy.

### Denture hygiene

We found insufficient evidence from RCTs to assess clinical effects on oropharyngeal candidiasis of mouth rinses, disinfectants, denture soaks, denture scrubbing, and microwave irradiation of dentures. Microwave treatment is not suitable for all dentures.

### Treatments in people with diabetes mellitus

We found no RCTs assessing treatments for oral candidiasis in people with diabetes mellitus.

**DEFINITION**  Oropharyngeal candidiasis is an opportunistic mucosal infection caused, in most cases, by *Candida albicans*. The four main types of oropharyngeal candidiasis are: (1) pseudomembranous (thrush), consisting of white discrete plaques on an erythematous background, located on the buccal mucosa, throat, tongue, or gingivae; (2) erythematous, consisting of smooth red patches on the hard or soft palate, dorsum of tongue, or buccal mucosa; (3) hyperplastic, consisting of white, firmly adherent patches or plaques, usually bilateral on the buccal mucosa; and (4) denture induced stomatitis, presenting as either a smooth or granular erythema confined to the denture bearing area of the hard palate and often associated with an angular cheilitis.[1] Symptoms vary, ranging from none to a sore and painful mouth with a burning tongue and altered taste. Oropharyngeal candidiasis can impair speech, nutritional intake, and quality of life.

**INCIDENCE/**  Candida species are commensals in the gastrointestinal tract. Transmission
**PREVALENCE**  occurs directly between infected people or on fomites (objects that can harbour pathogenic organisms). Candida is found in the mouth of 31–60% of healthy people.[2] Denture stomatitis associated with Candida is prevalent in 65% of denture wearers.[2] Oropharyngeal candidiasis affects 15–60% of people with haematological or oncological malignancies during periods of immunosuppression.[3] Oropharyngeal candidiasis occurs in 7–48% of people with HIV infection and in over 90% of those with advanced disease. In severely immunosuppressed people, relapse rates are high (30–50%) and usually occur within 14 days of stopping treatment.[4]

**AETIOLOGY/ RISK FACTORS** Risk factors associated with symptomatic oropharyngeal candidiasis include local or systemic immunosuppression, haematological disorders, broad spectrum antibiotic use, inhaled or systemic steroids, xerostomia, diabetes, and wearing dentures, obturators, or orthodontic appliances.[1,5] The same strain may persist for months or years in the absence of infection. In people with HIV infection, there is no direct correlation between the number of organisms and the presence of clinical disease. Symptomatic oropharyngeal candidiasis associated with *in vitro* resistance to fluconazole occurs in 5% of people with advanced HIV disease.[6] Resistance to azole antifungals is associated with severe immunosuppression ($\leq$ 50 CD4 cells/mm$^3$), more episodes treated with antifungal drugs, and longer median duration of systemic azole treatment.[7]

**PROGNOSIS** Untreated candidiasis persists for months or years unless associated risk factors are treated or eliminated. In neonates, spontaneous cure of oropharyngeal candidiasis usually occurs after 3–8 weeks.

Please refer to CD-ROM for full text and references.

# Halitosis

**Search date April 2003**

*Bazian Ltd*

## What are the effects of treatments in people with physiological halitosis? New

### LIKELY TO BE BENEFICIAL

**Single-use mouthwash (short term benefit only)**

Three small RCTs in people with confirmed halitosis found limited evidence that single-use mouthwash reduced odour unpleasantness and odour intensity between 1–8 hours after use compared with distilled water, saline rinse, or no treatment. One of these RCTs found no significant difference between single-use mouthwash and distilled water in odour unpleasantness or odour intensity after 24 hours.

### UNKNOWN EFFECTIVENESS

**Regular-use mouthwash**

We found no RCTs on the effects of the regular use of mouthwash.

**Artificial saliva; sugar free chewing gums; tongue cleaning, brushing, or scraping; zinc toothpastes**

We found no RCTs on the effects of these interventions.

| | |
|---|---|
| **DEFINITION** | Halitosis is an unpleasant odour emitted from the mouth. It can be because of oral conditions including poor oral hygiene and periodontal disease or extraoral conditions such as chronic sinusitis and bronchiectasis.[1,2] In this topic, we deal only with physiological halitosis, that is, confirmed persistent bad breath in the absence of systemic, periodontal, or gum disease. We have excluded halitosis due to underlying disease, which would require disease specific treatment, pseudo-halitosis (in people who believe they have bad breath but whose breath is not considered malodourous by others), and artificially induced halitosis (e.g. in studies requiring people to stop brushing their teeth). This topic is only applicable, therefore, to people in whom underlying causes have been ruled out, and in whom pseudo-halitosis has been excluded. There is no consensus regarding duration of bad breath for diagnosis of halitosis, although the standard organoleptic test🅖 for bad breath involves smelling the breath on at least two or three different days.[1] |
| **INCIDENCE/ PREVALENCE** | We found no reliable estimate of prevalence, although several studies report population prevalence of halitosis (physiological or because of underlying disease) to be about 50%.[1,3–5] One cross-sectional study of 491 people found that about 5% of people with halitosis have pseudo-halitosis and about 40% of people with halitosis have physiological bad breath not due to underlying disease.[6] We found no reliable data about age or sex distribution of physiological halitosis. |
| **AETIOLOGY/ RISK FACTORS** | We found no reliable data about risk factors for physiological bad breath. Mass spectrometric and gas chromatographic analysis of expelled air from the mouth of people with any type of halitosis have shown that the main malodourants are volatile sulphur compounds including hydrogen sulphide, methyl mercaptan, and dimethyl suphide.[7,8] |
| **PROGNOSIS** | We found no evidence on the prognosis of halitosis. |

Please refer to CD-ROM for full text and references.

Search date November 2002

*Andrew Smith*

## What are the effects of interventions to reduce postoperative pulmonary infections?

### BENEFICIAL

**Postoperative chest physiotherapy (deep breathing exercises)**
One systematic review and one subsequent RCT have found that deep breathing◉ exercises reduce postoperative pulmonary infections compared with control.

**Epidural anaesthesia**
Two systematic reviews have found that epidural anaesthesia with or without postoperative epidural analgesia reduces postoperative pulmonary infections compared with general anaesthesia with or without postoperative systemic analgesia. Neither review sought data on adverse effects. Subsequent and additional RCTs found inconsistent results.

### LIKELY TO BE BENEFICIAL

**Postoperative chest physiotherapy (incentive spirometry and intermittent positive pressure breathing)**
Two RCTs found that incentive spirometry◉ reduced pulmonary complications compared with control. One RCT found that intermittent positive pressure breathing◉ reduced postoperative pulmonary complications compared with control.

### UNKNOWN EFFECTIVENESS

**Advice to stop smoking preoperatively**
We found no RCTs about the effects of preoperative advice to stop cigarette smoking on postoperative pulmonary infections. Two observational studies found that people who smoked were more likely to develop postoperative pulmonary complications of all kinds than those who did not. One study suggested that people who had stopped smoking 6 months preoperatively reverted to the risk of those who had never smoked.

**DEFINITION**     A working diagnosis of postoperative pulmonary infection may be based on three or more new findings from: cough, phlegm, shortness of breath, chest pain, temperature above 38 °C, and pulse rate above 100/min.[1] In this topic, the diagnosis of pneumonia implies consolidation observed on a chest x ray.[2]

**INCIDENCE/**     Reported morbidity for chest complications depends on how carefully they are
**PREVALENCE**   investigated. One study found blood gas and chest radiograph abnormalities in about 50% of people after open cholecystectomy.[3] However, less than 20% of these had abnormal clinical signs and only 10% had a clinically significant chest infection. Another study estimated the incidence of pneumonia as 20%.[4] Another used a similarly strict definition and found the incidence has 23%.[5]

**AETIOLOGY/**     Risk factors include increasing age (> 50 years), cigarette smoking, obesity,
**RISK FACTORS** thoracic or upper abdominal operations, and pre-existing lung disease.[6] One multivariate analysis did not confirm the association with cigarette smoking but suggested that longer preoperative hospital stay and higher grading on the American Society of Anesthesiologists' physical status scale (> 2) increased the risk of postoperative pulmonary complications.[5] Depression of the immune system may also contribute.[7] ▶

# Postoperative pulmonary infections

**PROGNOSIS** In one large systematic review (search date 1997, 141 RCTs, 9559 people), 10% of people with postoperative pneumonia died.[8] If systemic sepsis ensues, mortality is likely to be substantial.[9] Pneumonia delays recovery from surgery and poor tissue oxygenation may contribute to delayed wound healing.

Please refer to CD-ROM for full text and references.

### Search date March 2003

*Michael Eddleston, Surjit Singh, and Nick Buckley*

## What are the effects of treatments for acute organophosphorus poisoning?

### LIKELY TO BE BENEFICIAL

**Atropine\***
Consensus supports atropine treatment. Many case series have found that it reverses the early muscarinic effects of acute organophosphorus poisoning. We found no RCTs comparing atropine versus placebo, but such an RCT would now be considered unethical.

**Benzodiazepines to control organophosphorus induced seizures\***
Consensus supports benzodiazepines for organophosphorus induced seizures. We found no RCTs comparing a benzodiazepine versus placebo or another anticonvulsant. It would now be unethical to conduct an RCT comparing benzodiazepines versus placebo.

**Glycopyrronium bromide (glycopyrrolate)\***
One small RCT found no significant difference in death or ventilation rates between glycopyrronium bromide and atropine, but it may have lacked power to detect clinically important differences. Glycopyrronium bromide (glycopyrrolate) has been used instead of atropine because it is thought to have fewer adverse effects on the central nervous system.

**Washing the poisoned person and removing contaminated clothes\***
Washing the poisoned person with warm water and soap and removing contaminated clothes after dermal and mucocutaneous exposure appears important and widely recommended, but this intervention has not been assessed in RCTs.

### UNKNOWN EFFECTIVENESS

**Gastric lavage**
We found no RCTs assessing the role of gastric lavage in acute organophosphorus poisoning. If the procedure cannot be performed in sedated and intubated patients, the risk of harm due to aspiration is likely to surpass its potential benefits.

**Milk or other home remedy immediately after ingestion**
We found no RCTs on the effect of giving a "home remedy" soon after the ingestion.

**Oximes**
One systematic review found insufficient evidence about the effects of oximes in acute organophosphorus poisoning.

**Activated charcoal (single or multiple dose); $\alpha_2$ adrenergic receptor agonists (clonidine); N-methyl-D-aspartate receptor antagonists; organophophorus hydrolases; sodium bicarbonate**
We found insufficient evidence about the effects of these interventions.

### LIKELY TO BE INEFFECTIVE OR HARMFUL

**Ipecacuanha (ipecac)\***
We found no RCTs on the effects of ipecacuanha in acute organophosphorus poisoning. The significant risk of harm, although not quantified, probably outweighs any potential benefits.

\*Based on consensus, RCTs would be considered unethical.

*Clin Evid Concise* 2003;10:307–308.

# Acute organophosphorus poisoning

**DEFINITION**      Acute organophosphorus poisoning occurs after dermal, respiratory, or oral exposure to either low volatility pesticides (e.g. chlorpyrifos, dimethoate) or high volatility nerve gases (e.g. sarin, tabun). Acetylcholinesterase🄖 inhibition at synapses results in accumulation of acetylcholine and over-activation of acetylcholine receptors at the neuromuscular junction and in the autonomic and central nervous systems.[1] Early clinical features mainly involve the parasympathetic system: bradycardia, bronchorrhoea, miosis, salivation, lachrymation, defecation, urination, and hypotension. Features of neuromuscular junction (muscle weakness and fasciculations) and central nervous system (seizures, coma) involvement are also common at this stage. An intermediate syndrome has been described (cranial nerve palsies and proximal muscle weakness with preserved distal muscle power after resolution of early cholinergic symptoms), but its definition, pathophysiology, and incidence are still unclear. A late motor or motor/sensory peripheral neuropathy may also develop after recovery from acute poisoning with some organophosphorus compounds.[1]

**INCIDENCE/**      Most cases occur in the developing world following occupational or deliberate
**PREVALENCE**      exposure to organophosphorus pesticides.[2] Although data are sparse, organophosphates appear to be the most important cause of death from deliberate self poisoning worldwide.[3] In Sri Lanka, at least 17 000 cases of organophosphorus or carbamate poisoning occurred in 1999, resulting in 1700 deaths. More than 80% were intentional.[4] Case fatality rates across the developing world are commonly greater than 20%.[3] In Central America, occupational poisoning is more common than intentional poisoning and deaths are fewer.[5] Extrapolating from limited data, the World Health Organization has estimated that each year more than 200 000 people worldwide die from pesticide poisoning,[6] but these figures are old and widely contested.[2] Most deaths occur in Asia and organophosphorus pesticides probably cause at least 50% of cases.[3] Deaths from organophosphorus nerve gases occurred in Iran during the Iran–Iraq war.[7] Military or terrorist action with these chemical weapons remains possible. Twelve people died in a terrorist attack in Tokyo and thousands probably died in Iran after military or terrorist exposure.

**AETIOLOGY/**      The widespread accessibility of pesticides in rural parts of the developing world
**RISK FACTORS**    makes them easy options for acts of self harm.[3] Occupational exposure is due to insufficient or inappropriate protective equipment in the use of toxic compounds.[2]

**PROGNOSIS**      There are no validated scoring systems for categorising severity or predicting outcome, although many have been proposed. The highly variable natural history and difficulty in determining ingested dose make predicting outcome for an individual inaccurate and potentially hazardous, because people admitted in good condition can deteriorate rapidly and require intubation and mechanical ventilation. Prognosis in acute self poisoning is likely to depend on dose and toxicity of the ingested organophosphorus (e.g. neurotoxicity potential, half life, rate of ageing🄖, whether activation to the toxic compound is required [propoison🄖], and whether dimethylated or diethylated).[8,9] Prognosis in occupational exposure is better because the dose is normally smaller and the route is dermal.

Please refer to CD-ROM for full text and references.

### Search date November 2002

*Nick Buckley and Michael Eddleston*

Poisoning

---

## What are the effects of treatments?

**BENEFICIAL**

### Acetylcysteine

One systematic review in people with established paracetamol induced liver failure found that acetylcysteine versus placebo significantly reduced mortality at day 21. One observational study found that people given early treatment with acetylcysteine were less likely to develop liver damage than untreated historical controls.

**LIKELY TO BE BENEFICIAL**

### Methionine

One systematic review found insufficient evidence on the effects of methionine on mortality. It found limited evidence that methionine reduced hepatotoxicity compared with supportive care.

**UNKNOWN EFFECTIVENESS**

### Activated charcoal (single or multiple dose)

One systematic review found no evidence on the effects of activated charcoal, whether in single or multiple dose regimens, in paracetamol poisoning.

### Gastric lavage

One systematic review found no evidence of the effects of gastric lavage in paracetamol poisoning.

### Ipecacuanha

One systematic review found no evidence on the clinical effects of ipecacuanha in paracetamol poisoning.

**DEFINITION**  Paracetamol poisoning occurs as a result of either accidental or intentional overdose with paracetamol (acetaminophen).

**INCIDENCE/ PREVALENCE**  Paracetamol is the most common drug used for self poisoning in the UK.[1] It is also a common means of self poisoning in the rest of Europe, North America, and Australasia. An estimated 41 200 cases of poisoning with products containing paracetamol occurred in 1989–1990 in England and Wales, with a mortality of 0.40% (95% CI 0.38% to 0.46%). Overdoses owing to paracetamol alone result in an estimated 150–200 deaths and 15–20 liver transplants each year in England and Wales.

**AETIOLOGY/ RISK FACTORS**  Most cases in the UK are impulsive acts of self harm in young people.[1,2] In one study of 80 people who had overdosed with paracetamol, 42 had obtained the tablets for the specific purpose of taking an overdose and 33 had obtained them less than 1 hour before the act.[2]

**PROGNOSIS**  People with blood paracetamol concentrations above the standard treatment line (defined in the UK as a line joining 200 mg/L at 4 hours and 30 mg/L at 15 hours on a semilogarithmic plot) have a poor prognosis without treatment.[3–5] In one study of 57 untreated people with blood concentrations above this line, 33 developed severe liver damage and three died.[4] People with a history of chronic alcohol misuse, use of enzyme inducing drugs, eating disorders, or multiple paracetamol overdoses may be at risk of liver damage with blood concentrations below this line.[6] In the USA, a lower line is used as an indication for treatment but we found no data relating this line to prognostic outcomes.[7] ▶

# Paracetamol (acetaminophen) poisoning

**Dose effect:** The dose ingested also indicates the risk of hepatotoxicity. People ingesting less than 125 mg/kg had no significant hepatotoxicity with a sharp dose dependent rise for higher doses.[8] The threshold for toxicity after acute ingestion may be higher in children, where a single dose of less than 200 mg/kg has not been reported to lead to death and rarely causes hepatotoxicity.[9] For people who present later than 24 hours or an unknown time after ingestion, several other prognostic indicators have been proposed, including half life, prothrombin time, and abnormal liver function tests.[10,11] These have not been validated prospectively.

Please refer to CD-ROM for full text and references.

### Search date November 2002

*Richmal M Oates-Whitehead*

## What are the effects of treatment for nausea and vomiting in early pregnancy?

### LIKELY TO BE BENEFICIAL

#### Antihistamines (H1 antagonists)
Systematic reviews found limited evidence that antihistamines reduce nausea and vomiting, with no evidence of teratogenicity.

#### Cyanocobalamin (vitamin B$_{12}$)
One systematic review has found that cyanocobalamin🅖 reduces vomiting episodes compared with placebo.

#### Ginger
Three RCTs found that ginger reduces nausea and vomiting in early pregnancy.

#### Pyridoxine (vitamin B$_6$)
Systematic reviews have found limited evidence that pyridoxine reduces nausea but no evidence on the effect on vomiting.

### UNKNOWN EFFECTIVENESS

#### Acupuncture
One RCT found that acupuncture improved nausea scores, retching, and wellbeing compared with no acupuncture, without increasing adverse effects. However, an improvement was found both with traditional acupuncture and sham acupuncture compared with no treatment after 3 weeks. A second RCT found that acupuncture had no more effect than sham acupuncture.

#### Dietary interventions (excluding ginger)
We found insufficient evidence to assess the effects of dietary interventions (excluding ginger).

#### P6 acupressure
One systematic review of small RCTs found limited evidence that P6 acupressure🅖 reduced morning sickness compared with sham acupressure or no intervention. Four additional RCTs found that P6 acupressure reduced duration, but not intensity, of nausea and vomiting. However, a further small RCT found acupressure🅖 bands to be less effective than placebo bands.

#### Phenothiazines
One systematic review found limited evidence that phenothiazines reduced the proportion of women with nausea and vomiting. However, results were not conclusive.

## What are the effects of treatments for hyperemesis gravidarum?

### UNKNOWN EFFECTIVENESS

#### Acupuncture *New*
One randomised, crossover RCT in women with hyperemesis gravidarum found a faster reduction of nausea, as measured on a visual analogue scale, after active ▶

# Nausea and vomiting in early pregnancy

acupuncture compared with sham acupuncture. Episodes of vomiting were also reduced. However, we were unable to draw reliable conclusions from this small study.

### Corticosteroids

One RCT found no significant improvement in persistent vomiting or readmission to hospital after 1 week of treatment with prednisolone compared with placebo in women with hyperemesis gravidarum. One RCT identified in two systematic reviews found no significant improvement in persistence of vomiting but found a reduction in admission to hospital compared with promethazine.

### Corticotropins New

One RCT found no significant improvement in nausea and vomiting with intramuscular corticotropin (adrenocorticotrophic hormone, ACTH).

### Diazepam

One systematic review has found insufficient evidence on the effects of diazepam in women with hyperemesis gravidarum.

### Dietary interventions (excluding ginger)

One crossover RCT in women with hyperemesis gravidarum found no significant difference in nausea and vomiting after 3 weeks between carob seed flour and placebo.

### Ginger

One systematic review has found insufficient evidence to assess the effects of ginger in hyperemesis gravidarum.

### Ondansetron

We found insufficient evidence to assess the effects of ondansetron in hyperemesis gravidarum.

**DEFINITION** **Nausea and vomiting** are both common in early pregnancy. Most women do not require treatment. However, persistent vomiting and severe nausea can progress to hyperemesis if the woman is unable to maintain adequate hydration, and fluid and electrolytes as well as nutritional status are jeopardised. **Hyperemesis gravidarum** is a diagnosis of exclusion, characterised by prolonged and severe nausea and vomiting, dehydration, and body weight loss.[1] Laboratory investigation may show elevated plasma ketone levels in the absence of acidosis, low serum levels of sodium (hyponatraemia), potassium (hypokalaemia), a low serum urea level (hypouricaemia), metabolic hypochloraemic alkalosis (excess base alkali in the body fluids caused by chloride loss) and ketonuria (excessive ketones in the urine).

**INCIDENCE/** Nausea and vomiting are both common in pregnancy, with nausea affecting
**PREVALENCE** about 70% and vomiting affecting about 60% of women.[1] Symptoms commence between the fourth and the seventh week in 70% of the affected women.[2] Symptoms before the first missed period affect < 10% of pregnant women.[3] Vomiting ceases by the sixteenth week of pregnancy in about 90% of women.[1–3] Nausea and vomiting can occur any time of the day and may be constant throughout the day, although it has been misleadingly termed "morning sickness"[1] The true incidence of hyperemesis gravidarum is not known. It has been documented to range from 0.3–2.0%; however, most authors report an incidence of 0.5%.[2]

**AETIOLOGY/** The causes of nausea and vomiting in pregnancy are unknown. One theory, that
**RISK FACTORS** they are caused by the rise in human chorionic gonadotrophin concentration, is compatible with the natural history of the condition, its severity in pregnancies affected by hydatidiform mole**G**, and its good prognosis (see prognosis ▶

below).[4] The aetiology of hyperemesis gravidarum is also uncertain. Again, endocrine and psychological factors are suspected, but evidence is inconclusive.[4]

**PROGNOSIS**  One systematic review (search date 1988, 11 studies) found that nausea and vomiting were associated with a reduced risk of miscarriage (6 studies, 14 564 women; OR 0.36, 95% CI 0.32 to 0.42), but found no association with perinatal mortality.[5] Nausea and vomiting and hyperemesis usually improve over the course of pregnancy, but one observational study (cross sectional) found that 13% of women reported that nausea and vomiting persisted beyond 20 weeks' gestation.[6]

Please refer to CD-ROM for full text and references.

# Pre-eclampsia and hypertension

**Search date August 2002**

*Lelia Duley*

---

## What are the effects of preventive interventions?

### BENEFICIAL

**Antiplatelet drugs**

One systematic review has found that, in women considered at risk of pre-eclampsia, antiplatelet drugs (mainly aspirin) versus placebo or no treatment significantly reduces the risk of pre-eclampsia, death of the baby and delivery before 37 weeks, with no significant difference in other important outcomes. One small subsequent RCT found similar results. The systematic review found no evidence that aspirin versus placebo increased the risk of bleeding in mother or baby.

**Calcium supplementation (in high risk women or those with low intake)**

One systematic review has found that calcium supplementation (mainly 2 g daily) versus placebo reduces the risk of pre-eclampsia and hypertension and reduces the risk of having a baby with birthweight under 2500 g. There was no significant effect on the risk of stillbirth or perinatal death before discharge from hospital, caesarean section, or preterm delivery.

### UNKNOWN EFFECTIVENESS

**Magnesium supplementation**

One systematic review found insufficient evidence about the effects of magnesium supplements on the risk of pre-eclampsia or its complications.

**Other pharmacological interventions**

Two RCTs comparing atenolol or glyceryl trinitrate patches versus placebo were too small to draw reliable conclusions.

**Salt restriction**

Limited evidence from one systematic review found no significant difference in the risk of pre-eclampsia with a low salt diet versus a normal diet.

**Vitamin C and E**

One RCT in high risk women found limited evidence that vitamins C and E versus placebo significantly reduced the risk of pre-eclampsia. However, we were unable to draw reliable conclusions about effects. We found insufficient evidence about effects on other clinical outcomes.

**Evening primrose oil; fish oil**

We found six RCTs of evening primrose and fish oil, which were too small to draw reliable conclusions.

---

## What are the effects of treatments?

### BENEFICIAL

**Magnesium sulphate for eclampsia (better than other anticonvulsants)**

Systematic reviews have found that magnesium sulphate versus phenytoin, diazepam, or lytic cocktail significantly reduces further fits in women with eclampsia. All reviews found trends towards reduced maternal mortality with magnesium sulphate, although the benefit was not significant.

# Pre-eclampsia and hypertension

◄ **Prophylactic magnesium sulphate in severe pre-eclampsia**

One systematic review and one large RCT have found that prophylactic magnesium sulphate halves the risk of eclampsia compared with placebo in women with severe pre-eclampisa. The trials found no evidence of a difference between magnesium sulphate and placebo for rate of stillbirth or perinatal mortality in babies born to women with severe pre-eclampsia. A quarter of women reported mild adverse effects, mainly flushing.

**LIKELY TO BE BENEFICIAL**

**Antihypertensive drugs for very high blood pressure (although insufficient evidence on best choice of agent)**

One systematic review and one subsequent RCT in women with blood pressures high enough to merit immediate treatment found no evidence of a difference in the control of blood pressure by various antihypertensive drugs. The studies were too small to draw any further conclusions about the relative effects of different agents.

**UNKNOWN EFFECTIVENESS**

**Aggressive versus expectant management for severe early onset pre-eclampsia**

One systematic review based on two small RCTs found no evidence that aggressive management significantly reduced stillbirth or perinatal death rates compared with expectant management in babies born to mothers with severe early onset pre-eclampsia. However, it found that aggressive management increased rates of admission to neonatal intensive care and increased the risk of necrotising enterocolitis and respiratory distress in the baby compared with expectant management. We found insufficient evidence about effects of aggressive versus expectant management in the mother.

**Antihypertensive drugs for mild to moderate hypertension**

Two systematic reviews have found that antihypertensive agents versus placebo, no antihypertensive drug, or another antihypertensive drug significantly reduce the chance of developing severe hypertension, but found no clear effect on pre-eclampsia and perinatal death. Systematic reviews found that angiotensin converting enzyme inhibitors used in pregnancy were associated with fetal renal failure, and that β blockers increased the risk of the baby being small for its gestational age.

**Antioxidants in severe pre-eclampsia**

One RCT found insufficient evidence about the effects of a combination of vitamin E, vitamin C, and allopurinol versus placebo.

**Bed rest for proteinuric hypertension**

One systematic review found insufficient evidence about the effects of bed rest in hospital versus normal ambulation in hospital.

**Bed rest/hospital admission**

We found insufficient evidence about hospital admission, bed rest, or day care versus outpatient care or normal activities in hospital.

**Choice of analgesia during labour with severe pre-eclampsia**

One RCT found that epidural analgesia during labour versus intravenous patient controlled analgesia significantly reduced mean pain scores, but the clinical importance of the difference was unclear.

**Hospital admission for non-proteinuric hypertension**

One systematic review found no significant difference in any major outcome with hospital admission versus outpatient clinic assessment.

# Pre-eclampsia and hypertension

### Plasma volume expansion in severe pre-eclampsia
One systematic review found insufficient evidence about the effects of plasma volume expansion versus no expansion.

### Prophylactic diazepam in severe pre-eclampsia
One systematic review found insufficient evidence to compare prophylactic diazepam versus no anticonvulsant treatment in women with severe pre-eclampsia.

**DEFINITION**     Hypertension during pregnancy may be associated with one of several conditions. **Pregnancy induced hypertension** is a rise in blood pressure, without proteinuria, during the second half of pregnancy. **Pre-eclampsia** is a multisystem disorder, unique to pregnancy, which is usually associated with raised blood pressure and proteinuria. It rarely presents before 20 weeks' gestation. **Eclampsia** is one or more convulsions in association with the syndrome of pre-eclampsia. **Pre-existing hypertension** is known hypertension before pregnancy or raised blood pressure before 20 weeks' gestation. It may be essential hypertension or, less commonly, secondary to underlying disease.[1]

**INCIDENCE/**     Pregnancy induced hypertension affects 10% of pregnancies and pre-
**PREVALENCE**    eclampsia complicates 2–8%.[2] Eclampsia occurs in about 1/2000 deliveries in developed countries.[3] In developing countries, estimates of the incidence of eclampsia vary from 1/100 to 1/1700.[4,5]

**AETIOLOGY/**     The cause of pre-eclampsia is unknown. It is likely to be multifactorial and may
**RISK FACTORS**  result from deficient placental implantation during the first half of pregnancy.[6] Pre-eclampsia is more common among women likely to have a large placenta, such as those with multiple pregnancy, and among women with medical conditions associated with microvascular disease, such as diabetes, hypertension, and collagen vascular disease.[7,8] Other risk factors include genetic susceptibility, increased parity, and older maternal age.[9] Cigarette smoking seems to be associated with a lower risk of pre-eclampsia, but this potential benefit is outweighed by an increase in adverse outcomes such as low birth weight, placental abruption, and perinatal death.[10]

**PROGNOSIS**     The outcome of pregnancy in women with pregnancy induced hypertension alone is at least as good as that for normotensive pregnancies.[7,11] However, once pre-eclampsia develops, morbidity and mortality rise for both mother and child. For example, perinatal mortality for women with severe pre-eclampsia is double that for normotensive women.[7] Perinatal outcome is worse with early gestational hypertension.[7,9,11] Perinatal mortality also increases in women with severe essential hypertension.[12]

Please refer to CD-ROM for full text and references.

*Bridgette Byrne and John J Morrison*

## What are the effects of treatments?

**BENEFICIAL**

### Antenatal corticosteroids

One systematic review in women with anticipated preterm delivery has found that antenatal treatment with corticosteroids reduces the risk of respiratory distress syndrome, neonatal mortality, and intraventricular haemorrhage in preterm infants compared with placebo or no treatment.

**LIKELY TO BE BENEFICIAL**

### Antibiotic treatment for premature rupture of the membranes (prolongs gestation and may reduce infection, but unknown effect on perinatal mortality)

One systematic review in women with preterm premature rupture of membranesG has found that antibiotics compared with placebo prolong pregnancy and reduce the risk of neonatal morbidity, such as neonatal infection, requirement for treatment with oxygen, and abnormal cerebral ultrasound. It found that co-amoxiclav (amoxicillin [amoxycillin] plus clavulanic acid) was associated with an increase in the incidence of neonatal necrotising enterocolitis.

### Prophylactic cervical cerclage for women at risk of cervical incompetence

One large RCT has found that, in women presumed to have cervical incompetence, prophylactic cervical cerclageG compared with no cerclage reduces preterm birth (< 33 weeks' gestation) but increases the risk of puerperal pyrexia. It found that 24 women would need to undergo cerclage to prevent one additional preterm delivery. A second RCT in women with cervix changes detected by ultrasound found that cerclage plus bed rest reduced deliveries before 34 weeks compared with bed rest alone. A third RCT found no significant difference in preterm birth between cerclage plus bed rest and bed rest alone when mid-trimester cervical change has been detected by transvaginal ultrasound.

**TRADE OFF BETWEEN BENEFITS AND HARMS**

### Tocolytic treatment in threatened preterm labour

One systematic review and one subsequent RCT have found that atosiban, $\beta_2$ agonists, indometacin (indomethacin), and ethanol prolong pregnancy compared with placebo or no tocolytic, but they do not significantly reduce perinatal mortality or neonatal morbidity. Two systematic reviews found no significant difference in prolongation of pregnancy when comparing magnesium sulphate versus placebo or no tocolytics. Tocolytics increase maternal adverse effects, such as chest pain, nausea and vomiting, and dyspnoea. One systematic review has found that calcium channel blockers (mainly $\beta_2$ agonists) reduce deliveries within 48 hours, withdrawals caused by maternal adverse effects, and neonatal morbidity compared with other tocolytics.

**UNKNOWN EFFECTIVENESS**

### Amnioinfusion for preterm rupture of the membranes

One systematic review found insufficient evidence about the effects of amnio-infusionG.

# Preterm birth

**Pregnancy and childbirth**

### Enhanced antenatal care programmes for socially deprived population groups/high risk groups

RCTs carried out in a range of countries found no significant difference between enhanced antenatal care❻ and usual care in reducing the risk of preterm delivery.

### Elective rather than selective caesarean delivery in preterm labour

One systematic review has found limited evidence that elective compared with selective caesarean delivery❻ in women with preterm labour increases the risk of maternal morbidity, without clear evidence of benefit in neonatal morbidity or mortality.

### Antibiotic treatment for preterm labour with intact membranes

One systematic review found that antibiotics do not prolong pregnancy and do not reduce perinatal mortality compared with placebo.

### Thyrotropin releasing hormone before preterm delivery

One systematic review in women at risk of preterm birth has found no significant difference between thyrotropin releasing hormone plus corticosteroids and corticosteroids alone in improving neonatal outcomes. Thyrotropin releasing hormone plus corticosteroids increased maternal and fetal adverse events compared with corticosteroids alone.

**DEFINITION**   Preterm or premature birth is defined by the World Health Organization as delivery of an infant before 37 completed weeks of gestation.[1] There is no set lower limit to this definition, but 23–24 weeks' gestation is widely accepted,[1] which approximates to an average fetal weight of 500 g.

**INCIDENCE/**   Preterm birth occurs in about 5–10% of all births in developed countries,[2–4]
**PREVALENCE**   but in recent years the incidence seems to have increased in some countries, particularly the USA.[5] We found little reliable evidence for less developed countries that used the exact definition of premature birth. The rate in northwestern Ethiopia has been reported to vary between 11–22% depending on the age group studied, being highest in teenagers.[6]

**AETIOLOGY/**   About 30% of preterm births are unexplained and spontaneous.[4,7,8] The two
**RISK FACTORS**   strongest risk factors for idiopathic preterm labour❻ are low socioeconomic status and previous preterm delivery. Multiple pregnancy accounts for about another 30% of cases.[4,7] Other known risk factors include genital tract infection, preterm premature rupture of the membranes❻, antepartum haemorrhage, cervical incompetence, and congenital uterine abnormalities, which collectively account for about 20–25% of cases. The remaining cases (15–20%) are attributed to elective preterm delivery secondary to hypertensive disorders of pregnancy, intrauterine fetal growth restriction, congenital abnormalities, and medical disorders of pregnancy.[4,5,7,8]

**PROGNOSIS**   Preterm labour usually results in preterm birth. One systematic review (search date not stated) of tocolysis compared with placebo found that about 27% of preterm labours spontaneously resolved and about 70% progressed to preterm delivery.[9] Observational studies have found that one preterm birth significantly raises the risk of another in a subsequent pregnancy.[10]

---

Please refer to CD-ROM for full text and references.

Search date February 2003

*Peter Wark*

## What are the effects of treatment in people without chronic respiratory disease? *New*

### TRADE OFF BETWEEN BENEFITS AND HARMS

**Antibiotics versus placebo**

One systematic review and one subsequent RCT have found that antibiotics modestly reduce cough at 1–2 weeks but found no significant difference in quality of life or impairment in normal activity compared with placebo. Antibiotics increased risk of adverse events such as nausea, vomiting, rash, headache, and vaginitis compared with placebo. Widespread antibiotic use may lead to bacterial resistance to antibiotics.

### UNKNOWN EFFECTIVENESS

**Antibiotics versus each other**

RCTs found no significant difference in clinical improvement or cure between cefuroxime and amoxicillin (amoxycillin) or amoxicillin/clavulanic acid; among different cefalosporins; between azithromycin and clarithromycin; or between roxithromycin and amoxicillin. Two RCTs found that adverse effects were less common with cefuroxime than with amoxicillin/clavulanic acid.

**Antihistamines**

We found insufficient evidence about the effects of antihistamines compared with placebo in people with acute bronchitis.

**β Agonists**

One systematic review found no significant difference in cough or ability to return to work between β agonists and placebo in people with acute bronchitis. It found limited evidence from one small RCT that β agonists reduce cough compared with erythromycin. The review found that β agonists increase shaking and tremor compared with placebo or erythromycin.

**Over the counter antitussives**

RCTs found no significant difference in cough severity between codeine or dextromethorphan and placebo in children or adults with acute bronchitis. We found limited evidence from one RCT that moguisteine modestly reduced cough severity compared with placebo in adults, but was associated with more adverse gastrointestinal effects

**Over the counter expectorants**

We found insufficient evidence about the effects of over the counter expectorants in people with acute bronchitis.

**DEFINITION** Acute bronchitis is transient inflammation of the trachea and major bronchi. Clinically, it is diagnosed on the basis of cough and occasionally sputum, dyspnoea, and wheeze. This review is limited to episodes of acute bronchitis in people with no pre-existing respiratory disease and excluding those with clinical or radiographic evidence of pneumonia.

**INCIDENCE/ PREVALENCE** Acute bronchitis affects 44/1000 adults (> 16 years old) per year, with 82% of episodes occurring in autumn or winter.[1] Acute bronchitis was the fifth most common reason to present to a general practitioner in Australia.[2]

© BMJ Publishing Group Ltd 2003

# Acute bronchitis

**AETIOLOGY/ RISK FACTORS**

Infection is believed to be the trigger for acute bronchitis. However, pathogens have been identified in fewer than 55% of people.[1] Community studies that attempted to isolate pathogens from the sputum of people with acute bronchitis found viruses in 8–23%, typical bacteria (*Streptococcus pneumoniae*, *Haemophilus influenzae*, *Moraxella catarrhalis*) in 45%, and atypical bacteria (*Mycobacterium pneumoniae*, *Chlamydia pneumoniae*, *Bordetella pertussis*) in 0–25%.[1,3,4]

**PROGNOSIS**

Acute bronchitis is regarded as a mild self limiting illness but there are limited data on prognosis and complications such as chronic cough or progression to chronic bronchitis or pneumonia. One prospective longitudinal study reviewed 653 previously well adults who presented to suburban general practices over a 12 month period with symptoms of acute lower respiratory tract infection.[1] It found that within the first month of the illness 20% of people re-present to their general practitioner with persistent or recurrent symptoms. One prospective study of 138 previously well adults found that 34% had symptoms consistent with either chronic bronchitis or asthma 3 years after initial presentation with acute bronchitis.[5] It is also unclear whether acute bronchitis plays a causal role in the progression to chronic bronchitis or is simply a marker of predisposition to chronic lung disease.

Please refer to CD-ROM for full text and references.

Respiratory disorders (acute)

Respiratory disorders (acute)

## What are the effects of treatments?

### BENEFICIAL

**Antibiotics (amoxicillin, cephalosporins, macrolides, penicillin, quinolones) in hospital**

RCTs that compared different oral or intravenous antibiotics in people admitted to hospital found clinical cure or improvement in 73–96% of people. Four RCTs found no significant difference in clinical cure or improvement among different antibiotics, and two RCTs found that quinolones may increase clinical cure compared with co-amoxiclav (amoxicillin plus clavulanic acid) or cephalosporins. However, most trials were small and were designed to show equivalence between treatments rather than superiority of one over another.

**Antibiotics (amoxicillin, cephalosporins, macrolides, penicillin, quinolones) in outpatient settings**

One systematic review that evaluated different oral antibiotics in outpatient settings has found clinical cure or improvement in over 90% of people regardless of antibiotic taken. Another systematic review found that azithromycin significantly reduced clinical failures over 6–21 days compared with other macrolides, cephalosporins, or penicillin. A third systematic review and a subsequent RCT found no significant difference in clinical cure or improvement between quinolones and amoxicillin, cephalosporins, or macrolides. Most trials were designed to show equivalence between treatments rather than superiority of one over another.

### LIKELY TO BE BENEFICIAL

**Prompt versus delayed administration of antibiotics in people severely ill with community acquired pneumonia**

Retrospective studies found that prompt administration of antibiotics improved survival. It probably would be unethical to perform an RCT of delayed antibiotic treatment.

### UNKNOWN EFFECTIVENESS

**Bottle blowing**

One unblinded RCT in people receiving antibiotics and usual medical care found that bottle blowing physiotherapy plus early mobilisation plus encouragement to regularly sit up and take deep breaths reduced mean hospital stay compared with early mobilisation alone. It found no significant difference in duration of fever.

**Different antibiotic combinations in intensive care settings**

We found no RCTs comparing one combination of antibiotics versus another in intensive care units.

**Guidelines for treating pneumonia (for clinical outcomes)**

One systematic review that compared a guideline that incorporated early switch from intravenous to oral antibiotics and early discharge strategies (or both) versus usual care found no significant difference in clinical outcomes.

▶

# Community acquired pneumonia

**UNLIKELY TO BE BENEFICIAL**

## Intravenous versus oral antibiotics in immunocompetent people in hospital without life threatening illness

Two RCTs in immunocompetent people admitted to hospital who did not have life threatening illness found no significant difference in clinical cure or mortality between intravenous and oral antibiotics (co-amoxiclav [amoxicillin plus clavulanic acid] or cefuroxime). The RCTs found that intravenous antibiotics may increase the length of hospital stay compared with oral antibiotics.

## What are the effects of preventive interventions?

**BENEFICIAL**

## Pneumococcal vaccine in immunocompetent adults

One systematic review found that pneumococcal vaccination reduced pneumonia in immunocompetent people compared with no vaccination.

**LIKELY TO BE BENEFICIAL**

## Influenza vaccine in elderly people

We found no RCTs that assessed the effects of influenza vaccine in preventing community acquired pneumonia. Observational studies suggest that influenza vaccine may reduce the incidence of pneumonia and may reduce mortality.

**UNKNOWN EFFECTIVENESS**

## Pneumococcal vaccine in chronically ill, immunosuppressed, or elderly people

One systematic review found no significant difference between pneumococcal vaccination and no vaccination in the incidence of pneumonia in elderly people or people likely to have an impaired immune system.

**DEFINITION**     Community acquired pneumonia is pneumonia contracted in the community rather than in hospital. It is defined by clinical symptoms and signs, with radiological confirmation.

**INCIDENCE/**     In the northern hemisphere, community acquired pneumonia affects about
**PREVALENCE**     12/1000 people a year, particularly during winter and at the extremes of age (incidence: < 1 year old 30–50/1000 people a year; 15–45 years 1–5/1000 people a year; 60–70 years 10–20/1000 people a year; 71–85 years 50/1000 people a year).[1–6]

**AETIOLOGY/**     Over 100 microorganisms have been implicated in community acquired pneu-
**RISK FACTORS**     monia, but most cases are caused by *Streptococcus pneumoniae* ❶.[4–7] Smoking is probably an important risk factor.[8] One large cohort study in Finland (4175 people aged ≥ 60 years) suggested that risk factors for pneumonia in the elderly included alcoholism (RR 9.0, 95% CI 5.1 to 16.2), bronchial asthma (RR 4.2, 95% CI 3.3 to 5.4), immunosuppression (RR 3.1, 95% CI 1.9 to 5.1), lung disease (RR 3.0, 95% CI 2.3 to 3.9), heart disease (RR 1.9, 95% CI 1.7 to 2.3), institutionalisation (RR 1.8, 95% CI 1.4 to 2.4), and increasing age (≥ 70 years *v* 60–69 years; RR 1.5, 95% CI 1.3 to 1.7).[9]

**PROGNOSIS**     Severity varies from mild to life threatening illness within days of the onset of symptoms. One systematic review of prognosis studies for community acquired pneumonia (search date 1995, 33 148 people) found overall mortality to be 13.7%, ranging from 5.1% for ambulant people to 36.5% for people requiring intensive care.[9] The following prognostic factors were significantly associated with mortality: male sex (OR 1.3, 95% CI 1.2 to 1.4); pleuritic chest pain (OR

0.5, 95% CI 0.3 to 0.8, i.e. lower mortality); hypothermia (OR 5.0, 95% CI 2.4 to 10.4); systolic hypotension (OR 4.8, 95% CI 2.8 to 8.3); tachypnoea (OR 2.9, 95% CI 1.7 to 4.9); diabetes mellitus (OR 1.3, 95% CI 1.1 to 1.5); neoplastic disease (OR 2.8, 95% CI 2.4 to 3.1); neurological disease (OR 4.6, 95% CI 2.3 to 8.9); bacteraemia (OR 2.8, 95% CI 2.3 to 3.6); leucopenia (OR 2.5, 95% CI 1.6 to 3.7); and multilobar radiographic pulmonary infiltrates (OR 3.1, 95% CI 1.9 to 5.1).

Please refer to CD-ROM for full text and references.

# Spontaneous pneumothorax

**Search date December 2002**

*John Cunnington*

## What are the effects of treatments?

UNKNOWN EFFECTIVENESS

### Chest tube drainage

We found no RCTs comparing chest tube drainage versus observation. RCTs provided insufficient evidence to compare chest tube drainage versus needle aspiration.

### Chest tube drainage plus suction

One small RCT found no significant difference in the rate of resolution whether chest tube drainage bottles were connected to suction or not, but the trial was too small to exclude a clinically important difference.

### Needle aspiration

RCTs provided insufficient evidence to compare needle aspiration versus observation or chest tube drainage.

### One way valves on chest tubes versus bottles with underwater seal

One RCT found no significant difference in rates of resolution between one way valves and drainage bottles with underwater seals, but it is likely to have been too small to detect a clinically important difference. It found that people treated with one way valves used less analgesia and spent less time in hospital than people treated with drainage bottles.

### Small versus standard sized chest tubes

We found no RCTs comparing small versus standard sized chest tubes.

## What are the effects of interventions to prevent recurrence?

TRADE OFF BETWEEN BENEFITS AND HARMS

### Chemical pleurodesis

Two RCTs have found that adding chemical pleurodesis to chest tube drainage reduces the rate of recurrence of spontaneous pneumothorax compared with chest tube drainage alone, but one of the RCTs found that treatment can be painful. The RCTs found no significant difference in length of hospital stay. We found no RCTs comparing chemical versus surgical pleurodesis.

### Surgical pleurodesis

One RCT found that thoracoscopic surgery with talc instillation reduced the rate of recurrence at 5 years compared with chest tube drainage. Another RCT found that video-assisted thoracoscopic surgery reduced hospital stay compared with thoracotomy. It found no significant difference in the rate of recurrence after 3 years, but the limited evidence cannot exclude a clinically important difference. We found no RCTs comparing surgical versus chemical pleurodesis.

UNKNOWN EFFECTIVENESS

### Optimal timing of pleurodesis (after first, second, or third spontaneous pneumothorax)

We found no RCTs or good cohort studies assessing whether pleurodesis should take place after the first, second, or subsequent episodes of spontaneous pneumothorax.

**DEFINITION**

A pneumothorax is air in the pleural space. A spontaneous pneumothorax occurs when there is no provoking factor, such as trauma, surgery, or diagnostic intervention. It implies a leak of air from the lung parenchyma through the visceral pleura into the pleural space.

**INCIDENCE/ PREVALENCE**

In a survey in Minnesota, USA, the incidence of spontaneous pneumothorax was 7/100 000 men and 1/100 000 for women.[1] Smoking increases the likelihood of spontaneous pneumothorax by 22 times for men and eight times for women. A dose–response relationship has been observed.[2]

**AETIOLOGY/ RISK FACTORS**

Spontaneous pneumothorax can be primary (typically in young fit people and thought to be because of a congenital abnormality of the visaral pleura) or secondary (caused by underlying lung disease, typically occurring in older people with emphysema or pulmonary fibrosis).

**PROGNOSIS**

Death from spontaneous pneumothorax is rare. Morbidity with pain and shortness of breath is common. Published recurrence rates vary. One cohort study in Denmark found that, after a first episode of primary spontaneous pneumothorax, 23% of people suffered a recurrence within 5 years, most within a year.[3] Recurrence rates had been thought to increase substantially after the first recurrence, but one retrospective case control study (147 military personnel) found that 28% of men with a first spontaneous pneumothorax had a recurrence; 23% of the 28% had a second recurrence; and 14% of that 23% had a third recurrence, giving a total recurrence rate of 35%.[4]

Please refer to CD-ROM for full text and references.

# Upper respiratory tract infection

**Search date February 2003**

*Chris Del Mar and Paul Glasziou*

## What are the effects of treatments?

### BENEFICIAL

**Analgesia/anti-inflammatory drugs for symptom relief**

One systematic review has found that analgesics or anti-inflammatory drugs reduce sore throat at 1–5 days compared with placebo.

**Antibiotics for preventing (rare) complications of β haemolytic streptococcal pharyngitis**

One systematic review has found that antibiotics prevent non-suppurative complications of β haemolytic streptococcal pharyngitis compared with no antibiotics, but in industrialised countries such complications are rare.

### LIKELY TO BE BENEFICIAL

**Antibiotics for reducing time to recovery in people with proven infection with *Haemophilus influenzae*, *Moraxella catarrhalis*, or *Streptococcus pneumoniae***

In a minority of people, upper respiratory tract infection is found to be caused by *H influenzae*, *M catarrhalis*, or *S pneumoniae*. One RCT found that, in these people, antibiotics increased recovery at 5 days compared with placebo. However, we have no methods currently of easily identifying this subgroup at first consultation.

**Antihistamines for runny nose and sneezing**

One systematic review has found that antihistamines reduce runny nose and sneezing after 2 days compared with placebo, but the clinical benefit is small.

**Decongestants for short term relief of congestive symptoms**

One systematic review found that a single dose of decongestant reduced nasal congestion over 3–10 hours compared with placebo.

**Vitamin C**

One systematic review found that vitamin C slightly reduced the duration of cold symptoms compared with placebo, but the benefit was small and may be explained by publication bias.

### TRADE OFF BETWEEN BENEFITS AND HARMS

**Antibiotics for reducing time to recovery in people with acute sore throat**

One systematic review has found that antibiotics slightly improve symptoms at 6–8 days compared with placebo. Adverse effects (nausea, vomiting, headache, rash, vaginitis) were more common with antibiotics.

### UNKNOWN EFFECTIVENESS

**Echinacea for prevention**

One systematic review found that, compared with no treatment, echinacea reduced the proportion of people who had one infection episode, but found insufficient evidence about the effects of echinacea compared with placebo.

**Echinacea for treatment**

Systematic reviews found limited evidence that some preparations of echinacea may improve symptoms compared with placebo, but we found insufficient evidence about the effects of any specific product.

◀ **Steam inhalation**

One systematic review found insufficient evidence about the effects of steam inhalation.

**Zinc (intranasal gel or lozenges)**

Two RCTs found that zinc intranasal gel reduced the mean duration of cold symptoms compared with placebo, but the difference was significant in only one of the RCTs. Two systematic reviews found limited evidence that zinc gluconate or acetate lozenges may reduce duration of symptoms at 7 days compared with placebo.

## LIKELY TO BE INEFFECTIVE OR HARMFUL

**Antibiotics in people with colds**

Systematic reviews found no significant difference between antibiotics and placebo in cure or general improvement at 6–14 days.

**Decongestants for long term relief of congestive symptoms**

One systematic review found insufficient evidence to assess the effects of longer use of decongestants. One case control study found weak evidence that phenylpropanolamine may increase the risk of haemorrhagic stroke.

**DEFINITION**    Upper respiratory tract infection involves inflammation of the respiratory mucosa from the nose to the lower respiratory tree, but not including the alveoli. In addition to malaise, it causes localised symptoms that constitute several overlapping syndromes: sore throat (pharyngitis), rhinorrhoea (common cold), facial fullness and pain (sinusitis — see acute sinusitis, p 103), and cough (bronchitis — see acute bronchitis, p 319).

**INCIDENCE/**    Upper respiratory tract infections, nasal congestion, throat complaints, and
**PREVALENCE**  cough are responsible for 11% of general practice consultations in Australia.[1] Each year, children suffer about five such infections and adults two to three infections.[1–3]

**AETIOLOGY/**    Infective agents include over 200 viruses (with 100 rhinoviruses) and several
**RISK FACTORS** bacteria. Transmission is mostly through hand to hand contact with subsequent passage to the nostrils or eyes rather than, as commonly perceived, through droplets in the air.[4] A systematic review of the risk factors for developing prolonged illness (especially tiredness) after infectious mononucleosis of five cohort studies of 531 adults showed that this occurred in 2–56% of people. The best predictor for tiredness was poor physical functioning immediately after the start of the illness; previous psychological factors were identified as unimportant in four studies and predictive in one.[5]

**PROGNOSIS**    Upper respiratory tract infections are usually self limiting. Although they cause little mortality or serious morbidity, upper respiratory tract infections are responsible for considerable discomfort, lost work, and medical costs. Clinical patterns vary and overlap between infective agents. In addition to nasal symptoms, half of sufferers experience sore throat and 40% experience cough. Symptoms peak within 1–3 days and generally clear by 1 week, although cough often persists.[4]

Please refer to CD-ROM for full text and references.

# Asthma

## Search date September 2002

*J Mark FitzGerald and Bazian Ltd*

---

## What are the effects of treatments for chronic and acute asthma?

### BENEFICIAL

#### Adding inhaled long acting $\beta_2$ agonists to inhaled corticosteroids in poorly controlled mild to moderate, persistent asthma (for symptom control)

RCTs have found that, in people with asthma that is poorly controlled with inhaled corticosteroids, adding regular long acting inhaled $\beta_2$ agonists significantly improves symptoms and lung function compared with adding placebo or a leukotriene antagonist. One systematic review and one additional RCT have found that adding regular doses of long acting inhaled $\beta_2$ agonists significantly improves lung function and symptoms and reduces rescue medication compared with increasing the dose of inhaled corticosteroids. However, one further RCT found that increasing inhaled corticosteroid dose reduced exacerbations compared with adding long acting inhaled $\beta_2$ agonists.

#### Inhaled corticosteroids for acute asthma (better than placebo)

One systematic review has found that inhaled corticosteroids versus placebo given in the emergency department significantly reduces hospital admission rates in adults. One systematic review found no significant difference in relapse rates for oral versus inhaled steroids at 7–10 days.

#### Inhaled plus oral corticosteroid for acute asthma (as effective as oral corticosteroid alone)

One systematic review found no significant difference in relapse rates for inhaled plus oral corticosteroid versus oral corticosteroids up to 24 days.

#### Inhaled short acting $\beta_2$ agonists as needed for symptom relief (as effective as regular use) in adults with mild or to moderate, persistent asthma

One systematic review and one subsequent RCT have found no significant difference between regular and as needed inhaled short acting $\beta_2$ agonists for clinically important outcomes.

#### Ipratropium bromide added to $\beta_2$ agonists for acute exacerbations

Two systematic reviews and one subsequent RCT have found that ipratropium bromide plus salbutamol⊖ versus salbutamol alone improves lung function and is likely to reduce hospital admission in people with severe acute asthma.

#### Low dose, inhaled corticosteroids in mild, persistent asthmaa

Systematic reviews and RCTs have found that, in people with mild, persistent asthma, low doses of inhaled corticosteroids significantly improve symptoms and lung function compared with placebo or regular inhaled $\beta_2$ agonists.

#### Short courses of oral systemic corticosteroids for acute exacerbations

Two systematic reviews and one subsequent RCT have found that early treatment with systemic corticosteroids reduces admission and relapse rates compared with placebo in people with acute asthma. One systematic review found no significant difference between oral and inhaled steroids for relapse rates at 7–10 days in adults with acute asthma.

◄ **Spacer devices for delivering inhaled medications from pressurised metered dose inhalers in acute asthma (as good as nebulisers)**

One systematic review in people with acute, but not life threatening exacerbations of asthma found no significant difference with $\beta_2$ agonists delivered by spacer device/holding chamber versus nebulisers in rates of hospital admission, time spent in the emergency department, peak expiratory flow rate, or forced expiratory volume in 1 second©.

## LIKELY TO BE BENEFICIAL

**Adding leukotriene antagonists in people with mild to moderate, persistent asthma (v no added treatment)**

RCTs in people taking $\beta_2$ agonists alone have found that leukotriene antagonists versus placebo significantly reduce asthma symptoms and $\beta_2$ agonist use. One systematic review and subsequent RCTs have found that adding leukotriene antagonists increased exacerbations, reduced lung function and were less effective for symptom control compared with inhaled corticosteroids. Two RCTs have found that an inhaled corticosteroid plus a long acting $\beta_2$ agonist significantly improved symptoms, lung function, and exacerbations compared with a leukotriene antagonist at 12 weeks.

**Education about acute asthma**

One systematic review and one subsequent RCT found that education to facilitate self management of asthma in adults versus usual care significantly reduced hospital admission, unscheduled visits to the doctor, and days off work. However, a second subsequent RCT found no significant effect of asthma education for quality of life or social functioning at 6 months.

**Magnesium sulphate for people with severe acute asthma**

One systematic review and three subsequent RCTs found no significant difference between intravenous magnesium sulphate and placebo for hospital admission rates. However, we found limited evidence from one systematic review and two subsequent RCTs that intravenous magnesium versus placebo improved lung function compared with placebo in people with severe acute asthma.

**Mechanical ventilation for people with severe acute asthma\***

We found no RCTs comparing mechanical ventilation with or without inhaled $\beta_2$ agonists versus no mechanical ventilation in people with severe acute asthma. Evidence from cohort studies support its use, although observational studies suggest that ventilation is associated with a high level of morbidity.

**Oxygen supplementation for acute asthma\***

We found no systematic review or RCTs of oxygen in acute asthma. However, consensus opinion and pathophysiology suggest that its role is vital in acute asthma.

**Specialist versus generalist care for acute exacerbations**

One systematic review found limited evidence that specialist versus generalist care improved outcomes in adults and children.

\*Highly likely to be effective. RCTs unlikely to be conducted.

## UNLIKELY TO BE BENEFICIAL

**Continuous versus intermittent nebulised short acting $\beta_2$ agonists for acute asthma**

One systematic review and one RCT have found no significant difference between continuous and intermittent nebulised short acting $\beta_2$ agonists for hospital admission rates in adults.

# Asthma

## Intravenous versus nebulised delivery of short acting $\beta_2$ agonists for acute asthma

One systematic review found that intravenous delivery of short acting $\beta_2$ agonists was no more effective than nebulised delivery in improving peak expiratory flow rate❻ at 60 minutes.

### UNKNOWN EFFECTIVENESS

## Adding leukotriene antagonists plus inhaled corticosteroids in people with mild to moderate, persistent asthma

One systematic review in people taking inhaled corticosteroids found no significant difference between leukotriene antagonists and placebo for exacerbation rates at 4–16 weeks. We found limited evidence from two RCTs that, in people with asthma that is poorly controlled with inhaled corticosteroids, adding a leukotriene antagonist was less effective for symptoms and lung function compared with adding a long acting $\beta_2$ agonist.

## Helium–oxygen mixture for acute asthma

One systematic review found no significant difference for helium–oxygen mixture versus air or oxygen in pulmonary function tests at 60 minutes in adults and children with acute asthma.

**DEFINITION**   Chronic asthma Acute asthma Asthma is characterised by variable airflow obstruction and airway hyperresponsiveness. Symptoms include dyspnoea, cough, chest tightness, and wheezing. The normal diurnal variation❻ of peak expiratory flow rate is increased in people with asthma❶. Chronic asthma is defined here as asthma requiring maintenance treatment. Asthma is classified differently in the USA and UK❶. Where necessary, the text specifies the system of classification used.[1,2] Acute asthma is defined here as an exacerbation of underlying asthma requiring urgent treatment.

**INCIDENCE/ PREVALENCE**   Reported prevalence of asthma is increasing worldwide. About 10% of people have suffered an attack of asthma.[3–5] Epidemiological studies have also found marked variations in prevalence in different countries.[6,7]

**AETIOLOGY/ RISK FACTORS**   Most people with asthma are atopic. Exposure to certain stimuli initiates inflammation and structural changes in airways causing airway hyperresponsiveness and variable airflow obstruction, which in turn cause most asthma symptoms. There are a large number of such stimuli; the more important include environmental allergens, occupational sensitising agents, and respiratory viral infections.[8,9]

**PROGNOSIS**   **Chronic asthma:** In people with mild asthma, prognosis is good and progression to severe disease is rare. However, as a group, people with asthma lose lung function faster than those without asthma, although less quickly than people without asthma who smoke.[10] People with chronic asthma can improve with treatment. However, for reasons not clearly understood, some people (possibly up to 5%) have severe disease that responds poorly to treatment. These people are most at risk of morbidity and death from asthma. **Acute asthma:** About 10–20% of people presenting to the emergency department with asthma are admitted to hospital. Of these, fewer than 10% receive mechanical ventilation,[11,12] although previous ventilation is associated with a 19-fold increased risk of ventilation for a subsequent episode.[13] It is unusual for people to die unless they have suffered respiratory arrest before reaching hospital.[14] One prospective study of 939 people discharged from emergency care found that 17% (95% CI 14% to 20%) relapsed by 2 weeks.[15]

Please refer to CD-ROM for full text and references.

## What are the effects of pharmacological treatments in people with bronchiectasis but without cystic fibrosis?

### UNKNOWN EFFECTIVENESS

**Bromhexine**

One systematic review found insufficient evidence to compare the effects of bromhexine versus placebo.

**Inhaled steroids**

One systematic review found insufficient evidence from two small RCTs about the effects of inhaled steroids versus placebo in people with bronchiectasis not due to a specific congenital disease.

**Long acting $\beta_2$ agonists**

One systematic review found no RCTs comparing long acting $\beta_2$ agonists versus placebo or other treatments in people with non-cystic fibrosis bronchiectasis.

**Oral steroids**

One systematic review found no RCTs comparing oral steroids versus placebo, no steroids, or other treatments in people with non-cystic fibrosis bronchiectasis.

**Recombinant human deoxyribonuclease**

One systematic review found insufficient evidence to compare the effects of recombinant human deoxyribonuclease versus those of placebo

**DEFINITION**      Bronchiectasis is defined as irreversible widening of medium sized airways (bronchi) in the lung. It is characterised by inflammation, destruction of bronchial walls, and chronic bacterial infection. The condition may be limited to a single lobe or lung segment, or it may affect one or both lungs more diffusely. Clinically, the condition manifests as chronic cough and chronic overproduction of sputum (up to about 500 mL daily), which is often purulent.[1] People with severe bronchiectasis may have life threatening haemoptysis and may develop features of chronic obstructive airways disease, such as wheezing, chronic respiratory failure, pulmonary hypertension, and right sided heart failure.

**INCIDENCE/**      We found few reliable data. Incidence has declined over the past 50 years and
**PREVALENCE**   prevalence is low in higher income countries. Prevalence is much higher in poorer countries and is a major cause of morbidity and mortality.

**AETIOLOGY/**      Bronchiectasis is most commonly a long term complication of previous lower
**RISK FACTORS** respiratory infections such as measles pneumonitis, pertussis, and tuberculosis. Foreign body inhalation and allergic, autoimmune, and chemical lung damage also predispose to the condition.[2] Underlying congenital disorders such as cystic fibrosis, cilial dysmotility syndromes, $\alpha_1$ antitrypsin deficiency, and congenital immunodeficiencies may also predispose to bronchiectasis and may be of greater aetiological importance than respiratory infection in higher income countries. Cystic fibrosis is the most common congenital cause.

© BMJ Publishing Group Ltd 2003

# Bronchiectasis

**PROGNOSIS**  Bronchiectasis is a chronic condition with frequent relapses of varying severity. Long term prognosis is variable. Data on morbidity and mortality are sparse.[3] Bronchiectasis frequently coexists with other respiratory disease, making it difficult to distinguish prognosis for bronchiectasis alone.

Please refer to CD-ROM for full text and references.

Topic search date October 2002

*Huib Kerstjens and Dirkje Postma*

## What are the effects of maintenance drug treatment in stable chronic obsructive pulmonary disease?

We found no evidence about effects of most interventions on progression of chronic obstructive pulmonary disease (measured by decline in lung function). However, we found good evidence from RCTs that inhaled corticosteroids do not prevent progression.

### BENEFICIAL

#### Inhaled anticholinergics

RCTs have found that inhaled anticholinergics versus placebo significantly improve forced expiratory volume in 1 second ($FEV_1$)🅖, exercise capacity, and symptoms. One large RCT found that adding ipratropium to a smoking cessation programme had no significant impact on decline in $FEV_1$ over 5 years. One RCT found that inhaled tiotropium (a long acting anticholinergic drug) reduced exacerbation and admission rates compared with placebo at 1 year.

#### Inhaled anticholinergics plus $\beta_2$ agonists

RCTs have found that combining a $\beta_2$ agonist with an anticholinergic drug for 2–12 weeks modestly but significantly improves $FEV_1$ compared with either drug alone. One RCT found that, when combined with an anticholinergic drug, a long acting $\beta_2$ agonist improved $FEV_1$ and peak expiratory flow🅖 rate significantly more than a short acting $\beta_2$ agonist.

#### Inhaled $\beta_2$ agonists

RCTs found that inhaled $\beta_2$ agonists improve $FEV_1$🅖 and symptoms compared with placebo after 1 week to 6 months' treatment.

### LIKELY TO BE BENEFICIAL

#### Inhaled anticholinergics versus $\beta_2$ agonists

RCTs have found that 3 months of a short acting inhaled anticholinergic significantly improved $FEV_1$ compared with short acting $\beta_2$ agonists. One RCT found that 6 months of a long acting inhaled anticholinergic significantly improved $FEV_1$ and quality of life compared with a long acting inhaled $\beta_2$ agonist. RCTs have found inconsistent evidence about effects of short acting inhaled anticholinergics versus long acting $\beta_2$ agonists over 3 months.

#### Long term domiciliary oxygen

RCTs found limited evidence that domiciliary oxygen versus no oxygen improved survival over 2 years in people with chronic obstructive pulmonary disease and hypoxaemia.

#### Mucolytics*

We found evidence from two systematic reviews that mucolytics versus placebo for 3–24 months may reduce the frequency and duration of exacerbations in people with chronic bronchitis. However, it is not clear whether these effects are generalisable to people with chronic obstructive pulmonary disease.

*Extrapolated from studies of different types of pulmonary disease, including chronic obstructive pulmonary disease. ▶

**Chronic obstructive pulmonary disease**

**TRADE OFF BETWEEN BENEFITS AND HARMS**

### Inhaled corticosteroids

RCTs have found no significant difference between inhaled corticosteroids and placebo in lung function ($FEV_1$) over 10 days to 10 weeks. However, large RCTs lasting at least 6 months suggested that inhaled steroids increased $FEV_1$ during the first 3–6 months of use, but we found evidence of no effect on subsequent decline in lung function. One systematic review found that long term inhaled steroids versus placebo reduced the frequency of exacerbations. Long term inhaled steroids may predispose to adverse effects, including osteoporosis, skin bruising, and oral candidiasis.

### Theophyllines

One systematic review has found a slight but significant improvement in $FEV_1$ with theophyllines compared with placebo after 3 months. One large RCT has found that theophyllines significantly improve $FEV_1$ compared with placebo after 12 months of treatment. The usefulness of these drugs is limited by adverse effects and the need for monitoring of blood concentrations.

**UNKNOWN EFFECTIVENESS**

### $\alpha_1$ Antitrypsin infusion

One RCT in people with $\alpha_1$ antitrypsin deficiency and moderate emphysema found no significant difference with $\alpha_1$ antitrypsin infusion versus placebo in the decline in $FEV_1$ after 1 year.

### Antibiotics

Two poor quality RCTs found no significant difference with antibiotics in frequency of exacerbations or decline in lung function over 5 years compared with placebo.

### Deoxyribonuclease

We found no RCTs comparing long term effects of deoxyribonuclease versus placebo.

**UNLIKELY TO BE BENEFICIAL**

### Oral corticosteroids

We found no evidence on long term benefits. One systematic review has found that oral corticosteroids for 2–4 weeks significantly improve lung function compared with placebo. Long term oral corticosteroids are associated with serious adverse effects, including osteoporosis and diabetes.

### Oral versus inhaled corticosteroids

Three RCTs provided insufficient evidence about effects of oral versus inhaled corticosteroids over 2 weeks. Systemic corticosteroids are associated with serious adverse effects, including osteoporosis and diabetes.

**DEFINITION**     Chronic obstructive pulmonary disease is characterised by chronic bronchitis or emphysema. Emphysema is abnormal permanent enlargement of the air spaces distal to the terminal bronchioles, accompanied by destruction of their walls and without obvious fibrosis. Chronic bronchitis is chronic cough or mucus production for at least 3 months in at least two successive years when other causes of chronic cough have been excluded.[1]

**INCIDENCE/**     Chronic obstructive pulmonary disease mainly affects middle aged and elderly
**PREVALENCE**     people. It is one of the leading causes of morbidity and mortality worldwide. In the USA, it affects about 14 million people and is the fourth leading cause of death. Both morbidity and mortality are rising. Estimated prevalence in the USA has risen by 41% since 1982, and age adjusted death rates rose by 71% between 1966 and 1985. All cause age adjusted mortality declined over the ▶

same period by 22% and mortality from cardiovascular diseases by 45%.[1] In the UK, physician diagnosed prevalence was 2% in men and 1% in women between 1990 and 1997.[2]

**AETIOLOGY/ RISK FACTORS**  Chronic obstructive pulmonary disease is largely preventable. The main cause is exposure to cigarette smoke. The disease is rare in lifelong non-smokers (estimated incidence 5% in 3 large representative US surveys from 1971–1984), in whom "passive" exposure to environmental tobacco smoke has been proposed as a cause.[3,4] Other proposed causes include airway hyperresponsiveness, air pollution, and allergy.[5–7]

**PROGNOSIS**  Airway obstruction is usually progressive in those who continue to smoke, resulting in early disability and shortened survival. Smoking cessation reverts the rate of decline in lung function to that of non-smokers.[8] Many people will need medication for the rest of their lives, with increased doses and additional drugs during exacerbations.

Please refer to CD-ROM for full text and references.

# Lung cancer

Search date January 2003

*Alan Neville*

## What are the effects of treatments for non-small cell lung cancer?

### BENEFICIAL

**Palliative chemotherapy with cisplatin or docetaxel containing regimens in stage 4 non-small cell lung cancer**

Systematic reviews in people with stage 4 non-small cell lung cancer have found that adding chemotherapy regimens containing cisplatin to best supportive care increases survival at 1 year compared with supportive care alone. Limited evidence from RCTs suggests that the adding chemotherapy to best supportive care may improve quality of life compared with best supportive care alone.

**Thoracic irradiation plus chemotherapy versus irradiation alone in unresected stage 3 non-small cell lung cancer**

Systematic reviews and one subsequent RCT in people with unresectable stage 3 non-small cell lung cancer have found that adding chemotherapy to irradiation improves survival at 2–5 years compared with irradiation alone. Another subsequent RCT has found no significant difference in median survival between radical radiotherapy plus chemotherapy and radiotherapy alone.

### UNKNOWN EFFECTIVENESS

**Hyperfractionated radiation treatment versus conventional radiotherapy in unresectable stage 3 non-small cell lung cancer**

One systematic review in people with stage 3 non-small cell lung cancer found no significant difference between standard hyperfractionation and conventional radiotherapy in survival at 2 years. One RCT in people with stage 1–3B non-small cell lung cancer found that continuous, hyperfractionated, accelerated radiotherapy⊙ significantly increased survival at 2 years compared with conventional radiotherapy.

**Newer single drug or combined drug regimens in stage 4 non-small cell lung cancer (not clearly better than cisplatin or docetaxel based regimens)**

One systematic review and subsequent RCTs in people with stage 3 and 4 non-small cell lung cancer found inconclusive evidence on the effects of single compared with combined chemotherapy. RCTs in people with stage 3 and 4 non-small cell lung cancer found no significant difference in survival at 1 year between first line platinum based and non-platinum based chemotherapy.

**Preoperative chemotherapy in people with resectable stage 3 non-small cell lung cancer**

One systematic review of small, weak RCTs and one subsequent RCT provided inconclusive evidence about the effects of preoperative chemotherapy in people with resectable stage 3 disease.

### UNLIKELY TO BE BENEFICIAL

**Postoperative chemotherapy in people with resected stage 1–3 non-small cell lung cancer**

Systematic reviews and subsequent RCTs in people with completely resected stage 1–3 non-small cell lung cancer have found no significant difference in survival at 5 years between postoperative cisplatin based chemotherapy and surgery with or without concomitant radiotherapy, although subgroup analysis in one RCT ▶

◄ suggests that postoperative chemotherapy may increase survival in people with stage 3 disease. One systematic review found that postoperative alkylating agents increased mortality compared with no postoperative chemotherapy.

---

## What are the effects of treatments for small cell lung cancer?

### BENEFICIAL

**Chemotherapy plus thoracic irradiation versus chemotherapy alone in limited stage small cell lung cancer**

Two systematic reviews in people with limited stage small cell lung cancer have found that adding thoracic irradiation to chemotherapy improves survival at 3 years. However, one of these reviews has found that chemotherapy plus thoracic irradiation increases deaths related to treatment.

### LIKELY TO BE BENEFICIAL

**Prophylactic cranial irradiation for people in complete remission with limited or extensive stage small cell lung cancer**

One systematic review in people in with small cell lung cancer in complete remission has found that, compared with no irradiation, prophylactic cranial irradiation improves survival at 3 years and reduces the risk of developing brain metastases. While long term cognitive dysfunction following cranial irradiation has been described in non-randomised studies, RCTs have not found a cumulative increase in neuropsychological dysfunction.

### UNKNOWN EFFECTIVENESS

**Dose intensive chemotherapy versus standard chemotherapy**

While one systematic review found limited evidence that intensifying chemotherapy dose by either increasing the number of chemotherapy cycles, increasing chemotherapy dose, or increasing dose intensity per cycle may modestly improve survival compared with standard chemotherapy, additional RCTs have found inconclusive evidence about the effects of dose intensification on survival.

### LIKELY TO BE INEFFECTIVE OR HARMFUL

**Oral etoposide in extensive stage small cell lung cancer**

Two RCTs in people with extensive stage small cell lung cancer found that oral etoposide reduced survival compared with combination chemotherapy at 1 year. One RCT, in people with extensive stage small cell lung cancer who had not responded to induction combination chemotherapy, found no significant difference between oral etoposide and no further treatment in mortality at 3 years, although overall mortality was lower in people taking etoposide. RCTs found that etoposide may reduce nausea, alopecia and numbness in the short term compared with combination chemotherapy, but found no evidence that it offered better quality of life overall.

**DEFINITION**    Lung cancer (bronchogenic carcinoma) is an epithelial cancer arising from the bronchial surface epithelium or bronchial mucous glands❶.

**INCIDENCE/**    Lung cancer is the leading cause of cancer death in both men and women,
**PREVALENCE** affecting about 100 000 men and 80 000 women annually in the USA, and about 40 000 men and women in the UK. Small cell lung cancer constitutes about 20–25% of all lung cancers, the remainder being non-small cell lung cancers, of which adenocarcinoma is now the most prevalent form.[1]

▶

# Lung cancer

**AETIOLOGY/**
**RISK FACTORS**
Smoking remains the major preventable risk factor, accounting for about 80–90% of all cases. Other respiratory tract carcinogens have been identified that may enhance the carcinogenic effects of tobacco smoke, either in the workplace (e.g. asbestos and polycyclic aromatic hydrocarbons) or in the home (e.g. indoor radon).[3]

**PROGNOSIS**
Lung cancer has an overall 5 year survival rate of 10–12%.[2] At the time of diagnosis, 10–15% of people with lung cancer have localised disease. Of these, half will have died at 5 years despite potentially curative surgery. Over half of people have metastatic disease at the time of diagnosis. People with non-small cell cancer who undergo surgery have a 5 year survival of 60–80% for stage 1 disease and 25–50% for stage 2 disease.[2] In people with small cell cancer, those with limited stage disease who undergo combined chemotherapy and mediastinal irradiation have a median survival of 18–24 months, whereas those with extensive stage disease who are given palliative chemotherapy have a median survival of 10–12 months.[2] About 5–10% of people with small cell lung cancer present with central nervous system involvement, and half develop symptomatic brain metastases by 2 years. Of these, only half respond to palliative radiation, and their median survival is less than 3 months.[2]

Please refer to CD-ROM for full text and references.

## What are the effects of antibacterial treatments?

Bacterial vaginosis may resolve spontaneously.

### BENEFICIAL

#### Antibacterial treatment in symptomatic non-pregnant women

One systematic review found no significant difference between oral and intravaginal antibacterial drugs in cure rates after 5–10 days or at 4 weeks. Another systematic review has found that a 7 day course of twice daily oral metronidazole increases cure rates at 3–4 weeks compared with a single 2 g dose. Limited evidence from RCTs found no significant difference in cure rates with oral clindamycin versus oral metronidazole twice daily for 7 days, and no significant difference between once and twice daily dosing with intravaginal metronidazole gel. One RCT found no significant difference in cure rates at 35 days between intravaginal clindamycin ovules for 3 days and intravaginal clindamycin cream for 7 days.

### LIKELY TO BE BENEFICIAL

#### Antibacterial treatment (except intravaginal clindamycin) in pregnant women who have had a previous preterm birth

Limited evidence from a subgroup analysis in pregnant women with bacterial vaginosis who had a previous preterm birth found that oral antibacterial treatment reduced the risk of premature delivery compared with placebo. One small RCT in women with bacterial vaginosis who had a previous labour or midtrimester abortion found a higher rate of preterm birth with oral metronidazole compared with placebo, but the group receiving metronidazole had higher previous antibacterial use and asymptomatic bacteriuria at baseline.

#### Oral antibacterial treatment before surgical abortion

RCTs consistently found that oral antibacterial treatment in women with bacterial vaginosis about to undergo surgical abortion was associated with a lower risk of pelvic inflammatory disease compared with placebo, but the difference was only significant in the largest RCT.

### UNKNOWN EFFECTIVENESS

#### Antibacterial treatment before gynaecological procedures (other than abortion)

We found no RCTs on the effects of antibacterial treatment in women with bacterial vaginosis about to undergo gynaecological procedures other than abortion.

#### Antibacterial treatment (except intravaginal clindamycin) in low risk pregnancy

Two systematic reviews of antibacterial treatment versus placebo found no significant difference in the risk of preterm delivery.

### LIKELY TO BE INEFFECTIVE OR HARMFUL

#### Treating pregnant women with intravaginal clindamycin cream

Four RCTs found that intravaginal clindamycin cream versus placebo was associated with an increased risk of preterm delivery and low birth weight, but the increase was not significant. ▶

# Bacterial vaginosis

◄ **Treating pregnant women without bacterial vaginosis**

Subgroup analysis in two RCTs of pregnant women without bacterial vaginosis found that both intravaginal clindamycin cream and oral metronidazole plus erythromycin were associated with an increased risk of preterm delivery before 34 weeks' gestation compared with placebo, although the difference was significant in only one of the RCTs.

## What are the effects of interventions to prevent recurrence?

**LIKELY TO BE INEFFECTIVE OR HARMFUL**

**Treating a woman's one steady male sexual partner with metonidazole or clindamycin**

One systematic review has found that, in women being treated with antibacterial agents, who have one steady male sexual partner, treating the partner with oral oral metronidazole or clindamycin does not reduce the woman's risk of recurrence.

**DEFINITION**  Bacterial vaginosis is a microbial disease characterised by an alteration in the bacterial flora of the vagina from a predominance of *Lactobacillus* species to high concentrations of anaerobic bacteria. Diagnosis requires three out of four features: the presence of clue cells; a homogenous discharge adherent to the vaginal walls; pH of vaginal fluid greater than 4.5; and a "fishy" amine odour of the vaginal discharge before or after addition of 10% potassium hydroxide. The condition is asymptomatic in 50% of infected women. Women with symptoms have an excessive white to grey, or malodorous vaginal discharge, or both; the odour may be particularly noticeable during sexual intercourse.

**INCIDENCE/**  Bacterial vaginosis is the most common infectious cause of vaginitis, being
**PREVALENCE**  about twice as common as candidiasis.[1] Prevalences of 10–61% have been reported among unselected women from a range of settings.[2] Data on incidence are limited but one study found that, over a 2 year period, 50% of women using an intrauterine contraceptive device had at least one episode, as did 20% of women using oral contraceptives.[3] Bacterial vaginosis is particularly prevalent in lesbians.[4]

**AETIOLOGY/**  The cause is not fully understood. Risk factors include new or multiple sexual
**RISK FACTORS**  partners[1,3,5] and early age of sexual intercourse,[6] but no causative microorganism has been shown to be transmitted between partners. Use of an intrauterine contraceptive device[3] and douching[5] have also been reported as risk factors. Infection seems to be most common around the time of menstruation.[7]

**PROGNOSIS**  The course of bacterial vaginosis varies and is poorly understood. Without treatment, symptoms may persist or resolve in both pregnant and non-pregnant women. Recurrence after treatment occurs in about a third of women. The condition is associated with complications of pregnancy: low birth weight; preterm birth (pooled OR from 10 cohort studies: 1.8, 95% CI 1.5 to 2.6);[8] preterm labour; premature rupture of membranes; late miscarriage; chorioamnionitis (48% v 22%, OR 2.6, 95% CI 1.0 to 6.6);[9] endometritis after normal delivery (8.2% v 1.5%, OR 5.6, 95% CI 1.8 to 17.2);[10] endometritis after caesarean section (55% v 17%, OR 5.8, 95% CI 3.0 to 10.9);[11] and surgery to the genital tract. Women who have had a previous premature delivery are especially at risk of complications in pregnancy, with a sevenfold increased risk of preterm birth (AR 24/428 [6%] in all women v 10/24 [42%] in women with a previous preterm birth).[12] Bacterial vaginosis can also enhance HIV acquisition and transmission.[13]

Please refer to CD-ROM for full text and references.

### Search date September 2002
*Nicola Low and Frances Cowan*

## What are the effects of antibiotic treatment for men and non-pregnant women with uncomplicated genital chlamydial infection?

Short term microbiological cure is the outcome used in most RCTs, but this may not mean eradication of *Chlamydia trachomatis*. Long term cure rates have not been studied extensively because of high default rates and difficulty in distinguishing persistent infection from reinfection due to re-exposure.

### BENEFICIAL

**Doxycycline, teracycline, rosaramicin (multiple dose regimens)**
Small RCTs with short term follow up and high withdrawal rates found that multiple dose regimens of tetracyclines (doxycycline, tetracycline) and macrolides (rosaramicin) achieve micrological cure in at least 95% of people with genital chlamydia.

### LIKELY TO BE BENEFICIAL

**Azithromycin (single dose)**
One systematic review of short term RCTs hasfound no significant difference in microbiological cure of *Chlamydia trachomatis* between a single dose of azithromycin versus a 7 day course of doxycycline, although the RCTs may have lacked power to detect a clinically important difference. Rates of adverse effects were similar.

**Erythromycin (multiple dose regimens)**
Three small RCTs found that erythromycin achieved microbiological cure in 77–100% of people, with the highest cure rate with a 2 g versus a 1 g daily dose.

### UNKNOWN EFFECTIVENESS

**Ofloxacin, trovafloxacin, minocycline, lymecycline, clarithromycin, ampicillin, rifampicin (multiple dose regimens)**
We found insufficient evidence on these regimens.

### UNLIKELY TO BE BENEFICIAL

**Ciprofloxacin (multiple dose)**
Two RCTs found that ciprofloxacin cured 63–92% of people. Meta-analysis found that ciprofloxacin versus doxycycline significantly increased microbiological failure.

## What are the effects of antibiotic treatment for pregnant women with uncomplicated genital chlamydial infection?

### LIKELY TO BE BENEFICIAL

**Azithromycin (single v multiple dose antibiotics)**
One systematic review has found that a single dose of azithromycin versus a 7 day course of erythromycin significantly increases microbiological cure. Two subsequent unblinded RCTs found no significant difference in cure rate between single dose azithromycin versus multiple dose amoxicillin.

# Genital chlamydial infection

### ◄ Erythromycin, amoxicillin (multiple dose regimens)

One systematic review of one small RCT has found erythromycin versus placebo significantly increased microbiological cure. The review found no significant difference between erythomycin and amoxicillin in microbiological cure, and high cure rates with both drugs.

## UNKNOWN EFFECTIVENESS

### Clindamycin (multiple dose)

One small RCT has found no significant difference in cure rates between clindamycin versus erythromycin.

| | |
|---|---|
| **DEFINITION** | Uncomplicated genital chlamydia is a sexually transmitted infection of the urethra in men and of the endocervix, urethra (or both) in women that has not ascended to the upper genital tract. Infection is asymptomatic in up to 80% of women, but may cause non-specific symptoms, including vaginal discharge and intermenstrual bleeding. Infection in men causes urethral discharge and urethral irritation or dysuria, but may also be asymptomatic in up to half of cases.[1] Complicated chlamydia infection includes spread to the upper genital tract (causing pelvic inflammatory disease [see pelvic inflammatory disease, p 350] in women and epididymo-orchitis in men) and extra genital sites, such as ocular infection. |
| **INCIDENCE/ PREVALENCE** | Genital chlamydia is the most common bacterial sexually transmitted infection in developed countries. In the USA, over 642 000 cases of chlamydia were reported in the year 2000.[2] The prevalence of uncomplicated genital chlamydia in women attending general practice surgeries in the UK is reported to be 3–5%.[3] Prevalence is highest in young adults. Reported rates in 16–19 year old women are about 940/100 000 in the UK,[4] 1000/100 000 in Sweden,[1] and 2500/100 000 in the USA.[5] |
| **AETIOLOGY/ RISK FACTORS** | Infection is caused by the bacterium *C trachomatis* serotypes D–K. It is transmitted primarily through sexual intercourse. |
| **PROGNOSIS** | In women, untreated chlamydial infection that ascends to the upper genital tract causes pelvic inflammatory disease in an estimated 30–40% of women.[6] Tubal infertility has been found to occur in about 11% of women after a single episode of pelvic inflammatory disease, and the risk of ectopic pregnancy is increased six- to sevenfold.[7] Ascending infection in men causes epididymitis, but evidence that this causes male infertility is limited.[8] Maternal to infant transmission can lead to neonatal conjunctivitis and pneumonitis in 30–40% of cases.[1] Chlamydia may coexist with other genital infections and may facilitate transmission and acquisition of HIV infection.[1] Untreated chlamydial infection persists symptomatically in most women for at least 60 days and for a shorter period in men.[9] Spontaneous remission also occurs but data are insufficient to determine the rate of clearance.[9] |

Please refer to CD-ROM for full text and references.

**Search date November 2002**

*Bazian Ltd*

## What are the effects of treatments?

### BENEFICIAL

#### Daily oral antiviral treatment in people with high rates of recurrence

RCTs have found that daily maintenance treatment with oral antiviral compared with placebo reduces the frequency of recurrences and improves psychosocial morbidity agents in people with frequent recurrence.

#### Oral antiviral treatment in first episodes

RCTs in people with a first episode of genital herpes have found that oral antiviral treatment versus placebo reduces the duration of symptoms, lesions, and viral shedding but found no significant difference in the time to recurrence or frequency of subsequent recurrences.

#### Oral antiviral treatment taken at the start of a recurrence

One systematic review and one subsequent RCT have found that oral antiviral treatment taken at the start of a recurrence reduces the duration of lesions, symptoms and viral shedding compared with placebo in people with recurrent genital herpes. RCTs found no significant differences among different antiviral agents.

### UNKNOWN EFFECTIVENESS

#### Oral antiviral treatment in immunocompromise people with HIV infection

We found no RCTs evaluating antiviral treatment for genital herpes in people immunocompromised with HIV infection.

#### Psychotherapy to reduce recurrence

One systematic review found insufficient evidence on the effects of psychotherapy on genital herpes recurrence.

## What are the effects of interventions to prevent transmission?

### LIKELY TO BE BENEFICIAL

#### Male condom use to prevent sexual transmission to women*

Limited evidence from a prospective cohort study suggested that male condom use reduced the transmission of herpes simplex virus type 2 to women who had sexual partners with herpes simplex virus 2.

*Categorisation based on observational evidence.

### UNKNOWN EFFECTIVENESS

#### Abdominal delivery in women with genital lesions at term

We found insufficient evidence of the effects of abdominal delivery on mother to baby transmission of genital herpes. The procedure carries the risk of increased maternal morbidity and mortality.

#### Antiviral treatment to prevent sexual transmission

We found no good evidence on the effects of antiviral treatments to prevent sexual transmission.

© BMJ Publishing Group Ltd 2003

# Genital herpes

◀ **Daily oral antiviral treatment in late pregnancy (36 or more wks of gestation) in women with a history of genital herpes**

We found insufficient direct evidence about effects on neonatal infection. One systematic review and one subsequent RCT found that aciclovir reduced the rate of genital lesions at term in women with first or recurrent episodes of genital herpes simplex virus during pregnancy.

## Female condoms

We found no good evidence on the effects of female condoms to prevent transmission.

## Male condoms to prevent sexual transmission to men

One prospective cohort study found no significant difference between male condom use versus no condom use in preventing transmission of herpes simplex virus type 2 to men who had sexual partners with genital herpes.

## Serological screening and counselling in late pregnancy

The highest risk of mother to baby transmission is in women newly infected with genital herpes in late pregnancy. We found insufficient evidence of the effects of interventions to prevent infection in late pregnancy (such as serological screening and counselling).

### UNLIKELY TO BE BENEFICIAL

## Recombinant glycoprotein vaccine (gB2 and gD2)

One RCT found no significant difference between glycoprotein vaccine versus placebo in acquisition rates of herpes simplex virus 2. We found no good evidence on other forms of immunisation.

**DEFINITION** Genital herpes is an infection with herpes simplex virus type 1 or type 2, causing ulceration in the genital area. Herpes simplex virus infections can be defined on the basis of virological and serological findings. Types of infection include **first episode primary infection**, which is herpes simplex virus in a person without prior herpes simplex virus type 1 or type 2 antibodies; **first episode non-primary infection**, which is herpes simplex virus type 2 in a person with prior herpes simplex virus type 1 antibodies or vice versa; **first recognised recurrence**, which is herpes simplex virus type 2 (or type 1) in a person with prior herpes simplex virus type 2 (or type 1) antibodies; and **recurrent genital herpes**, which is caused by reactivation of latent herpes simplex virus.

**INCIDENCE/ PREVALENCE** Genital herpes infections are among the most common sexually transmitted diseases. Seroprevalence studies show that 22% of adults in the USA have herpes simplex virus type 2 antibodies.[1] A UK study found that 23% of adults attending sexual medicine clinics and 7.6% of blood donors in London had antibodies to herpes simplex virus type 2.[2] However, herpes simplex type 2 can cause other herpes infections such as ocular herpes.

**AETIOLOGY/ RISK FACTORS** Both herpes simplex virus type 1 and 2 can cause a first episode of genital infection, but herpes simplex virus type 2 is more likely to cause recurrent disease.[3] Most people with herpes simplex virus type 2 infection are not aware that they have genital herpes, as their symptoms are mild. However, these people can pass on the infection to sexual partners and newborns.[4,5]

**PROGNOSIS** Sequelae of herpes simplex virus infection include neonatal herpes simplex virus infection, opportunistic infections in immunocompromised people, recurrent genital ulceration, and psychosocial morbidity. Herpes simplex virus type 2 infection is associated with an increased risk of HIV transmission and acquisition.[6] The most common neurological complications are aseptic meningitis (reported in about 25% of women during primary infection) and urinary ▶

retention. The absolute risk of neonatal infection is high (41%, 95% CI 26% to 56%) in babies born to women who acquire infection near the time of labour[7,8] and low (< 3%) in women with established infection, even in those who have a recurrence at term. About 15% of neonatal infections result from postnatal transmission from oral lesions.

Please refer to CD-ROM for full text and references.

# Gonorrhoea

**Search date January 2003**

*John Moran*

---

## What are the effects of treatments?

**BENEFICIAL**

**Single dose regimens using selected cephalosporins or spectinomycin in uncomplicated infection in pregnant women**

One systematic review has found that antibiotic treatment (amoxicillin [amoxycillin] plus probenecid, spectinomycin, ceftriaxone, and cefixime) is effective for curing gonorrhoea in pregnant women. We found no reports of serious adverse effects.

**Single dose regimens using selected fluoroquinolones, selected cephalosporins, or spectinomycin in uncomplicated infection in men and non-pregnant women***

One systematic review found limited evidence by combining cure rates across different arms of RCTs. It found that single dose regimens (ceftriaxone, ciprofloxacin, gatifloxacin, spectinomycin, azithromycin, ofloxacin, cefixime) achieve cure rates of 95% or higher in urogenital or rectal infection. Cure rates were lower ($\leq 80\%$) for pharyngeal infection. Resistance to penicillins, tetracyclines, and sulphonamides is now widespread, and resistance to fluoroquinolones has become common in some geographic areas.

**LIKELY TO BE BENEFICIAL**

**Selected injectable fluoroquinolones or selected injectable cephalosporins in disseminated infection****

We found no RCTs assessing treatments for disseminated gonococcal infection published in the past 20 years, but there is strong consensus that multidose regimens using injectable cephalosporins or quinolones (except where quinolone-resistant *Neisseria gonorrhoeae* have been reported) are the most effective treatment. We found no reports of treatment failures with these regimens.

**UNKNOWN EFFECTIVENESS**

**Dual treatment for gonorrhoea and chlamydia infections in all people diagnosed with gonorrhoea**

Dual treatment for gonorrhoea and chlamydia infections is based on theory and expert opinion rather than on evidence from RCTs. The balance between benefits and harms will vary with the prevalence of coinfection in each population.

*Based on comparisons of results across arms of different trials.
**Based only on non-RCT evidence and consensus.

**DEFINITION**    Gonorrhoea is caused by infection with *Neisseria gonorrhoeae*. In men, uncomplicated urethritis is the most common manifestation, with dysuria and urethral discharge. Less typically, signs and symptoms are mild and indistinguishable from chlamydial urethritis. In women, the most common manifestation is cervicitis, which produces symptoms (e.g. vaginal discharge, lower abdominal discomfort, and dyspareunia) in only half of the women. Coinfection with chlamydia is reported in 20–40% of people.[1,2]

**INCIDENCE/** Between 1975 and 1997 the incidence of reported gonorrhoea in the USA fell
**PREVALENCE** by 74%, reaching a nadir of 122/100 000 people. Since 1997 between 128 and 133 cases have been reported per 100 000 people each year.[3] Rates are highest in younger people. In 2001 the incidence was highest in women aged ▶

15–19 years (703/100 000) and men aged 20–24 years (564/100 000). In England, Wales, and Northern Ireland, diagnoses of gonorrhoea have increased since 1994, reaching 256/100 000 for 20–24 year old males and 196/100 000 for 16–19 year old females in 2001.[4]

**AETIOLOGY/ RISK FACTORS**  Most infections result from penile–vaginal, penile–rectal, or penile–pharyngeal contact. An important minority of infections are transmitted from mother to child during birth, which can cause ophthalmia neonatorum. Less common are ocular infections in older children and adults as a result of sexual exposure, poor hygiene, or the medicinal use of urine.

**PROGNOSIS**  The natural history of untreated gonococcal infection is spontaneous resolution after weeks or months of unpleasant symptoms. During this time, there is a substantial likelihood of transmission to others and of complications developing in the infected individual.[5] In many women, the lack of readily discernible signs or symptoms of cervicitis means that infections go unrecognised and untreated. An unknown proportion of untreated infections causes local complications, including lymphangitis, periurethral abscess, bartholinitis, and urethral stricture; epididymitis in men; and in women involvement of the uterus, fallopian tubes, or ovaries causing pelvic inflammatory disease (see pelvic inflammatory disease, p000). Gonorrhoea is associated with pelvic inflammatory disease. One review found N gonorrhoeae was cultured from 8% to 32% of women with acute pelvic inflammatory disease in 11 European studies and from 27% to 80% of women in eight US studies.[6] The proportion of N gonorrhoeae infections in women that lead to pelvic inflammatory disease has not been well studied. However, one study of women exposed to men with gonorrhoea found that five out of 19 culture-positive women had pelvic inflammatory disease and another four of the 19 had uterine adnexal tenderness.[7] Pelvic inflammatory disease may lead to infertility (see pelvic inflammatory disease, p000). In some people, localised gonococcal infection may disseminate. A US study estimated the risk of dissemination to be 0.6% to 1.1% among women, whereas a European study estimated it to be 2.3–3%.[8,9] The same European study found a lower risk in men, estimated to be 0.4–0.7%.[9] When gonococci disseminate, they cause petechial or pustular skin lesions; asymmetrical arthropathies, tenosynovitis or septic arthritis; and, rarely, meningitis or endocarditis.

Please refer to CD-ROM for full text and references.

# Partner notification

## Search date November 2002

*Catherine Mathews, Nicol Coetzee, Merrick Zwarenstein, and Sally Guttmacher*

---

## What are the effects of different partner notification strategies in different groups of people and what are the effects of interventions to improve patient referral?

We found no good evidence on the effects of partner notification on relationships between patients and partners and, in particular, on the rate of violence, abuse, and abandonment of patient or partner.

We found no studies comparing the effects of an intervention across different groups, such as people with different diseases or combinations of diseases, or people from different settings.

### LIKELY TO BE BENEFICIAL

**Contract referral (as effective as provider referral in people with syphilis)**

One systematic review of one large RCT comparing different partner notification strategies in people with syphilis found no significant difference in the proportion of partners notified between provider referral🜨 and contract referral🜨, when people receiving the contract referral option were given 2 days to notify their partners.

**Offering a choice between provider and patient referral (v patient referral) in people with HIV**

One systematic review of one RCT comparing different partner notification strategies found that in people with HIV, offering a choice between provider referral (where the identity of the index patient was not revealed) and patient referral was improved notification rates compared with offering patient referral alone.

**Provider referral, or contract referral (v patient referral) in people with gonorrhoea or non-gonococcal urethritis (mainly chlamydia)**

One systematic review, has found that, for people with gonorrhoea, contract referral compared with patient referral increased the rate of partners presenting for treatment. For people with non-gonococcal urethritis, one systematic review found that provider versus patient referral increased the proportion of partners notified and of positive partners detected per patient.

### UNKNOWN EFFECTIVENESS

**Adding telephone reminders and contract cards to patient referral; educational videos; information pamphlets; patient referral by different types of healthcare professionals; patient referral in HIV**

We found insufficient evidence about the effects of these interventions in improving partner notification.

**DEFINITION**   Partner notification is a process whereby the sexual partners of people with a diagnosis of sexually transmitted infection are informed of their exposure to infection. The main methods are patient referral🜨, provider referral🜨, contract referral🜨, and outreach assistance🜨.

**INCIDENCE/**   A large proportion of people with sexually transmitted infections will have
**PREVALENCE**   neither symptoms nor signs of infection. For example, 22–68% of men with gonorrhoea who were identified through partner notification were asymptomatic.[1] Partner notification is one of the two strategies to reach such ▶

individuals, the other strategy being screening. Managing infection in people with more than one current sexual partner is likely to have the greatest impact on the spread of sexually transmitted infections.[2]

**PROGNOSIS**    We found no studies showing that partner notification results in a health benefit, either to the partner or to future partners of infected partners. Obtaining such evidence would be technically and ethically difficult. One RCT in asymptomatic women compared identifying, testing, and treating women at increased risk for cervical chlamydial infection versus usual care. It found these reduced incidence of pelvic inflammatory disease (RR 0.44, 95% CI 0.2 to 0.9).[3] This evidence suggests that partner notification, which also aims to identify and treat people who are largely unaware of infection, would provide a direct health benefit to partners who are infected.

Please refer to CD-ROM for full text and references.

*Sexual health*

# Pelvic inflammatory disease

**Search date December 2002**

*Jonathan Ross*

---

## What are the effects of treatments?

### LIKELY TO BE BENEFICIAL

**Antibiotics (for symptoms and microbiological clearance in women with confirmed pelvic inflammatory disease)**

One systematic review of observational studies and RCTs has found that several different antibiotic regimens (including parenteral clindamycin plus oral aminoglycoside; parenteral cefalosporin plus oral doxycycline with or without probenecid, ofloxacin, and co-amoxiclav) are similarly effective in relieving the symptoms of pelvic inflammatory disease (PID), and achieve high rates of clinical and microbiological cure.

### UNKNOWN EFFECTIVENESS

**Different durations of antibiotic treatment**

Systematic reviews found no good evidence on the optimal duration of treatment.

**Empirical antibiotic treatment versus treatment guided by test results**

We found no RCTs comparing empirical treatment with antibiotics (before receiving results of microbiological tests) versus treatment that is guided by test results.

**Oral versus parenteral antibiotics**

Two RCTs found no significant difference between oral ofloxacin and parenteral cefoxitin plus doxycycline.

**Outpatient versus inpatient antibiotic treatment**

One RCT found no significant difference between outpatient treatment with intramuscular cefoxitin plus probenecid plus oral doxycycline versus inpatient treatment with parenteral antibiotics for recurrence, infertility, or ectopic pregnancy at 35 months.

**Routine antibiotic prophylaxis before intrauterine device insertion in women at high risk**

We found no good evidence about antibiotic prophylaxis before intrauterine device insertion in women at high risk.

### UNLIKELY TO BE BENEFICIAL

**Routine antibiotic prophylaxis before intrauterine device insertion in women at low risk**

One systematic review found no significant difference between routine prophylaxis with doxycycline versus placebo before intrauterine contraceptive device insertion in PID in women at low risk of PID.

**DEFINITION** PID is inflammation and infection of the upper genital tract in women, typically involving the fallopian tubes, ovaries, and surrounding structures.

**INCIDENCE/ PREVALENCE** The exact incidence of PID is unknown because the disease cannot be diagnosed reliably from clinical symptoms and signs.[1-3] Direct visualisation of the fallopian tubes by laparoscopy is the best single diagnostic test, but it is invasive and not used routinely in clinical practice. PID is the most common gynaecological reason for admission to hospital in the USA, accounting for 49/10 000 recorded hospital discharges. A diagnosis of PID is made in 1/62 (1.6%) women aged 16–45 years attending their primary care physician in ▶

England and Wales.[4] However, because most PID is asymptomatic, this figure underestimates the true prevalence.[1,5] A crude marker of PID in developing countries can be obtained from reported hospital admission rates, where it accounts for 17–40% of gynaecological admissions in sub-Saharan Africa, 15–37% in Southeast Asia, and 3–10% in India.[6]

**AETIOLOGY/ RISK FACTORS** Factors associated with PID mirror those for sexually transmitted infections: young age, reduced socioeconomic circumstances, African/Afro-Caribbean ethnicity, lower educational attainment, and recent new sexual partner.[2,7,8] Infection ascends from the cervix, and initial epithelial damage caused by bacteria (especially *Chlamydia trachomatis* and *Neisseria gonorrhoeae*) allows the opportunistic entry of other organisms. Many different microbes, including *Mycoplasma hominis* and anaerobes, may be isolated from the upper genital tract.[9] The spread of infection to the upper genital tract may be increased by vaginal douching and instrumentation of the cervix, but reduced by the barrier method and oral contraceptives compared with other forms of contraception.[10–13]

**PROGNOSIS** PID has a high morbidity; about 20% of affected women become infertile, 20% develop chronic pelvic pain, and 10% of those who conceive have an ectopic pregnancy.[2] We found no placebo controlled trials of antibiotic treatment. Uncontrolled observations suggest that clinical symptoms and signs resolve in a significant proportion of untreated women.[14] Repeated episodes of PID are associated with a four to six times increase in the risk of permanent tubal damage.[15] One case control study (76 cases and 367 controls) found that delaying treatment by even a few days is associated with impaired fertility (OR 2.6, 95% CI 1.2 to 5.9).[16]

Please refer to CD-ROM for full text and references.

# Cellulitis and erysipelas

**Search date February 2003**

*Andrew Morris*

Skin disorders

---

## What are the effects of treatments?

### Antibiotics

We found no RCTs comparing antibiotics versus placebo. RCTs comparing different single antibiotic regimens found clinical cure in 50–100% of people at 4–30 days.

### Different antibiotic regimens

RCTs comparing different antibiotic regimens were designed to test equivalence rather than to detect a clinically significant difference in cure rates between antibiotics.

### Oral versus intravenous antibiotics; short versus long courses of antibiotics

We found no RCTs comparing oral antibiotics versus intravenous antibiotics, or different durations of antibiotics.

### Treatment of predisposing factors to prevent recurrence

We found no RCTs or observational studies on the effects of treating predisposing factors for recurrence of cellulitis or erysipelas.

**DEFINITION**     Cellulitis is a spreading bacterial infection of the dermis and subcutaneous tissues. It causes local signs of inflammation such as warmth, erythema, pain, lymphangitis, and frequently systemic upset with fever and raised white blood cell count. Erysipelas is a form of cellulitis and is characterised by pronounced superficial inflammation. The lower limbs are by far the most common sites, but any area can be affected. The term erysipelas is commonly used when the face is affected.

**INCIDENCE/**     We found no specific data on the incidence of cellulitis, but cellulitis and
**PREVALENCE**     abscess infections were responsible for 158 consultations per 10 000 person years at risk in the UK in 1991.[1] In 1985 in the UK, skin and subcutaneous tissue infections resulted in 29 820 hospital admissions and a mean occupancy of 664 hospital beds each day.[2]

**AETIOLOGY/**     The most common infective organisms for cellulitis and erysipelas in adults are
**RISK FACTORS**     streptococci (particularly *Streptococcus pyogenes*) and *Staphylococcus aureus*.[3] In children, *Haemophilus influenzae* is a frequent cause. Several risk factors for cellulitis and erysipelas have been identified in a case control study (167 cases and 294 controls): lymphoedema (OR 71.2, 95% CI 5.6 to 908.0), leg ulcer (OR 62.5, 95% CI 7.0 to 556.0), toe web intertrigo (OR 13.9, 95% CI 7.2 to 27.0), and traumatic wounds (OR 10.7, 95% CI 4.8 to 23.8).[4]

**PROGNOSIS**     Cellulitis can spread through the bloodstream and lymphatic system. A retrospective case study of people admitted to hospital with cellulitis found that systemic symptoms such as fever and raised white blood cell count were present in up to 42% of cases at presentation.[5] Lymphatic involvement can lead to obstruction and damage the lymphatic system that predisposes to recurrent cellulitis. Recurrence can occur rapidly or after months or years. One study found that 29% of people with erysipelas had a recurrent episode within ▶

3 years.[6] Local necrosis and abscess formation can also occur. It is not known whether the prognosis of erysipelas differs from that of cellulitis. We found no evidence about factors that predict recurrence, or a better or worse outcome. We found no good evidence on the prognosis of untreated cellulitis.

Please refer to CD-ROM for full text and references.

# Head lice

### Search date February 2003

*Ian Burgess*

## What are the effects of treatments?

### LIKELY TO BE BENEFICIAL

**Insecticide based pharmaceutical products**

One systematic review has found that permethrin and malathion both increase lice eradication rates compared with placebo. Limited evidence from another systematic review suggested that permethrin increased eradication rates compared with lindane.

### UNKNOWN EFFECTIVENESS

**Essential oils and other chemicals used as repellents**

We found insufficient evidence on the effects of these interventions.

**Herbal treatments**

We found no RCTs that compared herbal treatment with placebo. One RCT found no significant difference in eradication rates between a herbal product (coconut, anise, and ylang ylang) and insecticide (permethrin, malathion, and piperonyl butoxide). However, results may not generalise to different concentrations of these components or to different herbal preparations.

**Mechanical removal of lice or viable eggs by combing**

We found inconclusive evidence from three RCTs about effects of combing instead of or in addition to insecticides.

| | |
|---|---|
| **DEFINITION** | Head lice are obligate ectoparasites of socially active humans. They infest the scalp and attach their eggs to the hair shafts. Itching, resulting from multiple bites, is not diagnostic but may increase the index of suspicion. Infestation can be diagnosed only by finding living lice. Eggs glued to hairs, whether hatched (nits) or unhatched, are not proof of active infection, because eggs may retain a viable appearance for weeks after death. |
| **INCIDENCE/ PREVALENCE** | We found no studies on incidence and no recent published prevalence results from any developed country. Anecdotal reports suggest that prevalence has increased in the past few years in most communities in the UK and USA. |
| **AETIOLOGY/ RISK FACTORS** | Observational studies indicate that infections occur most frequently in school children, although there is no proof of a link with school attendance.[1,2] We found no evidence that lice prefer clean hair to dirty hair. |
| **PROGNOSIS** | The infection is almost harmless. Sensitisation reactions to louse saliva and faeces may result in localised irritation and erythema. Secondary infection of scratches may occur. Lice have been identified as primary mechanical vectors of scalp pyoderma caused by streptococci and staphylococci usually found on the skin.[3] |

Please refer to CD-ROM for full text and references.

Skin disorders

## What are the effects of preventive interventions?

**LIKELY TO BE BENEFICIAL**

**Oral antiviral agents**
Limited evidence from RCTs suggests that prophylactic oral antiviral agents may reduce the frequency and severity of attacks compared with placebo, but the optimal timing and duration of treatment is uncertain.

**Sunscreen**
We found limited evidence from two small crossover RCTs that ultraviolet sunscreen may reduce herpes recurrence compared with placebo.

**UNKNOWN EFFECTIVENESS**

**Topical antiviral agents**
We found no RCTs on the effects of topical antiviral agents used as prophylaxis.

## What are the effects of treatments?

**LIKELY TO BE BENEFICIAL**

**Oral aciclovir for first attack**
One small RCT in children found that oral aciclovir reduced the mean duration of pain compared with placebo. Another small RCT in children found that oral aciclovir reduced the median time to healing compared with placebo.

**Oral aciclovir for recurrent attack**
Two RCTs found that oral aciclovir (if taken early in the attack) marginally reduced the duration of symptoms and pain compared with placebo.

**Topical antiviral agents for recurrent attacks**
We found limited evidence from RCTs that topical penciclovir or aciclovir reduced the duration of pain and symptoms compared with placebo.

**UNKNOWN EFFECTIVENESS**

**Topical anaesthetic agents**
One small RCT found limited evidence that topical tetracaine reduced the mean time to scab loss compared with placebo. However, the clinical importance of this result is unclear.

**Topical antiviral agents for first attack**
We found no RCTs on the effects of topical antiviral agents.

**Zinc oxide cream**
One small RCT found limited evidence that zinc oxide cream reduced time to healing compared with placebo but found that it increased the risk of skin irritation.

**DEFINITION**  Herpes labialis is a mild self limiting infection with herpes simplex virus type 1. It causes pain and blistering on the lips and perioral area (cold sores); fever and constitutional symptoms are rare. Most people have no warning of an attack, but some experience a recognisable prodrome.

**INCIDENCE/**  Herpes labialis accounts for about 1% of primary care consultations in the UK
**PREVALENCE**  each year; 20–40% of people have experienced cold sores at some time.[1]  ▶

# Herpes labialis

**AETIOLOGY/ RISK FACTORS**   Herpes labialis is caused by herpes simplex virus type 1. After the primary infection, which usually occurs in childhood, the virus is thought to remain latent in the trigeminal ganglion.[2] A variety of factors, including exposure to bright sunlight, fatigue, or psychological stress, can precipitate a recurrence.

**PROGNOSIS**   In most people, herpes labialis is a mild, self limiting illness. Recurrences are usually shorter and less severe than the initial attack. Healing is usually complete in 7–10 days without scarring.[3] Rates of reactivation are unknown. Herpes labialis can cause serious illness in immunocompromised people.

Please refer to CD-ROM for full text and references.

# Malignant melanoma (non-metastatic)

**Search date February 2003**

*Philip Savage, Thomas Crosby, and Malcolm Mason*

## What are the effects of preventive interventions and treatments?

### LIKELY TO BE BENEFICIAL

**High dose adjuvant alfa interferon**

One RCT has found that high dose alfa interferon extends the time to relapse at median follow up of 6.9 years compared with no adjuvant treatment, and may improve overall survival. However, another RCT found no significant difference in relapse rates or overall survival between high dose interferon and no adjuvant treatment. Toxicity (myelosuppression, hepatotoxicity and neurotoxicity) and withdrawal rates were high.

### UNKNOWN EFFECTIVENESS

**Adjuvant vaccines in people with malignant melanoma**

Four RCTs found no significant difference in survival between adjuvant vaccines and surgery alone or surgery plus placebo vaccine in people with malignant melanoma, but they may have been underpowered to detect a clinically important difference.

**Low dose adjuvant alfa interferon**

RCTs found inconsistent evidence on the effects of low dose alfa interferon compared with no adjuvant treatment or relapse free and overall survival. Toxicity occurred in 10% of people.

**Sunscreens in prevention**

We found no RCTs about the preventive effects of sunscreens. One systematic review of case control studies found inconclusive evidence about the effects of sunscreen for preventing malignant melanoma. However, consensus suggests that the appropriate use of sunscreen (to reduce excessive exposure to sunlight rather than to prolong the time spent in the sun) may reduce the risk of developing melanoma.

**Surveillance to prevent recurrence**

We found no RCTs of surveillance to prevent recurrence of malignant melanoma.

### UNLIKELY TO BE BENEFICIAL

**Prophylactic lymph node dissection**

One systematic review found no significant difference in survival at 5 years between elective lymph node dissection and delayed or no lymph node dissection in people with melanoma without clinically detectable lymph node metastases.

**Wide primary excision (no better than narrower excision)**

RCTs found no significant difference in local recurrence rates or overall survival over 4–10 years between more radical local surgery (4–5 cm excision margins) and less radical surgery (1–2 cm excision margins). One RCT found that wide compared with narrow excision increased the need for skin grafting and the length of hospital stay.

**DEFINITION**    Cutaneous malignant melanoma is a tumour derived from melanocytes in the basal layer of the epidermis. After undergoing malignant transformation, it becomes invasive by penetrating into and beyond the dermis. ▶

# Malignant melanoma (non-metastatic)

**INCIDENCE/ PREVALENCE**
Incidence in developed countries has increased by 50% in the past 20 years. Incidence varies in different populations❶ and is about 10-fold higher in white than in non-white populations. Despite the rise in incidence, death rates have flattened and even fallen in some populations (e.g. in women and young men in Australia).[1,2] During the same period there has been a sixfold increase in the incidence of melanoma *in situ*, suggesting earlier detection.

**AETIOLOGY/ RISK FACTORS**
The number of common, atypical, and dysplastic naevi on a person's body correlates closely with the risk of developing malignant melanoma. A genetic predisposition probably accounts for 5–10% of all cases. Although the risk of developing malignant melanoma is higher in fair skinned populations living close to the equator, the relation between sun exposure, sunscreen use, and skin type is not clear cut. Exposure to excessive sunlight and severe sunburn in childhood are associated with an increased risk of developing malignant melanoma in adult life. However, people do not necessarily develop tumours at sites of maximum exposure to the sun.

**PROGNOSIS**
The prognosis of early malignant melanoma (stages I–III)❶ relates to the depth of invasion of the primary lesion, the presence of ulceration, and involvement of the regional lymph nodes, with the prognosis worsening with the number of nodes involved.[3] A person with a thin lesion (Breslow thickness❻ < 0.75 mm) and without lymph node involvement has a 3% risk of developing metastases and a 95% chance of surviving 5 years.[4] If regional lymph nodes are macroscopically involved there is a 20–50% chance of surviving 5 years. Most studies have shown a better prognosis in women and in people with lesions on the extremities compared with those with lesions on the trunk.

---

Please refer to CD-ROM for full text and references.

## What are the effects of treatments?

### BENEFICIAL

#### Permethrin
One systematic review has found that permethrin increases clinical and parasitic cure after 28 days compared with crotamiton. The systematic review found conflicting results with permethrin versus lindane. One subsequent RCT found limited evidence that permethrin increased clinical cure at 14 days compared with ivermectin.

### LIKELY TO BE BENEFICIAL

#### Crotamiton
One systematic review found that crotamiton was less successful in terms of clinical and parasite cure after 28 days compared with permethrin. One systematic review identified one RCT that found no significant difference between crotamiton and lindane in clinical cure rates at 28 days.

#### Oral ivermectin
One systematic review identified one RCT that found that ivermectin increased clinical cure rates after 7 days compared with placebo. Another small RCT identified by the review found no significant difference between ivermectin and benzyl benzoate in clinical cure rates at 30 days. One subsequent RCT found that, compared with benzyl benzoate, ivermectin increased clinical cure rates at 30 days. One systematic review identified one small RCT that found no significant difference between ivermectin and lindane in cure rates at 15 days. One subsequent RCT found no significant difference between ivermectin and lindane in failed clinical cure rates at 2 weeks, but it found that ivermectin decreased failed cure rates at 4 weeks. One RCT found limited evidence that ivermectin reduced clinical cure rates at 14 days compared with permethrin. Experience suggests oral ivermectin is safe in younger adults being treated for onchocerciasis, but no such experience exists for children, and there have been reports of increased risk of death in elderly people.

### TRADE OFF BETWEEN BENEFITS AND HARMS

#### Lindane
One systematic review identified one RCT that found no significant difference between lindane and crotamiton in clinical cure rates at 28 days. The systematic review found conflicting results between lindane and permethrin after 28 days. Another small RCT identified by the review found no significant difference between lindane and ivermectin in cure rates at 15 days. One subsequent RCT found no significant difference between lindane and ivermectin in failed clinical cure rates at 2 weeks, but it found a higher proportion of people with failed clinical cure between lindane and ivermectin at 4 weeks. We found reports of rare, serious adverse effects such as convulsions.

### UNKNOWN EFFECTIVENESS

#### Benzyl benzoate
One systematic review identified one small RCT that found no significant difference between benzyl benzoate and ivermectin in clinical cure rates at 30 days. One subsequent RCT found that benzyl benzoate reduced clinical cure at 30 days ▶

# Scabies

compared with ivermectin. One systematic review identified one RCT that found no significant difference with benzyl benzoate versus sulphur ointment in clinical cure at 8 or 14 days.

## Malathion

One systematic review found no RCTs on the effects of malathion. Case series have reported cure rates in scabies of over 80%.

## Sulphur compounds

One systematic review identified one RCT that found no significant difference with sulphur ointment versus benzyl benzoate in clinical cure at 8 or 14 days.

**DEFINITION**  Scabies is an infestation of the skin by the mite *Sarcoptes scabiei*.[1] Typical sites of infestation are skin folds and flexor surfaces. In adults, the most common sites are between the fingers and on the wrists, although infection may manifest in elderly people as a diffuse truncal eruption. In infants and children, the face, scalp, palms, and soles are also often affected.

**INCIDENCE/ PREVALENCE**  Scabies is a common public health problem with an estimated prevalence of 300 million cases worldwide, mostly affecting people in developing countries where prevalence can exceed 50%.[2] In industrialised countries, it is most common in institutionalised communities. Case studies suggest that epidemic cycles occur every 7–15 years and that these partly reflect the population's immune status.

**AETIOLOGY/ RISK FACTORS**  Scabies is particularly common where there is social disruption, overcrowding with close body contact, and limited access to water.[3] Young children, immobilised elderly people, people with HIV/AIDS, and other medically and immunologically compromised people are predisposed to infestation and have particularly high mite counts.[4]

**PROGNOSIS**  Scabies is not life threatening, but the severe, persistent itch and secondary infections may be debilitating. Occasionally, crusted scabies develops. This form of the disease is resistant to routine treatment and can be a source of continued reinfestation and spread to others.

Please refer to CD-ROM for full text and references.

# Squamous cell carcinoma of the skin (non-metastatic)

## Search date May 2003

*Adèle Green and Robin Marks*

## What are the effects of preventive interventions?

### LIKELY TO BE BENEFICIAL

### Sunscreen in prevention (daily v discretionary use)

One RCT in adults in a subtropical community in Queensland, Australia found that daily compared with discretionary use of sunscreen on the head, neck, arms, and hands reduced the incidence of squamous cell carcinoma after 4.5 years.

### Sunscreens to prevent development of new solar keratoses (v placebo)

One RCT in people aged over 40 years living in Victoria, Australia who had previous solar keratoses (a risk factor for squamous cell carcinoma) found that daily sunscreen reduced the incidence of new solar keratoses after 7 months compared with placebo.

## What are the effects of treatments?

### UNKNOWN EFFECTIVENESS

### Micrographically controlled surgery (compared with standard surgical excision)

We found no RCTs or observational studies of sufficient quality comparing the effects of micrographically controlled surgery◉ versus standard primary surgical excision on local recurrence rates.

### Optimal primary excision margin

We found no RCTs or observational studies of sufficient quality relating size of primary excision margin to local recurrence rate.

### Radiotherapy after surgery (compared with surgery alone)

We found no RCTs or observational studies of sufficient quality comparing the effects of radiotherapy after surgery versus surgery alone on local recurrence rates.

**DEFINITION** Cutaneous squamous cell carcinoma is a malignant tumour of keratinocytes arising in the epidermis, showing histological evidence of dermal invasion.

**INCIDENCE/ PREVALENCE** Incidence rates are often derived from surveys because few cancer registries routinely collect notifications of squamous cell carcinoma of the skin. Incidence rates on exposed skin vary markedly around the world according to skin colour and latitude, and range from negligible rates in black populations and white populations living at high latitudes to rates of about 1000/100 000 in white residents of tropical Australia.[1]

**AETIOLOGY/ RISK FACTORS** People with fair skin colour who sunburn easily without tanning, people with xeroderma pigmentosum◉,[2–4] and those who are immunosuppressed[5] are susceptible to squamous cell carcinoma. The strongest environmental risk factor for squamous cell carcinoma is chronic sun exposure. Cohort and case control studies have found that the risk of squamous cell carcinoma is three times greater in people with fair skin colour, a propensity to burn on initial exposure to sunlight, or a history of multiple sunburns. Clinical signs of chronic ▶

# Squamous cell carcinoma of the skin (non-metastatic)

skin damage, especially solar keratoses, are also risk factors for cutaneous squamous cell carcinoma.[3,4] In people with multiple solar keratoses (> 15), the risk of squamous cell carcinoma is 10–15 times greater than in people with no solar keratoses.[3,4]

**PROGNOSIS**   Prognosis is related to the location and size of tumour, histological pattern, depth of invasion, perineural involvement, and immunosuppression.[6,7] A world-wide review of 95 case series, each comprising at least 20 people, found that the overall metastasis rate for squamous cell carcinoma on the ear was 11% and on the lip 14%, compared with an average for all sites of 5%.[7] A review of 71 case series found that lesions less than 2 cm in diameter compared with lesions greater than 2 cm have less than half the local recurrence rate (7% v 15%), and less than a third of the rate of metastasis (9% v 30%).[7]

Please refer to CD-ROM for full text and references.

### Search date January 2003

*Mike Bigby, Sam Gibbs, Ian Harvey, and Jane Sterling*

## What are the effects of treatments?

### BENEFICIAL

#### Topical treatments containing salicylic acid

One systematic review has found that simple topical treatments containing salicylic acid increase complete wart clearance, successful treatment, or loss of one or more warts after 6–12 weeks compared with placebo. The review identified two RCTs, which found no significant difference between cryotherapy and salicylic acid in wart clearance at 3–6 months.

### LIKELY TO BE BENEFICIAL

#### Cryotherapy

One systematic review of two small RCTs found no significant difference between cryotherapy❻ and placebo in wart clearance after 2–4 months. However, the RCTs may have been too small to detect a clinically important difference. Meta-analysis of two larger RCTs found limited evidence of equivalence between cryotherapy and salicylic acid in wart clearance at 3–6 months. One RCT found that aggressive cryotherapy compared with gentle cryotherapy increased wart clearance after 1–3 months.

#### Contact immunotherapy (dinitrochlorobenzene)

One systematic review has found that contact immunotherapy❻ with dinitrochlorobenzene increases wart clearance compared with placebo.

### UNKNOWN EFFECTIVENESS

#### Carbon dioxide laser

One systematic review identified no RCTs about the effects of carbon dioxide laser.

#### Cimetidine

Three small RCTs found insufficient evidence about the effects of cimetidine compared with placebo for wart clearance after 12 weeks, and one RCT found insufficient evidence about the effects of cimetidine versus local treatments. One RCT found that levamisole plus cimetidine increased wart clearance compared with cimetidine alone.

#### Distant healing

One RCT found insufficient evidence about the effects of distant healing on wart clearance.

#### Hypnotic suggestion

We found no RCTs on the effects of hypnotic suggestion in clearance of warts.

#### Inosine pranobex

One RCT found insufficient evidence about the effects of inosine pranobex on wart clearance.

#### Intralesional bleomycin

RCTs found conflicting evidence about the effects of intralesional bleomycin. ▶

# Warts

### Levamisole

Two RCTs and one CCT found insufficient evidence about the effects of levamisole compared with placebo on the clearance of warts. One RCT found that levamisole plus cimetidine significantly increased wart clearance at 12 weeks compared with cimetidine alone.

### Photodynamic treatment

RCTs found insufficient evidence about the effects of photodynamic treatment⊙ on wart clearance.

### Pulsed dye laser

One RCT found insufficient evidence about the effects of pulsed dye laser in number of warts cured.

### Surgical procedures

One systematic review identified no RCTs about the effects of surgical procedures on wart clearance.

### Systemic interferon α

We found no RCTs of sufficient quality about systemic interferon α.

## UNLIKELY TO BE BENEFICIAL

### Homeopathy

Two RCTs found no significant difference between homeopathy and placebo in with wart clearance after 8–18 weeks.

**DEFINITION**  Non-genital warts are an extremely common, benign, and usually self limiting skin disease. Infection of epidermal cells with the human papillomavirus results in cell proliferation and a thickened, warty papule on the skin. Any area of skin can be infected but the commonest sites involved are the hands and feet. Genital warts are not covered in this review.

**INCIDENCE/**  There are few reliable, population based data on the incidence and preva-
**PREVALENCE**  lence of common warts. Prevalence probably varies widely between different age groups, populations, and periods of time. Two large population based studies found prevalence rates of 0.84% in the USA[1] and 12.9% in Russia.[2] Prevalence rates are highest in children and young adults, and two studies in school populations have shown prevalence rates of 12% in 4–6 year olds in the UK[3] and 24% in 16–18 year olds in Australia.[4]

**AETIOLOGY/**  Warts are caused by human papillomavirus, of which there are over 70 different
**RISK FACTORS**  types. They are most common at sites of trauma such as the hands and feet, and probably result from inoculation of virus into minimally damaged areas of epithelium. Warts on the feet can be acquired from common bare foot areas. One observational study (146 adolescents) found that the prevalence of warts on the feet was 27% in those that used a communal shower room compared with 1.3% in those that used the locker room.[5] Hand warts are also an occupational risk for butchers and meat handlers. One cross-sectional survey (1086 people) found that the prevalence of hand warts was 33% in abattoir workers, 34% in retail butchers, 20% in engineering fitters, and 15% in office workers.[6] Immunosuppression is another important risk factor. One observational study in immunosuppressed renal transplant recipients found that, at 5 years or longer after transplantation, 90% had warts.[7]

**PROGNOSIS**  Non-genital warts in immunocompetent people are harmless and usually resolve spontaneously as a result of natural immunity within months or years. The rate of resolution is highly variable and probably depends on several factors including host immunity, age, human papillomavirus type, and site of infection. One cohort study (1000 children in long stay accommodation) found that two ▶

◄ thirds of warts resolved without treatment within a 2 year period.[8] One systematic review (search date 2000, 17 RCTs) comparing local treatments versus placebo found that about 30% of people taking placebo (range 0–73%) had no warts after about 10 weeks (range 4–24 weeks).[9]

Please refer to CD-ROM for full text and references.

# Wrinkles

Search date April 2003

*Miny Samuel, Rebecca Brooke, and Christopher Griffiths*

## What are the effects of preventive interventions?

### UNKNOWN EFFECTIVENESS

**Sunscreens; vitamins (vitamin C and vitamin E)**
We found no RCTs on the effects of these interventions in preventing wrinkles.

## What are the effects of treatments?

### BENEFICIAL

**Tazarotene (0.1% strength more beneficial than lower strength or placebo)**
Two RCTs in people with moderately photodamaged skin found that tazarotene cream improved fine wrinkling compared with placebo at 24 weeks. One RCT found no significant difference between tazarotene cream and tretinoin in fine wrinkling at 24 weeks.

**Tretinoin (for fine wrinkles after 6 months)**
RCTs in people with mild to moderate photodamage found that topical tretinoin applied for up to 48 weeks improved fine wrinkles compared with vehicle cream, but the effect on coarse wrinkles differed among studies. Three RCTs in people with moderate to severe photodamage found that topical tretinoin (0.01–0.02%) applied for 6 months improved fine and coarse wrinkles on the face compared with vehicle cream. Common short term adverse effects with tretinoin included itching, burning, and erythema. Skin peeling was the most common persistent adverse effect, which was most frequent and severe at 12–16 weeks.

### TRADE OFF BETWEEN BENEFITS AND HARMS

**Isotretinoin**
In people with mild to severe photodamage, two RCTs found that isotretinoin cream improved fine and coarse wrinkles after 36 weeks compared with vehicle cream. Severe facial irritation occurred in 5–10% of people using isotretinoin.

### UNKNOWN EFFECTIVENESS

**Carbon dioxide laser**
We found no RCTs comparing carbon dioxide laser versus placebo or no treatment. We found insufficient evidence from small RCTs about the effects of carbon dioxide laser compared with dermabrasion, chemical peel, or other laser treatments.

**Dermabrasion**
We found no RCTs comparing dermabrasion versus placebo or no treatment. Three small RCTs in women with perioral wrinkles found no significant difference between dermabrasion and carbon dioxide laser in improvement in wrinkles at 4–6 months. Adverse effects were commonly reported. Erythema was reported in all three RCTs, two of which found that erythema was more common with laser than with dermabrasion.

**Facelift**
We found no RCTs on the effects of facelifts.

◀ **Oral natural cartilage polysaccharides**

One RCT found no significant difference between an oral preparation of cartilage polysaccharide and placebo in wrinkle appearance at 3 months. Smaller RCTs found that oral cartilage polysaccharide reduced fine, moderate, or severe wrinkles compared with placebo. However, these studies were small and of limited reliability. We found limited evidence that some preparations may be more effective than others.

**Retinyl esters**

We found no systematic review or RCTs of retinyl esters that evaluated clinical outcomes.

**Topical antioxidants (ascorbic acid)**

One poor quality RCT found limited evidence that an ascorbic acid formulation compared with a vehicle cream applied daily to the face for 3 months improved fine and coarse wrinkles. Stinging and erythema were common but were not analysed by treatment group. We were unable to draw reliable conclusions from this study.

**Topical natural cartilage polysaccharides**

One small RCT found that a topical commercial preparation of natural cartilage polysaccharide reduced the number of fine and coarse wrinkles at 120 days compared with placebo. However, we were unable to draw reliable conclusions from this study.

**DEFINITION**    Wrinkles, also known as rhytides, are visible creases or folds in the skin. Wrinkles less than 1 mm in width and depth are defined as fine wrinkles and those greater than 1 mm are coarse wrinkles. Most RCTs have studied wrinkles on the face, forearms, and hands.

**INCIDENCE/**    We found no information on the incidence of wrinkles alone, only on the
**PREVALENCE**    incidence of skin photodamage❻, which includes a spectrum of features such as wrinkles, hyperpigmentation, tactile roughness, and telangiectasia. The incidence of ultraviolet light associated skin disorders increases with age and develops over several decades. One Australian study (1539 people aged 20–55 years living in Queensland) found moderate to severe photoageing in 72% of men and 47% of women under 30 years of age.[1] The severity of photoageing was significantly greater with increasing age, and was independently associated with solar keratoses ($P < 0.01$) and skin cancer ($P < 0.05$). Wrinkling was more common in people with white skin, especially skin phototypes I and II. One study reported that the incidence of photodamage in European and North American populations with Fitzpatrick skin types I, II, and III❻ is about 80–90%.[2] We found few reports of photodamage in black skin (phototypes V and VI).

**AETIOLOGY/**    Wrinkles may be caused by intrinsic factors (e.g. ageing, hormonal status, and
**RISK FACTORS**    intercurrent diseases) and by extrinsic factors (e.g. exposure to ultraviolet radiation and cigarette smoke). These factors contribute to epidermal thinning, loss of elasticity, skin fragility, and creases and lines in the skin. The severity of photodamage varies with skin type, which includes skin colour and the capacity to tan.[3] One review of five observational studies found that facial wrinkles in men and women were more common in smokers than in non-smokers.[4] It also found that the risk of moderate to severe wrinkles in lifelong smokers was more than twice that in current smokers (RR 2.57, 95% CI 1.83 to 3.06). Oestrogen deficiency may contribute to wrinkles in postmenopausal women.[5]

**PROGNOSIS**    Although wrinkles cannot be considered a medical illness requiring intervention, concerns about ageing may commonly affect quality of life. Such concerns are likely to be influenced by geographical differences, culture, and personal values. In some cases concerns about physical appearance can lead to ▶

**Skin disorders** ◄

# Wrinkles

difficulties with interpersonal interactions, occupational functioning, and self esteem.[6] In societies in which the ageing population is growing and a high value is placed on the maintenance of a youthful appearance, there is a growing preference for interventions that ameliorate the visible signs of ageing.

Please refer to CD-ROM for full text and references.

## What are the effects of non-drug treatments in older people?

### LIKELY TO BE BENEFICIAL

#### Exercise programmes

One systematic review identified one small RCT. It found that sleep quality improved following a 16 week programme of regular, moderate intensity exercise four times weekly versus no treatment.

### UNKNOWN EFFECTIVENESS

#### Cognitive behavioural therapy

One systematic review identified one small RCT, which found that individual or group cognitive behavioural therapy⊕ improved sleep quality more than no treatment at 3 months, although mean sleep quality scores were consistent with continuing insomnia both with and without treatment.

#### Timed exposure to bright light

One systematic review found no RCTs about the effects of timed bright light exposure versus other treatments or no treatment.

| | |
|---|---|
| **DEFINITION** | Insomnia is defined by the US National Institutes of Health as experience of poor quality sleep, with difficulty in initiating or maintaining sleep, waking too early in the morning, or failing to feel refreshed. Chronic insomnia is defined as insomnia occurring for at least three nights per week for 1 month or more.[1] Primary insomnia is defined as chronic insomnia without specific underlying medical or psychiatric disorders such as sleep apnoea, depression, or dementia. |
| **INCIDENCE/ PREVALENCE** | Across all adult age groups, up to 40% of people have insomnia.[2] However, prevalence increases with age, with estimates ranging from 31–38% in people aged 18–64 years to 45% in people aged 65–79 years.[3] |
| **AETIOLOGY/ RISK FACTORS** | The aetiology of insomnia is uncertain. The risk of primary insomnia increases with age and may be related to age associated changes in circadian rhythms. Psychological factors and lifestyle changes may exacerbate perceived effects of age associated changes in sleep patterns, leading to reduced satisfaction with sleep.[4] Other risk factors in all age groups include hyperarousal, chronic stress, and daytime napping.[1,5] |
| **PROGNOSIS** | We found few reliable data on long term morbidity and mortality in people with primary insomnia. Primary insomnia is a chronic and relapsing condition.[6] Likely consequences include reduced quality of life and increased risk of accidents due to daytime sleepiness. People with primary insomnia may be at greater risk of dependence on hypnotic medication, depression, dementia, and falls, and may be more likely to require residential care.[6,7] |

Please refer to CD-ROM for full text and references.

# Sleep apnoea

Search date December 2002

*Michael Hensley and Cheryl Ray*

## What are the effects of treatments?

### BENEFICIAL

#### Nasal continuous positive airway pressure in moderate to severe obstructive sleep apnoea-hypopnoea syndrome (OSAHS)

Systematic reviews and subsequent RCTs have found that nasal continuous positive airway pressure reduces daytime sleepiness, improves vigilance and cognitive functioning, and reduces depression in people with moderate to severe obstructive sleep apnoea-hypopnoea syndrome after 3–9 months compared with placebo, oral appliances❸, or no treatment.

### LIKELY TO BE BENEFICIAL

#### Nasal continuous positive airway pressure in mild OSAHS

One systematic review of four RCTs in people with mild OSAHS found no significant difference between nasal continuous positive airway pressure and conservative treatment or placebo tablets in daytime sleepiness, but found significant improvement in some measures of cognitive performance at about 4 weeks. One subsequent RCT found no significant difference between nasal continuous positive pressure plus conservative treatment and conservative treatment alone for daytime sleepiness or functional or cognitive outcomes, but found significant improvement in sleep apnoea-hypopnoea related symptoms at 3 and 6 months.

#### Oral appliance in mild OSAHS

One RCT found that oral appliances that produce mandibular advancement reduced apnoea❸ and hypopnoea❸, but had no significant effect on daytime sleepiness or quality of life compared with uvulopalatopharyngoplasty in people with mild OSAHS.

#### Oral appliance in moderate to severe OSAHS

RCTs have found that oral appliances that produce anterior advancement of the mandible reduce daytime sleepiness and sleep disordered breathing❸ at 1–4 weeks in people with moderate to severe obstructive sleep apnoea-hypopnoea syndrome compared with no treatment or control oral appliances.

### UNKNOWN EFFECTIVENESS

#### Weight loss in mild OSAHS

One systematic review found no RCTs on the effects of weight loss in people with mild OSAHS.

#### Weight loss in moderate to severe OSAHS

One systematic review found no RCTs on the effects of weight loss in people with moderate to severe OSAHS.

**DEFINITION**   Obstructive sleep apnoea-hypopnoea syndrome (OSAHS) is abnormal breathing during sleep that causes recurrent arousals, sleep fragmentation, and nocturnal hypoxaemia. It is associated with daytime sleepiness, impaired vigilance and cognitive functioning, and reduced quality of life.[1,2] Criteria for the diagnosis of significant sleep disordered breathing have not been rigorously assessed, but have been set by consensus and convention.[3,4] Diagnostic criteria have variable sensitivity and specificity. For example, an apnoea/hypopnoea index❸ of 5–20 episodes an hour is often used to define borderline to mild OSAHS, 20–35 to define moderate OSAHS, and more than ▶

35 to define severe OSAHS.[5] However, people with upper airway resistance syndrome🅖 have an index below 5 episodes an hour,[6] and many healthy elderly people have an index greater than five episodes an hour.[7] In an effort to obtain an international consensus, new criteria have been proposed but have not been widely used.[8] The most pragmatic test for clinically significant OSAHS is to show clinical improvement in daytime symptoms after treatment for sleep disordered breathing. In this topic, the criteria for OSAHS include apnoeas and hypopnoeas caused by upper airway obstruction. Central sleep apnoea and sleep associated hypoventilation syndromes are not covered here.

**INCIDENCE/ PREVALENCE** The Wisconsin Sleep Cohort Study of over 1000 people (mean age 47 years) in North America found a prevalence of apnoea/hypopnoea index greater than five episodes an hour in 24% of men and 9% of women, and of OSAHS with an index greater than five plus excessive sleepiness in 4% of men and 2% of women.[9] There are international differences in the occurrence of OSAHS, for which obesity is considered to be an important determinant.[10] Ethnic differences in prevalence have also been found after adjustment for other risk factors.[7,10] Little is known about the burden of illness in developing countries.

**AETIOLOGY/ RISK FACTORS** The site of the upper airway obstruction in the OSAHS is around the level of the tongue, soft palate, or epiglottis. Disorders that predispose to either narrowing of the upper airway or reduction in its stability (e.g. obesity, certain craniofacial abnormalities, vocal cord abnormalities, and enlarged tonsils) have been associated with an increased risk of OSAHS. It has been estimated that a $1 \text{ kg/m}^2$ increase in body mass index (3.2 kg for a person 1.8 m tall) leads to a 30% increase (95% CI 13% to 50%) in the relative risk of developing abnormal sleep disordered breathing (apnoea/hypopnoea index $\geq 5$/hour) over a period of 4 years.[10] Other strong associations include increasing age and sex (male to female ratio is 2 : 1). Weaker associations include menopause, family history, smoking, and night time nasal congestion.[10]

**PROGNOSIS** The long term prognosis of people with untreated severe OSAHS is poor with respect to quality of life, likelihood of motor vehicle accidents, hypertension, and possibly cardiovascular disease and premature mortality.[11] Unfortunately, the prognosis of both treated and untreated OSAHS is unclear.[7] The limitations in the evidence include bias in the selection of participants, short duration of follow up, and variation in the measurement of confounders (e.g. smoking, alcohol use, and other cardiovascular risk factors). Treatment is widespread, making it difficult to find evidence on prognosis for untreated OSAHS. Observational studies support a causal association between OSAHS and systemic hypertension, which increases with the severity of OSAHS (OR 1.21 for mild OSAHS to 3.07 for severe OSAHS).[11] OSAHS increases the risk of motor vehicle accidents three- to sevenfold.[11,12] It is associated with increased risk of premature mortality, cardiovascular disease, and impaired neurocognitive functioning.[11]

Please refer to CD-ROM for full text and references.

Search date January 2003

*Stephen Johnston and Justin Stebbing*

---

## What are the effects of treatments?

BENEFICIAL

*Chemotherapy*

### Anthracycline based regimens (CAF) containing doxorubicin as first line treatment

RCTs have found that combination chemotherapy⊙, regimens containing an anthracycline, such as doxorubicin (CAF)⊙, versus other regimens as first line treatment⊙ increase response rates, time to progression and survival.

### Classical combination chemotherapy (CMF)

One systematic review has found that classical combination chemotherapy as first line treatment increases response rate and survival compared with modified CMF⊙ regimens.

### First line chemotherapy plus monoclonal antibody (in women with overexpressed HER2 neu oncogene)

One RCT found that, in women whose tumours overexpress HER2, standard chemotherapy⊙ plus the monoclonal antibody trastuzumab as first line treatment increased the time to disease progression, objective response⊙, and overall survival compared with standard chemotherapy alone.

*Hormone treatment*

### Selective aromatase inhibitors as first line hormonal treatment⊙ in postmenopausal women

RCTs have found that the aromatase inhibitor ⊙, anastrozole as first line treatment in metastatic postmenopausal breast cancer is at least as effective as tamoxifen⊙, in reducing time to disease progression, and found that the aromatase inhibitor letrozole was superior to tamoxifen in reducing time to disease progression.

### Selective aromatase inhibitors as second line hormonal treatment in postmenopausal women

RCTs in postmenopausal women who have relapsed during or after treatment with tamoxifen have found that the selective aromatase inhibitors anastrozole, letrozole, and exemestane increase overall survival at 2–3 years, and are associated with fewer adverse effects compared with progestins⊙, or the non-selective aromatase inhibitor aminoglutethamide. Two RCTs found that anastrozole was as effective as fulvestrant for delaying progression.

### Tamoxifen as first line treatment in oestrogen receptor positive disease

RCTs have found that antioestrogens such as tamoxifen prolong remission in women with oestrogen receptor positive metastatic breast cancer.

*Radiotherapy*

### Radiotherapy for spinal cord compression*

We found no RCTs. Retrospective analyses found that early radiotherapy improved outcomes, but fewer than 10% of people walked again if severe deterioration of motor function occurred before radiotherapy.

◀ **Radiotherapy plus appropriate analgesia for bone metastases***

We found no RCTs comparing radiotherapy versus no treatment or versus bisphos-phonates. We found limited evidence from non-randomised studies that persistent and localised bone pain can be treated successfully in over 80% of women with radiotherapy plus concomitant appropriate analgesia (from non-steroidal anti-inflammatory drugs to morphine and its derivatives). RCTs found no evidence that short courses are less effective for pain relief than long courses of radiotherapy. One RCT found that different fractionation schedules can be used to treat neuropathic bone pain effectively.

## Radiotherapy plus high dose steroids in spinal cord compression*

One small RCT found that adding high dose steroids to radiotherapy improved the chance of walking after 6 months.

### LIKELY TO BE BENEFICIAL

## Bisphosphonates for bone metastases

RCTs in women receiving standard chemotherapy for bone metastases secondary to metastatic breast cancer found that adding bisphosphonates⊕ reduced and delayed skeletal complications compared with adding placebo. None of the RCTs found an impact on overall survival.

## Combined gonadorelin analogues and tamoxifen as first line treatment in premenopausal women

RCTs (in premenopausal women with oestrogen receptor positive metastatic breast cancer) have found that first line treatment with gonadorelin analogues⊕ plus tamoxifen improves response rates, overall survival, and progression free survival⊕ compared with gonadorelin analogues alone.

## Radiotherapy to control cerebral and choroidal metastases*

We found no RCTs. Retrospective studies suggest that whole brain radiation improves general neurological function in some women with brain metastases secondary to breast cancer, and that radiotherapy benefits some women with choroidal metastases.

## Taxanes for anthracycline resistant disease

We found limited evidence that taxanes⊕ may improve response rates compared with CMF or continued doxorubicin, especially in anthracycline resistant disease⊕. One RCT found no significant difference in progression or overall survival between docetaxel and 5-fluorouracil plus vinorelbine given as second line chemothera-py⊕.

## Taxane based chemotherapy as first line treatment (compared with single agent) *New*

One RCT found that doxorubicin-paclitaxel (AT) improved response rate compared with either doxorubicin or paclitaxel alone, but found no significant difference in overall survival. One RCT found no significant difference between AT and doxorubicin-cyclophosphamide in survival or response rate.

### UNKNOWN EFFECTIVENESS

## Capecitabine for anthracycline resistant disease

One RCT found no significant difference in progression or response rate between capecitabine and paclitaxel following anthracycline failure.

## Semisynthetic vinca alkaloids for anthracycline resistant disease

One RCT found no significant difference in survival or quality of life between vinorelbine plus docetaxel versus vinorelbine alone. One RCT found no significant difference in progression or overall survival between docetaxel and 5-fluorouracil ▶

# Breast cancer (metastatic)

plus vinorelbine given as second line chemotherapy. One RCT found that second line vinorelbine improved survival and reduced progression compared with melphalan.

## TRADE OFF BETWEEN BENEFITS AND HARMS

### Ovarian ablation as first line treatment in premenopausal women (v tamoxifen)

One systematic review and one subsequent RCT in premenopausal women found no significant difference in response rate, duration of response, or survival with ovarian ablation (surgery or irradiation) versus tamoxifen as first line treatment. Ovarian ablation is associated with substantial adverse effects such as hot flushes and "tumour flare".

### Progestins (v tamoxifen, beneficial as first line treatment in women with bone pain or anorexia)

RCTs found no significant difference in response rates, remission rates, or survival between progestins and tamoxifen as first line treatment, but found that progestins increased adverse effects, including nausea, weight gain, and exacerbations of hypertension. One RCT found that medroxyprogesterone versus tamoxifen improved bone pain. Observational evidence suggests that progestins may increase appetite, weight gain, and well being.

## LIKELY TO BE INEFFECTIVE OR HARMFUL

### High dose chemotherapy (v conventional chemotherapy) as first line treatment

One systematic review found no significant difference in overall survival or progression free survival between high dose chemotherapy (requiring haematopoeitic cell transplant) and standard dose chemotherapy. It found that high dose chemotherapy increased treatment related morbidity and mortality compared with standard chemotherapy.

### Progestins (v aromatase inhibitors) as second line treatment

RCTs have found that, in postmenopausal women with metastatic breast cancer who have relapsed on adjuvant tamoxifen or progressed during first line treatment with tamoxifen, the selective aromatase inhibitors anastrozole, letrozole, and exemestane prolong survival compared with progestins or aminoglutethimide, with minimal adverse effects.

*Not based on RCT evidence.

**DEFINITION** Metastatic or advanced breast cancer is the presence of disease at distant sites such as the bone, liver, or lung. It is not treatable by primary surgery and is currently considered incurable. However, young people with good performance status may survive for 15 to 20 years.[1] Symptoms may include pain from bone metastases, breathlessness from spread to the lung, and nausea or abdominal discomfort from liver involvement.

**INCIDENCE/ PREVALENCE** Breast cancer is the second most frequent cancer in the world (1.05 million people) and is by far the most common malignant disease in women (22% of all new cancer cases). Worldwide, the ratio of mortality to incidence is about 36%. It ranks fifth as a cause of death from cancer overall (although it is the leading cause of mortality in women — the 370 000 annual deaths represent 13.9% of cancer deaths in women). In the USA, metastatic breast cancer causes 46 000 deaths, and in the UK causes 15 000 deaths.[2] It is the most prevalent cancer in the world today and there are an estimated 3.9 million women alive who have had breast cancer diagnosed in the past 5 years (compared, for example, with lung cancer, where there are 1.4 million alive).

Women's health

The true prevalence of metastatic disease is high because some women live with the disease for many years. Since 1990, there has been an overall increase in incidence rates of about 1.5% annually.[3]

**AETIOLOGY/ RISK FACTORS**
The risk of metastatic disease relates to known prognostic factors in the original primary tumour. These factors include oestrogen receptor negative disease, primary tumours 3 cm or more in diameter, and axillary node involvement — recurrence occurred within 10 years of adjuvant chemotherapy for early breast cancer🅖 in 60–70% of node positive women and 25–30% of node negative women in one large systematic review.[4]

**PROGNOSIS**
Prognosis depends on age, extent of disease, and oestrogen receptor status. There is also evidence that overexpression of the product of the HER2/neu oncogene, which occurs in about a third of women with metastatic breast cancer, is associated with a worse prognosis.[5] A short disease free interval🅖 (e.g. < 1 year) between surgery for early breast cancer and developing metastases suggests that the recurrent disease is likely to be resistant to adjuvant treatment🅖.[6] In women who receive no treatment for metastatic disease, the median survival from diagnosis of metastases is 12 months.[7] The choice of first line treatment🅖 (hormonal or chemotherapy) is based on a variety of clinical factors 🅣.[8–11] In many countries, such as USA, Canada and some countries in Europe, there is evidence of a decrease in death rates in recent years. This probably reflects improvements in treatment (and therefore improved survival) as well as earlier diagnosis.[2,12]

---

Please refer to CD-ROM for full text and references.

# Breast cancer (non-metastatic)

**Search date October 2002**

*J Michael Dixon, Kate Gregory, Stephen Johnston, and Alan Rodger*

## What are the effects of treatments for ductal carcinoma in situ?

### LIKELY TO BE BENEFICIAL

**Radiotherapy after breast conserving surgery (reduces recurrence)**

RCTs found that radiotherapy🟢 reduced the risk of local recurrence and invasive carcinoma, with no evidence of an effect on survival.

**Tamoxifen plus radiotherapy after breast conserving surgery (reduces recurrence)**

One RCT has found that adjuvant🟢 tamoxifen🟢 significantly reduces breast cancer events in women who have undergone wide excision and radiotherapy, but found no significant difference in overall survival at about 6 years.

## What are the effects of treatments for operable breast cancer?

### BENEFICIAL

**Adjuvant chemotherapy**

One systematic review has found that adjuvant chemotherapy versus no chemotherapy significantly reduces rates of recurrence and improves survival at 10 years. The benefit seems to be independent of nodal or menopausal status, although the absolute improvements are greater in women with node positive disease, and probably greater in younger women.

**Adjuvant tamoxifen**

One systematic review has found that adjuvant tamoxifen taken for up to 5 years reduces the risk of recurrence and death in women with oestrogen receptor positive tumours irrespective of age, menopausal status, nodal involvement, or the addition of chemotherapy. Tamoxifen slightly increases the risk of endometrial cancer, but we found no evidence of an overall adverse effect on non-breast cancer mortality.

**Anthracycline regimens as adjuvant chemotherapy**

One systematic review has found that adjuvant regimens containing an anthracycline🟢 significantly reduce recurrence, and significantly improve survival compared with a standard multidrug chemotherapy regimen (CMF🟢) at 5 years.

**Breast conserving surgery (similar survival to more extensive surgery)**

Systematic reviews and long term results from included RCTs have found that, providing all local disease is excised, more extensive surgery does not increase survival up to 20 years. More extensive local resection in breast conserving surgery🟢 gives worse cosmetic results.

**Chemotherapy plus tamoxifen**

One RCT found that adding chemotherapy (CMF) to tamoxifen significantly improves survival at 5 years.

**Ovarian ablation in premenopausal women**

One systematic review has found that in women less than 50 years of age, ovarian ablation🟢 versus no ablation significantly improves survival for at least 15 years. ▶

### Radiotherapy after breast conserving surgery (reduces local recurrence; no evidence of effect on survival)

One systematic review has found that adding radiotherapy to breast conserving surgery significantly reduces the risk of isolated local recurrence and loss of a breast, but does not increase survival at 10 years. Rates of survival and local recurrence are similar with radiotherapy plus either breast conserving surgery or mastectomy.

### Radiotherapy after mastectomy in women at high risk of local recurrence

RCTs in high risk women receiving adjuvant chemotherapy after mastectomy have found that radiotherapy versus no radiotherapy significantly reduces local recurrence and increases survival at 10–15 years. Radiotherapy may be associated with late adverse effects, which are rare, including pneumonitis, pericarditis, arm oedema, brachial plexopathy, and radionecrotic rib fracture.

## LIKELY TO BE BENEFICIAL

### Neoadjuvant chemotherapy (reduces mastectomy rates v adjuvant chemotherapy; no evidence of effect on survival)

RCTs have found that neoadjuvant⊕ versus adjuvant chemotherapy reduces mastectomy rates, but found no significant difference in survival at 4–10 years.

### Radiotherapy after mastectomy in node positive disease, large tumours, or where lymphovascular invasion is present

One systematic review has found that radiotherapy to the chest wall after mastectomy reduces the risk of local recurrence by about two thirds and the risk of death from breast cancer at 10 years, but found no evidence of effect on overall 10 year survival. One review of retrospective data found that greater axillary node involvement, larger tumour size, higher histological grade, presence of lymphovascular invasion, and involvement of tumour margins reduced the chance of successful treatment. Radiotherapy may be associated with late adverse effects, which are rare, including pneumonitis, pericarditis, arm oedema, brachial plexopathy, and radionecrotic rib fracture.

### Total nodal radiotherapy in high risk disease

RCTs have found that, in women with high risk disease, total nodal irradiation⊕ versus no irradiation improves survival. An earlier systematic review found reduced locoregional recurrence, but no evidence of improved survival.

## TRADE OFF BETWEEN BENEFITS AND HARMS

### Axillary clearance (no evidence of survival benefit and increased morbidity compared with axillary sampling)

RCTs found no significant difference in survival at 5–10 years between axillary clearance versus axillary sampling⊕, axillary radiotherapy⊕, or sampling plus radiotherapy⊕ combined. One systematic review of mainly poor quality evidence found that the risk of arm lymphoedema was highest with axillary clearance plus radiotherapy, lower with axillary sampling plus radiotherapy, and lowest with sampling alone.

### Axillary radiotherapy

One systematic review has found that axillary radiotherapy versus axilliary clearance significantly reduces isolated local recurrence, and has found no significant difference in mortality or overall recurrence at 10 years. One systematic review of mainly poor quality evidence found that radiotherapy plus axillary surgery was associated with arm lymphoedema.

# Breast cancer (non-metastatic)

**Radiotherapy after mastectomy in women not at high risk of local recurrence**

One systematic review has found that radiotherapy to the chest wall after mastectomy reduces the risk of local recurrence by about two thirds and the risk of death from breast cancer at 10 years, but found no evidence of an effect on overall 10 year survival. Radiotherapy may be associated with later adverse effects, which are rare, including pneumonitis, pericarditis, arm oedema, brachial plexopathy, and radionecrotic rib fracture.

## UNKNOWN EFFECTIVENESS

**Radiotherapy to the internal mammary chain**

One RCT found no significant difference in overall survival or breast cancer specific survival at 2–3 years between radiotherapy versus no radiotherapy to the internal mammary chain. Treatment may increase radiation induced cardiac morbidity.

**Radiotherapy to the ipsilateral supraclavicular fossa**

We found insufficient evidence about the effects of irradiation of the ipsilateral supraclavicular fossa on survival. RCTs have found that radiotherapy reduces the risk of supraclavicular fossa nodal recurrence.

## UNLIKELY TO BE BENEFICIAL

**Enhanced dose regimens of adjuvant chemotherapy**

RCTs found no significant improvement from enhanced dose regimens.

**Prolonged chemotherapy (8–12 months v 4–6 months)**

One systematic review found no additional benefit from prolonging adjuvant chemotherapy from 4–6 to 8–12 months.

**Radical mastectomy (no greater survival than less extensive surgery)**

Systematic reviews and long term follow up of one RCT have found no significant difference between radical, total, supraradical❺, or simple mastectomy in survival up to 25 years. More extensive surgery results in greater mutilation.

---

## What are the effects of treatments for locally advanced breast cancer?

## LIKELY TO BE BENEFICIAL

**Radiotherapy**

For locally advanced breast cancer❺ that is rendered operable, small RCTs found that radiotherapy or surgery as sole local treatments have similar effects on response rates, duration of response, and overall survival.

**Radiotherapy after attempted curative surgery**

One RCT found weak evidence that radiotherapy after attempted curative surgery versus no further local treatment may reduce local and/or regional recurrence.

**Surgery**

For locally advanced breast cancer that is rendered operable, small RCTs found that surgery or radiotherapy as sole local treatments have similar effects on response rates, duration of response, and overall survival.

**Tamoxifen plus radiotherapy (v radiotherapy)**

One RCT found that hormone treatment plus radiotherapy versus radiotherapy alone significantly improved locoregional recurrence at 6 years and improved median survival at 8 years.

◀ **UNLIKELY TO BE BENEFICIAL**

## Chemotherapy (cyclophosphamide/methotrexate/fluorouracil or anthracycline based regimens)

We found no evidence that the cytotoxic, multidrug chemotherapy regimen (CMF) improves survival, disease free survival🅖, or long term locoregional control.

**DEFINITION**
Ductal carcinoma *in situ* is a non-invasive🅖 tumour characterised by the presence of malignant cells in the breast ducts but with no evidence that they breach the basement membrane and invade into periductal connective tissues. **Invasive breast cancer** can be separated into three main groups: early🅖 or operable breast cancer, locally advanced disease, and metastatic breast cancer (see p 372). **Operable breast cancer** is apparently restricted to the breast and sometimes to local lymph nodes and can be surgically removed. Although these women do not have overt metastases at the time of staging🅖, they remain at risk of local recurrence and of metastatic spread. They can be divided into those women with tumours greater than 4 cm or multifocal cancers that can be treated by mastectomy, and those with tumours less than 4 cm that are unifocal that can be treated by breast conserving surgery🅖. **Locally advanced breast cancer** is defined according to the TNM staging system of the UICC TNM🅣 system🅖[1] as stage III B (includes T4 a–d; N2 disease, but absence of metastases). It is a disease presentation with evidence (clinical or histopathological) of skin and/or chest wall involvement and/or axillary nodes matted together by tumour extension. **Metastatic breast cancer** is presented in a separate topic (see p 372).

**INCIDENCE/ PREVALENCE**
Breast cancer affects 1/10–1/11 women in the UK and causes about 21 000 deaths per year. Prevalence is about five times higher, with over 100 000 women living with breast cancer at any one time. Of the 15 000 new cases of breast cancer per annum in the UK, the majority will present with primary operable disease.[2]

**AETIOLOGY/ RISK FACTORS**
The risk of breast cancer increases with age, doubling every 10 years up to the menopause. Risk factors include an early age at menarche, older age at menopause, older age at birth of first child, family history, atypical hyperplasia, excess alcohol intake, radiation exposure to developing breast tissue, oral contraceptive use, postmenopausal hormone replacement therapy, and obesity. Risk in different countries varies fivefold. The cause of breast cancer in most women is unknown. About 5% of breast cancers can be attributed to mutations in the genes *BRCA1* and *BRCA2*.[3]

**PROGNOSIS**
**Primary carcinoma** of the breast is potentially curable. The risk of relapse depends on various clinico-pathological features, including axillary node involvement, oestrogen receptor status, and tumour size. Tumour size, axillary node status, histological grade, and oestrogen receptor status provide the most significant prognostic information. Seventy per cent of women with operable disease are alive 5 years after diagnosis and treatment (adjuvant drug treatment is given to most women after surgery). Risk of recurrence is highest during the first 5 years, but the risk remains even 15–20 years after surgery. Those with node positive disease have a 50–60% chance of recurrence within 5 years, compared with 30–35% for node negative disease. Recurrence within 10 years according to one large systematic review occurred in 60–70% of node positive women compared with 25–30% of node negative women.[4] The prognosis for a disease free survival🅖 at 5 years is worse for stage III B (33%) than that for stage III A (71%). Five year overall survival is 44% and 84%, respectively.[5] Poor survival and high rates of local recurrence characterise locally advanced breast cancer🅖.

Please refer to CD-ROM for full text and references.

# Breast pain

**Search date November 2002**

*Nigel Bundred*

## What are the effects of treatments?

### LIKELY TO BE BENEFICIAL

**Low fat, high carbohydrate diet**

One small RCT found that advice to follow a low fat, high carbohydrate diet compared with general dietary advice reduced breast swelling and breast tenderness at 6 months.

### TRADE OFF BETWEEN BENEFITS AND HARMS

**Danazol**

One RCT found that danazol compared with placebo reduced cyclical breast pain after 12 months, but increased adverse effects (weight gain, deepening of the voice, menorrhagia, and muscle cramps). It found no significant difference in pain relief between 6 months treatment with danazol and tamoxifen.

**Gestrinone**

One RCT found that gestrinone compared with placebo reduced breast pain after 3 months, but increased adverse effects (greasy skin, hirsutism, acne, reduction in breast size, headache, and depression).

**Tamoxifen**

Three RCTs found limited evidence that tamoxifen is more effective than placebo at reducing breast pain. Two of the RCTs found more hot flushes and vaginal discharge with tamoxifen compared with placebo. The third RCT did not report on adverse events. One RCT found no significant difference in pain relief between tamoxifen and danazol. One RCT found fewer adverse effects with a lower dose of 10 mg compared with a higher dose of 20 mg.

### UNKNOWN EFFECTIVENESS

**Lisuride maleate**

One RCT with weak methods found that lisuride maleate (a dopamine agonist) compared with placebo reduced breast pain over 2 months.

**Tibolone**

One small RCT found limited evidence that tibolone reduced breast pain after 1 year compared with hormone replacement therapy.

**Antibiotics; diuretics; evening primrose oil; gonadorelin analogues (luteinising hormone releasing hormone analogues); progestogens; pyridoxine; vitamin E**

We found no RCTs on the effects of these interventions.

### UNLIKELY TO BE BENEFICIAL

**Bromocriptine**

Two RCTs found limited evidence that bromocriptine (a dopamine agonist) compared with placebo reduced breast pain. Both RCTs found a higher incidence of adverse effects with bromocriptine compared with placebo. Adverse events included nausea, dizziness, postural hypotension, and constipation.

**Hormone replacement therapy**

One small RCT found limited evidence that women taking hormone replacement therapy had more breast pain after 1 year than women taking tibolone.

◄ **Progesterones**
Two small crossover RCTs found no significant difference between progesterones and placebo on breast pain.

| | |
|---|---|
| **DEFINITION** | Breast pain can be differentiated into cyclical mastalgia (worse before a menstrual period) or non-cyclical mastalgia (unrelated to the menstrual cycle).[1,2] Cyclical pain is often bilateral, usually most severe in the upper outer quadrants of the breast, and may be referred to the medial aspect of the upper arm.[1-3] Non-cyclical pain may be caused by true breast pain or chest wall pain located over the costal cartilages.[1,2,4] Specific breast pathology and referred pain unrelated to the breasts are not included in this definition. |
| **INCIDENCE/ PREVALENCE** | Up to 70% of women develop breast pain in their lifetime.[1,2] Of 1171 US women attending a gynaecology clinic, 69% suffered regular discomfort, which was judged as severe in 11% of women, and 36% had consulted a doctor about breast pain.[2] |
| **AETIOLOGY/ RISK FACTORS** | Breast pain is more common in women aged 30–50 years.[1,2] |
| **PROGNOSIS** | Cyclical breast pain resolves spontaneously within 3 months of onset in 20–30% of women.[5] The pain tends to relapse and remit, and up to 60% of women develop recurrent symptoms 2 years after treatment.[1] Non-cyclical pain responds poorly to treatment but may resolve spontaneously in about 50% of women.[1] |

Please refer to CD-ROM for full text and references.

# Candidiasis (vulvovaginal)

Search date March 2003

*Des Spence*

## What are the effects of treatments for acute vulvovaginal candidiasis in non-pregnant women?

### BENEFICIAL

#### Intravaginal imidazoles

RCTs found that intravaginal imidazoles (butoconazole, clotrimazole, miconazole, or terconazole) reduced persistent symptoms of vulvovaginal candidiasis after 9–38 days compared with placebo, and found no clear evidence that effects differ among the various intravaginal imidazoles. RCTs found no clear evidence of any difference in persistent symptoms between shorter and longer durations of treatment (1–14 days). RCTs found no significant difference in symptoms between and intravaginal imidazoles and oral fluconazole, itraconozole or ketoconazole. RCTs found that intravaginal imidazoles were associated with less nausea, headache, and abdominal pain but more vulvar irritation and vaginal discharge, than oral fluconazole or oral ketoconazole. Two RCTs provided insufficient evidence to compare intravaginal imidazoles versus intravaginal nystatin.

#### Oral fluconazole

We found no RCTs comparing oral fluconazole versus placebo or no treatment. One systematic review found no significant difference in persistent symptoms of vulvovaginal candidiasis over 1–12 weeks between oral fluconazole or oral itraconazole and intravaginal imidazoles, and found that oral fluconazole was associated with more nausea, headache, and abdominal pain but less vulvar irritation and vaginal discharge than intravaginal imidazoles. Two weak RCTs provided insufficient evidence to compare oral fluconazole versus oral itraconazole. One systematic review found no significant difference in persistent symptoms of vulvovaginal candidiasis or adverse effects between oral fluconazole and oral ketoconazole.

#### Oral itraconazole

One RCT found that oral itraconazole reduced persistent symptoms of vulvovaginal candidiasis at 1 week after treatment compared with placebo. One systematic review found no significant difference in persistent symptoms over 1–12 weeks between oral itraconazole or oral fluconazole and intravaginal imidazoles. One weak RCT provided insufficient evidence to compare oral itraconazole versus oral fluconazole.

### LIKELY TO BE BENEFICIAL

#### Intravaginal nystatin

One RCT found that intravaginal nystatin reduced the proportion of women with a poor symptomatic response after 14 days' treatment compared with placebo. Two RCTs provided insufficient evidence to compare intravaginal nystatin versus intravaginal imidazoles. We found no RCTs comparing intravaginal nystatin versus oral fluconazole, itraconazole, or ketoconazole.

### UNLIKELY TO BE BENEFICIAL

#### Oral ketoconazole

We found no RCTs comparing oral ketoconazole versus placebo or versus no treatment. RCTs found no significant difference between oral ketoconazole and intravaginal imidazoles in persistent symptoms of vulvovaginal candidiasis and found that oral ketoconazole may cause more nausea, fatigue and headaches but ▶

◀ less vulvar irritation. One systematic review found no significant difference in persistent symptoms or adverse effects between oral ketoconazole and oral itraconazole. Case reports have associated ketoconazole with a low risk of fulminant hepatitis (1/12 000 courses of treatment with oral ketoconazole).

---

## What are the effects of treatments for recurrent vulvovaginal candidiasis in non-pregnant women?

### LIKELY TO BE BENEFICIAL

**Regular prophylaxis with oral itraconazole**

One RCT found that regular prophylaxis with oral itraconazole reduced the rate of symptomatic recurrence of vulvovaginal candidiasis over 6 months compared with placebo.

### TRADE OFF BETWEEN BENEFITS AND HARMS

**Intermittent or continous prophylaxis with oral ketoconazole**

One RCT found that oral ketoconazole, reduced symptomatic recurrence of vulvovaginal candidiasis over 6 months compared with placebo. This benefit is associated with an increased risk of harms, including rare cases of fulminant hepatitis (1/12 000 courses of treatment with oral ketoconazole).

### UNKNOWN EFFECTIVENESS

**Regular prophylaxis with intravaginal imidazoles**

Two RCTs provided insufficient evidence about the effects of regular prophylaxis with intravaginal clotrimazole versus placebo in preventing recurrence of vulvovaginal candidiasis. One RCT found no significant difference in the number of episodes of symptomatic vaginitis over 6 months between regular prophylaxis with intravaginal clotrimazole and treatment as required, although women taking regular prophylaxis had fewer episodes. The RCT was too small to exclude a clinically important difference. More women preferred treatment as required. One RCT found insufficient evidence about the effects of regular prophylaxis with intravaginal clotrimazole versus oral itraconazole.

**Regular prophylaxis with oral fluconazole**

We found no RCTs about the effects of regular prophylaxis with oral fluconazole in preventing symptomatic recurrence of vulvovaginal candidiasis.

**Treating a male sexual partner**

Two RCTs found no significant difference between treating and not treating a woman's male sexual partner in the resolution of the woman's symptoms of vulvovaginal candidiasis over 1–4 weeks or in the rate of symptomatic recurrance. The women in the RCTs were not selected because of a history of recurrent vulvovaginal candidiasis.

**DEFINITION**   Vulvovaginal candidiasis is symptomatic vaginitis (inflammation of the vagina), which often involves the vulva, caused by infection with a *Candida* yeast. Predominant symptoms are vulvar itching and abnormal vaginal discharge (which may be minimal, a "cheese like" material, or a watery secretion). Differentiation from other forms of vaginitis requires the presence of yeast on microscopy of vaginal fluid. The definition of recurrent vulvovaginal candidiasis varies among RCTs, but it is commonly defined as four or more symptomatic episodes a year.[1] This review excludes studies of asymptomatic women with vaginal colonisation by *Candida* species.

# Candidiasis (vulvovaginal)

**INCIDENCE/ PREVALENCE**   Vulvovaginal candidiasis is the second most common cause of vaginitis (after bacterial vaginosis). Estimates of its incidence are limited, and often derived from women attending hospital clinics. At least one episode of vulvovaginal candidiasis occurs during the lifetime of 50–75% of all women. Vulvovaginal candidiasis is diagnosed in 5–15% of women attending sexually transmitted disease and family planning clinics.[1] About half of the women who have an episode develop recurrent vulvovaginal candidiasis.[2]

**AETIOLOGY/ RISK FACTORS**   *Candida albicans* accounts for 85–90% of cases of vulvovaginal candidiasis. Development of symptomatic vulvovaginal candidiasis probably represents increased growth of yeast that previously colonised the vagina without causing symptoms. Risk factors for vulvovaginal candidiasis include pregnancy (RR 2–10), diabetes mellitus, and systemic antibiotics. The evidence that different types of contraceptives are risk factors is contradictory. The incidence of vulvovaginal candidiasis rises with initiation of sexual activity, but we found no direct evidence that vulvovaginal candidiasis is sexually transmitted.[3-5]

**PROGNOSIS**   We found few descriptions of the natural history of untreated vulvovaginal candidiasis. Discomfort is the main complication and can include pain while passing urine or during sexual intercourse. Balanitis🅖 in male partners of women with vulvovaginal candidiasis can occur, but it is rare.

---

Please refer to CD-ROM for full text and references.

### Search date February 2003

*Michelle Proctor and Cynthia Farquhar*

Women's health

## What are the effects of treatments?

### BENEFICIAL

#### Non-steroidal anti-inflammatory drugs (other than aspirin)

Two systematic reviews have found that naproxen, ibuprofen, mefenamic acid, valdecoxib, and rofecoxib reduce pain compared with placebo. It remains unclear from direct comparisons which non-steroidal anti-inflammatory drugs have better efficacy or safety. One systematic review found that naproxen reduced pain more and was associated with fewer adverse effects than co-proxamol. It also found that mefenamic acid reduced symptoms more than co-proxamol.

### LIKELY TO BE BENEFICIAL

#### Aspirin, paracetamol, and compound analgesics

One systematic review found that aspirin was more effective for pain relief than placebo, but less effective than naproxen or ibuprofen. The review found no significant difference between paracetamol compared with placebo, aspirin, or ibuprofen in pain relief, although some of the RCTs may have been too small to rule out clinically important differences. It found limited evidence that co-proxamol◉ reduced pain compared with placebo.

#### Magnesium

One systematic review found limited evidence from two out of three small RCTs that magnesium reduced pain after 5–6 months compared with placebo. A third RCT found no significant difference.

#### Thiamine

One large RCT identified by a systematic review found that thiamine reduced pain after 60 days compared with placebo.

#### Toki-shakuyaku-san (herbal remedy)

One systematic review found limited evidence that toki-shakuyaku-san reduced pain after 6 months compared with placebo and that it reduced the need for additional medication with diclofenac.

#### Topical heat (about 39 °C)

One RCT found topical heat (about 39 °C) treatment to be as effective as ibuprofen and more effective than placebo in reducing pain.

#### Transcutaneous electrical nerve stimulation

One systematic review found limited evidence from small RCTs that high frequency transcutaneous electrical nerve stimulation◉ reduced pain compared with placebo transcutaneous electrical nerve stimulation. We found insufficient evidence from small RCTs to assess effects of low frequency transcutaneous electrical nerve stimulation compared with other or no treatment.

#### Vitamin E

One RCT found limited evidence that vitamin E reduced pain compared with placebo.

▶

# Dysmenorrhoea

◀ UNKNOWN EFFECTIVENESS

## Acupuncture
One systematic review of one small RCT found insufficient evidence to compare acupuncture with placebo or no treatment.

## Behavioural interventions
We found insufficient evidence from two poor quality RCTs about the effects of behavioural interventions⊖.

## Combined oral contraceptives
One systematic review found insufficient evidence about the effects of combined oral contraceptives versus placebo for pain relief.

## Fish oil
One small RCT identified by a systematic review and one additional RCT found limited evidence that fish oil reduced pain and symptoms after 1–3 months compared with placebo.

## Herbal remedies (other than toki-shakuyaku-san)
We found no RCTs of other herbal remedies.

## Surgical interruption of pelvic nerve pathways
One small RCT found limited evidence suggesting that laparoscopic uterine nerve ablation⊖ increased pain relief compared with diagnostic laparoscopy. Another RCT found that laparoscopic uterine nerve ablation reduced pain at 12 months compared with laparoscopic presacral neurectomy⊖. It found no significant difference in pain relief between treatments at 3 months. It also found increased constipation with laparoscopic uterine nerve ablation.

## Vitamin $B_{12}$
We found no RCTs that compared vitamin $B_{12}$ with placebo. One small RCT found insufficient evidence for vitamin $B_{12}$ compared with advice to follow a low fat vegetarian diet.

UNLIKELY TO BE BENEFICIAL

## Spinal manipulation
One systematic review has found inconclusive evidence on the effects of spinal manipulation compared with placebo or no treatment in pain relief.

**DEFINITION** Dysmenorrhoea is painful menstrual cramps of uterine origin. It is commonly divided into primary dysmenorrhoea (pain without organic pathology) and secondary dysmenorrhoea (pelvic pain associated with an identifiable pathological condition, such as endometriosis [see endometriosis p 388] or ovarian cysts). The initial onset of primary dysmenorrhoea is usually shortly after menarche (6–12 months) when ovulatory cycles are established. Pain duration is commonly 8–72 hours and is usually associated with the onset of menstrual flow. Secondary dysmenorrhoea can also occur at any time after menarche, but may arise as a new symptom during a woman's fourth and fifth decade, after the onset of an underlying causative condition.[1]

**INCIDENCE/ PREVALENCE** Variations in the definition of dysmenorrhoea make it difficult to determine prevalence precisely. However, various types of study have found a consistently high prevalence in women of different ages and nationalities. One systematic review (search date 1996) of the prevalence of chronic pelvic pain, summarising both community and hospital surveys, estimated prevalence to be 45–95%.[2] Reports focus on adolescent girls and generally include only primary dysmenorrhoea, although this is not always specified❶.

▶

**AETIOLOGY/ RISK FACTORS** A longitudinal study of a representative sample of women born in 1962 found that severity of dysmenorrhoea was significantly associated with duration of menstrual flow (average duration of menstrual flow was 5.0 days for women with no dysmenorrhoea and 5.8 days for women with severe dysmenorrhoea; where severe dysmenorrhoea was defined as pain that did not respond well to analgesics and clearly inhibited daily activity; P < 0.001; WMD −0.80, 95% CI −1.36 to −0.24); younger average menarcheal age (13.1 years in women without dysmenorrhoea v 12.6 years in women with severe dysmenorrhoea; P < 0.01; WMD 0.50, 95% CI 0.09 to 0.91); and cigarette smoking (41% of smokers and 26% of non-smokers experienced moderate or severe dysmenorrhoea).[9] There is also some evidence of a dose-response relationship between exposure to environmental tobacco smoke and increased incidence of dysmenorrhoea.[10]

**PROGNOSIS** Primary dysmenorrhoea is a chronic recurring condition that affects most young women. Studies of the natural history of this condition are sparse. One longitudinal study in Scandinavia found that primary dysmenorrhoea often improves in the third decade of a woman's reproductive life, and is also reduced after childbirth.[9] We found no studies that reliably examined the relationship between the prognosis of secondary dysmenorrhoea and the severity of underlying pathology such as endometriosis.

---

Please refer to CD-ROM for full text and references.

# Endometriosis

**Search date October 2002**

*Cynthia Farquhar*

---

## What are the effects of treatments in women with pain attributed to endometriosis?

We found no RCTs comparing medical and surgical treatments.

### BENEFICIAL

**Hormonal treatment at diagnosis (danazol, medroxyprogesterone, gestrinone, gonadorelin [gonadotrophin releasing hormone — GnRH] analogues)**

Small systematic reviews and small RCTs have found that hormonal treatments (except for dydrogesterone) reduce pain attributed to endometriosis, compared with placebo, and are all similarly effective.

### LIKELY TO BE BENEFICIAL

**Combined oral contraceptive pill**

One systematic review found that combined low dose oral contraceptive significantly reduced dysmenorrhoea compared with goserelin during 6 months of treatment, but all women improved 6 months after stopping treatment. Two RCTs found no significant difference with combined oral contraceptives in overall pain relief compared with gonadorelin analogues.

**Combined ablation of endometrial deposits and uterine nerve**

One RCT found that laparoscopic ablation of deposits plus laparoscopic uterine nerve ablation reduced pain more than diagnostic laparoscopy at 6 months.

**Cystectomy for ovarian endometrioma (better than drainage)**

One RCT found that cystectomy reduced pain caused by ovarian endometrioma at 2 years compared with drainage. Complication rates were similar.

**Postoperative hormonal treatment after conservative surgery**

RCTs have found that postoperative hormonal treatment with danazol or medroxyprogesterone for 6 months reduces pain and delays the recurrence of pain at 12 and 24 months compared with placebo. One RCT found no significant difference in recurrence of pain between combined oral contraceptives and placebo at 6 months. Adverse effects of hormonal treatment are common and include hot flushes and bone loss with gonadorelin analogues and androgenic adverse effects with danazol.

### UNKNOWN EFFECTIVENESS

**Dydrogesterone**

Systematic reviews have found no significant difference in pain at 6 months with dydrogesterone given at two different doses in the luteal phase compared with placebo.

**Laparoscopic ablation of endometrial deposits without ablation of the uterine nerve**

We found no systematic reviews or RCTs assessing the effects of laparoscopic ablation of endometrial deposits without ablation of the uterine nerve.

**Laparoscopic uterine nerve ablation**

One systematic review found insufficient evidence on the effects of laparoscopic uterine nerve ablation in women with pain attributed to endometriosis. ▶

◀ **Postoperative hormonal treatment after oophorectomy**

One RCT in women who previously had an oophorectomy found insufficient evidence on the effects of hormone replacement therapy in recurrence of endometriosis compared with no treatment.

**Preoperative hormonal treatment**

Two RCTs found insufficient evidence on the effects of preoperative hormonal treatments in pain attributed to endometriosis.

## What are the effects of treatments in women with subfertility attributed to endometriosis?

### LIKELY TO BE BENEFICIAL

#### Cystectomy for ovarian endometrioma (better than drainage)

One RCT found that cystectomy increased pregnancy rates compared with drainage in women with subfertility caused by ovarian endometrioma. Complication rates were similar.

#### Laparoscopic ablation/excision of endometrial deposits

One systematic review found that laparoscopic surgery increased cumulative pregnancy rates compared with diagnostic laparoscopy after 9–12 months. We found no RCTs comparing medical and surgical treatments.

### UNLIKELY TO BE BENEFICIAL

#### Hormonal treatment at diagnosis (danazol, medroxyprogesterone acetate, gonadorelin [GnRH] analogues)

One systematic review and one subsequent RCT found no significant difference between hormonal treatments and placebo in rates of pregnancy at 4–6 months.

#### Postoperative hormonal treatment (gonadorelin analogues and decapeptyl) after conservative surgery

RCTs found no significant difference between gonadorelin analogues and placebo after conservative surgery in rates of pregnancy or time to conception. Adverse effects of hormonal treatment are common and include hot flushes and bone loss with gonadorelin analogues and androgenic adverse effects with danazol.

**DEFINITION** Endometriosis is characterised by ectopic endometrial tissue, which can cause dysmenorrhoea, dyspareunia, non-cyclical pelvic pain, and subfertility. Diagnosis is made by laparoscopy. Most endometrial deposits are found in the pelvis (ovaries, peritoneum, uterosacral ligaments, pouch of Douglas, and rectovaginal septum). Extrapelvic deposits, including those in the umbilicus and diaphragm, are rare. Severity of endometriosis🅖 is defined by the American Fertility Society: this review uses the terms mild (stage I and II), moderate (stage III), and severe (stage IV).[1] Endometriomas are cysts of endometriosis within the ovary.

**INCIDENCE/ PREVALENCE** In asymptomatic women, the prevalence of endometriosis ranges from 2–22%, depending on the diagnostic criteria used and the populations studied.[2–5] In women with dysmenorrhoea, the incidence of endometriosis ranges from 40–60%, and in women with subfertility from 20–30%.[3,6,7] The severity of symptoms and the probability of diagnosis increase with age.[8] Incidence peaks at about 40 years of age.[9] Symptoms and laparoscopic appearance do not always correlate.[10]

# Endometriosis

**AETIOLOGY/ RISK FACTORS**   The cause of endometriosis is unknown. Risk factors include early menarche and late menopause. Embryonic cells may give rise to deposits in the umbilicus, whereas retrograde menstruation may deposit endometrial cells in the diaphragm.[11,12] Use of oral contraceptives reduces the risk of endometriosis, and this protective effect persists for up to 1 year after their discontinuation.[9]

**PROGNOSIS**   We found two RCTs in which laparoscopy was repeated in women treated with placebo.[13,14] Over 6–12 months, endometrial deposits resolved spontaneously in up to a third of women, deteriorated in nearly half, and were unchanged in the remainder.

Please refer to CD-ROM for full text and references.

# Fibroids (uterine myomatosis, leiomyomas)

## Search date August 2002

*Anne Lethaby and Beverley Vollenhoven*

## What are the effects of medical treatment alone?

### TRADE OFF BETWEEN BENEFITS AND HARMS

**Gonadorelin analogues (gonadotropin releasing hormone analogues [GnRHa]) alone**

RCTs have found that gonadorelin analogues reduce fibroid related symptoms compared with placebo, but are associated with important adverse effects. One RCT found that nafarelin versus placebo significantly increased amenorrhoea at 12 weeks. One systematic review found insufficient evidence to compare nafarelin versus buserelin. One RCT found that higher versus lower doses of nafarelin increased amenorrhoea at 16 weeks. Two RCTs found that nafarelin versus placebo significantly reduced bone density from baseline after 16 weeks' treatment, but that bone density returned to pretreatment levels 6 months after treatment was stopped. Two RCTs found that hot flushes were significantly more common with nafarelin versus placebo or buserelin.

**Gonadorelin analogues (GnRHa) plus progestogen**

One small RCT found that leuprorelin (leuprolide) acetate plus progesterone significantly reduced heavy bleeding compared with leuprorelin acetate alone. Two small RCTs found that gonadorelin analogue plus progesterone significantly reduced the proportion of women with hot flushes compared with gonadorelin analogue alone.

### UNKNOWN EFFECTIVENESS

**Gonadorelin analogue (GnRHa) plus tibolone**

One small RCT found no significant difference with gonadorelin analogue alone versus gonadorelin analogue plus tibolone on uterine and fibroid size and fibroid related symptoms.

**Gonadorelin analogues (GnRHa) plus combined oestrogen and progestogen**

We found insufficient evidence from one small RCT to compare effects on fibroid related symptoms of gonadorelin analogue plus combined oestrogen and progestogen versus gonadorelin analogues plus progesterone alone.

**Non-steroidal anti-inflammatory drugs**

We found insufficient evidence from two small RCTs about the effects of non-steroidal anti-inflammatory drugs on heavy menstrual bleeding in women with uterine fibroids.

**Gestrinone; levonorgestrel intrauterine system; mifepristone**

We found no RCTs on the effects of these interventions.

## What are the effects of preoperative medical interventions?

### LIKELY TO BE BENEFICIAL

**Gonadorelin analogues (GnRHa)**

One systematic review and one additional RCT have found that gonadorelin analogues versus placebo or no treatment given at least 3 months before fibroid surgery increase haemoglobin and haematocrit and reduce uterine and pelvic symptoms and blood loss during surgery. Women having hysterectomy are more ▶

# Fibroids (uterine myomatosis, leiomyomas)

likely to have a vaginal rather than an abdominal procedure after gonadorelin treatment. However, women are more likely to experience adverse hypo-oestrogenic effects from preoperative treatment.

## What are the effects of surgical interventions?

**BENEFICIAL**

### Laparoscopic myomectomy (compared to abdominal myomectomy)
One RCT found that laparoscopic myomectomy❻ versus abdominal myomectomy resulted in less postoperative pain, and a shorter recovery time.

**LIKELY TO BE BENEFICIAL**

### Abdominal hysterectomy*
We found no RCTs. There is consensus that abdominal hysterectomy is superior to no treatment in reducing fibroid related symptoms.

*Based on consensus.

**UNKNOWN EFFECTIVENESS**

### Laparoscopic assisted vaginal hysterectomy
We found no RCTs comparing long term effects of laparoscopic assisted vaginal hysterectomy versus other treatments. One small RCT found limited evidence that women having laparoscopically assisted vaginal hysterectomy had shorter recovery and less postoperative pain compared with women having total abdominal hysterectomy❻.

### Thermal balloon endometrial ablation
We found no RCTs comparing thermal balloon ablation❻ versus non-surgical treatment or versus hysterectomy. One RCT compared thermal balloon ablation versus rollerball endometrial ablation❻ in women with fibroids smaller than the average size of a 12 week pregnancy, all of whom had been pretreated with gonadorelin analogues. It found no significant difference between thermal balloon and rollerball ablation in hysterectomy rates, amenorrhoea rates, pictorial bleeding assessment chart score❻, or haemoglobin at 12 months. It found that thermal balloon ablation reduced operation time and intraoperative complication rate compared with rollerball ablation. About a third of women reported being "not very satisfied" with either operation.

**DEFINITION**  Fibroids (uterine leiomyomas) are benign tumours of the smooth muscle cells of the uterus. Women with fibroids can be asymptomatic or can present with menorrhagia (30%), dysmenorrhoea, pelvic pain, pressure symptoms, infertility, and recurrent pregnancy loss.[1] However, much of the data describing the relationship between the presence of fibroids and symptoms are based on uncontrolled studies that have assessed the effect of myomectomy on the presenting symptom.[2]

**INCIDENCE/**  The reported incidence of fibroids varies from 5.4–77% depending on the
**PREVALENCE**  method of diagnosis (the gold standard is histological evidence). A random sample of 335 Swedish women aged 25–40 years was reported to have an incidence of fibroids of 5.4% (95% CI 3.0% to 7.8%) based on transvaginal ultrasound examination. The prevalence of these tumours increased with age (age 25–32 years: 3.3%, 95% CI 0.7% to 6.0%; 33–40 years: 7.8%, 95% CI 3.6% to 12%).[3] Based on postmortem examination of women, 50% were found to have these tumours.[4] Gross serial sectioning at 2 mm intervals of 100 consecutive hysterectomy specimens revealed the presence of fibroids in 77%. These women were having hysterectomies for reasons other than ▶

fibroids.[5] The incidence of fibroids in black women is three times greater than that in white women, based on ultrasound or hysterectomy diagnosis.[6] Submucosal fibroids have been diagnosed in 6–34% of women having a hysteroscopy for abnormal bleeding, and in 2–7% of women having infertility investigations.[7]

**AETIOLOGY/ RISK FACTORS**  The cause of uterine fibroids is unknown. It is known that each fibroid is of monoclonal origin and arises independently.[8,9] Factors thought to be involved include the sex steroid hormones oestrogen and progesterone as well as the insulin-like growth factors, epidermal growth factor and transforming growth factor. Risk factors for fibroid growth include nulliparity and obesity. There is a risk reduction to a fifth with five term pregnancies, compared with nulliparous women ($P < 0.001$).[10] Obesity increases the risk of fibroid development by 21% with each 10 kg weight gain ($P = 0.008$).[10] Factors associated with reduced incidence of fibroids include cigarette smoking and hormonal contraception. Women who smoke 10 cigarettes a day have an 18% lowered risk of fibroid development compared with non-smokers ($P = 0.036$).[10] The combined oral contraceptive pill reduces the risk of fibroids with increasing duration of use compared with never users (users for 4–6 years: OR 0.8, 95% CI 0.5 to 1.2; users for ≥ 7 years: OR 0.5, 95% CI 0.3 to 0.9).[11] Women who have used injections containing 150 mg depot medroxyprogesterone acetate also have a reduced incidence compared with women who have never used (OR 0.44, 95% CI 0.36 to 0.55).[12]

**PROGNOSIS**  There are few data on the long term untreated prognosis of these tumours, particularly in women who are asymptomatic at diagnosis. One small case control study reported that in a group of 106 women treated with observation alone over 1 year there was no significant change in symptoms and quality of life over that time.[13]

---

Please refer to CD-ROM for full text and references.

Women's health

# Infertility and subfertility

**Search date October 2002**

*Kirsten Duckitt*

---

## What are the effects of treatments in women with infertility caused by ovulation disorders?

### LIKELY TO BE BENEFICIAL

#### Clomifene

One systematic review has found that clomifene significantly increases pregnancy rate compared with placebo in women who ovulate infrequently. Four other studies comparing clomifene versus tamoxifen have found no significant difference in ovulation or pregnancy rates. One RCT found that clomifene plus metformin significantly increased pregnancy rate compared with clomifene alone after 6 months' treatment.

### UNKNOWN EFFECTIVENESS

#### Cyclofenil

One RCT found no significant difference in pregnancy rates with cyclofenil versus placebo.

#### Gonadotrophins

One systematic review found no significant difference between human menopausal gonadotrophins and urofollitropin (urofollitrophin, urinary follicle stimulating hormone) in pregnancy rates. Two RCTs found no significant difference in cumulative pregnancy or live birth rates with follitropin (recombinant follicle stimulating hormone) versus urofollitropin. The review found that urofollitropin versus human menopausal gonadotrophins significantly reduced the risk of ovarian hyperstimulation syndrome❺, although this was confined to women who were not treated with concomitant gonadotrophin releasing hormone analogues. Observational evidence suggests that gonadotrophins may be associated with an increased risk of non-invasive ovarian tumours and multiple pregnancies.

#### Laparoscopic ovarian drilling

One systematic review and one subsequent small RCT found no significant difference in pregnancy rate with laparoscopic ovarian drilling❺ versus gonadotrophins, but found that laparoscopic ovarian drilling significantly reduced rates of multiple pregnancies.

#### Pulsatile gonadotrophin releasing hormone

One systematic review found insufficient evidence on the effects of pulsatile gonadotrophin releasing hormone treatment.

---

## What are the effects of treatments in women with tubal infertility?

### LIKELY TO BE BENEFICIAL

#### Tubal flushing with oil soluble media

One systematic review found that tubal flushing with oil soluble media versus no intervention increased pregnancy rate. The review found that tubal flushing with oil soluble media increased the live birth rate compared with flushing with water soluble media.

### ◄ Tubal surgery (before in vitro fertilisation)

One systematic review in women undergoing in vitro fertilisation has found that tubal surgery significantly increases pregnancy and live birth rates compared with no treatment or medical treatment. Another review found no significant difference in pregnancy rates between different types of tubal surgery. One systematic review found no significant difference in pregnancy rates with tubal surgery plus additional treatments versus tubal surgery alone to prevent adhesion formation (steroids, dextran, noxytioline).

### UNKNOWN EFFECTIVENESS

#### In vitro fertilisation

We found no RCTs of in vitro fertilisation versus no treatment. One RCT found that immediate versus delayed in vitro fertilisation❻ significantly increased numbers of pregnancies and live births. Three RCTs found no significant difference in numbers of live births with in vitro fertilisation versus intracytoplasmic sperm injection. Observational evidence suggests that adverse effects associated with in vitro fertilisation include multiple pregnancies and ovarian hyperstimulation syndrome.

#### Selective salpingography plus tubal catheterisation

We found no RCTs on the effects of selective salpingography plus tubal catheterisation.

#### Tubal flushing with water soluble media

One systematic review found no RCTs of tubal flushing with water soluble media versus no intervention. It found that tubal flushing with water soluble media decreased live birth rate compared with flushing with oil soluble media.

---

## What are the effects of interventions in women with infertility associated with endometriosis?

### LIKELY TO BE BENEFICIAL

#### Intrauterine insemination plus gonadotrophins

One RCT found that intrauterine insemination plus gonadotrophins significantly increased live birth rates compared with no treatment. A second RCT found no significant difference in birth rates between expectant management versus intrauterine insemination plus pituitary down regulation plus gonadotrophins. A third RCT found that intrauterine insemination plus gonadotrophins significantly increased pregnancy rates compared with intrauterine insemination alone after the first treatment cycle.

### UNKNOWN EFFECTIVENESS

#### In vitro fertilisation

We found no RCTs in women with endometriosis related infertility.

#### Laparoscopic surgical treatment

Two RCTs found inconsistent evidence about effects on pregnancy and live birth rates of laparoscopic surgery compared with diagnostic laparoscopy.

### LIKELY TO BE INEFFECTIVE OR HARMFUL

#### Drug-induced ovarian suppression

One systematic review found no significant difference in pregnancy rates between drugs that induce ovarian suppression versus placebo. The review found that ►

# Infertility and subfertility

ovulation suppression agents cause adverse effects, including weight gain, hot flushes, and osteoporosis, and that danazol may cause dose related weight gain and androgenic effects.

## What are the effects of interventions in couples with male factor infertility?

### BENEFICIAL

**Intrauterine insemination**

Two systematic reviews have found that intrauterine insemination significantly increases pregnancy rate compared with intracervical insemination or natural intercourse.

### UNKNOWN EFFECTIVENESS

**Donor insemination**

We found no good evidence on the effects of donor insemination.

**Intracytoplasmic sperm injection plus in vitro fertilisation**

One systematic review found insufficient evidence on the effects of intracytoplasmic sperm injection plus in vitro fertilisation versus in vitro fertilisation alone.

**In vitro fertilisation versus gamete intrafallopian transfer**

One RCT found insufficient evidence on the effects of in vitro fertilisation versus gamete intrafallopian transfer.

## What are the effects of interventions in couples with unexplained infertility?

### BENEFICIAL

**Intrauterine insemination (plus ovarian stimulation treatment)**

Two systematic reviews and one subsequent RCT in couples undergoing ovarian stimulation treatment have found that intrauterine insemination significantly increases pregnancy rates compared with timed intercourse or intracervical insemination. One systematic review found no significant difference with intrauterine insemination versus timed intercourse or intracervical insemination in pregnancy rates, but found that adding ovarian stimulation to any of the three interventions significantly increased pregnancy rate per cycle. One systematic review and one subsequent RCT have found that fallopian tube sperm perfusion significantly increased pregnancy rates compared with intrauterine insemination. One systematic review found no significant difference between intrauterine insemination with or without ovarian stimulation versus in vitro fertilisation for live birth rate.

### LIKELY TO BE BENEFICIAL

**Clomifene**

One systematic review found limited evidence that clomifene versus placebo significantly increased rates of pregnancy per cycle.

**Fallopian tube sperm perfusion (v intrauterine insemination)**

One systematic review and one subsequent RCT have found that fallopian tube sperm perfusion☉ significantly increases pregnancy rates compared with intrauterine insemination.

### Gamete intrafallopian transfer

We found no RCTs of gamete intrafallopian transfer versus no treatment. RCTs found conflicting effects on pregnancy rates of gamete intrafallopian transfer versus other treatments (intrauterine insemination, timed intercourse, and in vitro fertilisation).

### In vitro fertilisation

One systematic review found no significant difference between in vitro fertilisation and expectant management for pregnancy rate. It found no significant difference between in vitro fertilisation versus gamete intrafallopian transfer or versus intraterine insemination with or without ovarian stimulation for live birth rate.

**DEFINITION**
Normal fertility has been defined as achieving a pregnancy within 2 years by regular sexual intercourse.[1] However, many define infertility as the failure to conceive after 1 year of unprotected intercourse. Infertility can be primary, in couples who have never conceived, or secondary, in couples who have previously conceived. Infertile couples include those who are sterile (who will never achieve a natural pregnancy) and those who are subfertile (who could eventually achieve a pregnancy).

**INCIDENCE/ PREVALENCE**
Although there is no evidence of a major change in the prevalence of infertility, many more couples are seeking help than previously. Currently, about 1/7 couples in industrialised countries will seek medical advice for infertility.[2] Rates of primary infertility vary widely between countries, ranging from 10% in Africa to about 6% in North America and Europe.[1] Reported rates of secondary infertility are less reliable.

**AETIOLOGY/ RISK FACTORS**
In the UK, nearly a third of infertility cases are unexplained. The rest are caused by ovulatory failure (27%), low sperm count or quality (19%), tubal damage (14%), endometriosis (5%), and other causes (5%).[3]

**PROGNOSIS**
In developed countries, 80–90% of couples attempting to conceive are successful after 1 year and 95% after 2 years.[3] The chances of becoming pregnant vary with the cause and duration of infertility, the woman's age, the couple's previous pregnancy history, and the availability of different treatment options.[4,5] For the first 2–3 years of unexplained infertility, cumulative conception rates remain high (27–46%) but decrease with increasing age of the woman and duration of infertility. The background rates of spontaneous pregnancy in infertile couples can be calculated from longitudinal studies of infertile couples who have been observed without treatment.[4]

Please refer to CD-ROM for full text and references.

# Menopausal symptoms

**Search date November 2002**

*Edward Morris and Janice Rymer*

---

## What are the effects of medical treatments?

**BENEFICIAL**

### Progestogens (at high doses, in reducing vasomotor symptoms)

One systematic review and six additional RCTs have found that progestogens with or without oestrogens reduce vasomotor symptoms compared with placebo. We found no good quality evidence on other outcomes, including quality of life.

### Tibolone

RCTs have found that tibolone improves vasomotor symptoms and sexual function compared with placebo. Two RCTs found that tibolone improved sexual function compared with hormone replacement therapy, However, we found insufficient evidence from RCTs about effects on vasomotor symptoms and vaginal dryness compared with hormone replacement therapy.

**LIKELY TO BE BENEFICIAL**

### Phyto-oestrogens

We found limited evidence from RCTs that phyto-oestrogens reduced vasomotor symptoms compared with placebo.

**UNKNOWN EFFECTIVENESS**

### Antidepressants

We found no RCTs on the effects of antidepressants on menopausal symptoms.

### Clonidine

One small RCT found that transdermal clonidine reduced the number and intensity of hot flushes after 8 weeks compared with placebo. However, we were unable to draw reliable conclusions from that study.

### Testosterone

We found no reliable RCTs evaluating testosterone alone. We found limited evidence from RCTs that testosterone plus oestrogens may improve vasomotor symptoms compared with oestrogen alone. However, we were unable to draw reliable conclusions from these studies.

**TRADE OFF BETWEEN BENEFITS AND HARMS**

### Oestrogens

One systematic review and three subsequent RCTs have found that oestrogen with or without progestogens improves vasomotor symptoms. Two systematic reviews and four subsequent RCTs have found that oestrogen reduces the incidence of urinary tract infection and improves urogenital symptoms. One systematic review found that oestrogens reduced depressed mood. Four RCTs have found that oestrogen improves quality of life in the short term. Important adverse effects include breast cancer, endometrial cancer, stroke and thromboembolic disease.

**DEFINITION** Menopause is defined as the end of the last menstrual period. A woman is deemed to be postmenopausal 1 year after her last period. For practical purposes most women are diagnosed as menopausal after 1 year of amenorrhoea. Menopausal symptoms often begin in the perimenopausal years. ▶

| | |
|---|---|
| **INCIDENCE/ PREVALENCE** | In the UK the mean age for the start of the menopause is 50 years and 9 months. The median onset of the perimenopause is 45.5–47.5 years. One Scottish survey (6096 women aged 45–54 years) found that 84% of women had experienced at least one of the classic menopausal symptoms, with 45% finding one or more symptoms a problem.[1] |
| **AETIOLOGY/ RISK FACTORS** | Urogenital symptoms of menopause are caused by decreased oestrogen concentrations, but the cause of vasomotor symptoms and psychological effects is complex and remains unclear. |
| **PROGNOSIS** | Menopause is a physiological event. Its timing may be determined genetically. Although endocrine changes are permanent, menopausal symptoms such as hot flushes, which are experienced by about 70% of women, usually resolve with time.[2] Some symptoms, however, such as genital atrophy, may remain the same or worsen. |

Please refer to CD-ROM for full text and references.

# Menorrhagia

**Search date February 2003**

*Kirsten Duckitt and Keri McCully*

## What are the effects of treatments?

### BENEFICIAL

#### Endometrial thinning before hysteroscopic surgery

One systematic review has found that preoperative gonadorelin (gonadotrophin releasing hormone) analogues reduce moderate or heavy periods and increase amenorrhoea compared with placebo, no preoperative treatment, or preoperative danazol. We found insufficient evidence about effects of preoperative danazol or progestogens compared with placebo or no preoperative treatment.

#### Hysterectomy (v endometrial destruction) after medical failure

Systematic reviews have found that hysterectomy reduces menstrual blood loss and the number of women requiring further operations, and increases satisfaction compared with endometrial destruction. RCTs found no differences in effectiveness between different types of hysterectomy. One large cohort study reported major or minor complications in about a third of women undergoing hysterectomy.

#### Non-steroidal anti-inflammatory drugs

One systematic review has found that non-steroidal anti-inflammatory drugs reduce mean menstrual blood loss compared with placebo. One systematic review found no significant difference in menstrual blood loss between mefenamic acid and naproxen, or between non-steroidal anti-inflammatory drugs and oral progestogens, oral contraceptives, or progesterone releasing intrauterine devices.

#### Tranexamic acid

Systematic reviews have found that tranexamic acid reduces menstrual blood loss compared with placebo or other drugs (oral progestogens, mefenamic acid, etamsylate, flurbiprofen, and diclofenac). Adverse effects of tranexamic acid include leg cramps and nausea, which occur in about a third of women using this drug. One long term population based observational study found no evidence that tranexamic acid increases the risk of thromboembolism.

### LIKELY TO BE BENEFICIAL

#### Hysteroscopic versus non-hysteroscopic destruction after medical failure

One systematic review found that hysteroscopic methods of endometrial destruction increased amenorrhoea at 12 months compared with non-hysteroscopic methods. We found no consistent evidence of a difference in amenorrhoea or satisfaction rates among different types of hysteroscopic procedure. RCTs found that complications, such as infection, haemorrhage, or uterine perforation occurred in up to 15% of women undergoing endometrial destruction.

### TRADE OFF BETWEEN BENEFITS AND HARMS

#### Danazol

Systematic reviews found limited evidence that danazol reduced blood loss compared with placebo, luteal phase oral progestogens, mefenamic acid, naproxen, or oral contraceptives, but found that danazol increased adverse effects compared with either non-steroidal anti-inflammatory drugs or oral progestogens. ▶

## UNKNOWN EFFECTIVENESS

### Combined oral contraceptives

One systematic review found insufficient evidence about effects of oral contraceptives in women with menorrhagia.

### Endometrial resection versus medical treatment

One systematic review and one additional RCT found no consistent evidence of a difference in blood loss or satisfaction between transcervical endometrial resection🅖 and medical treatment. RCTs found that complications, such as infection, haemorrhage, or uterine perforation occurred in up to 15% of women undergoing endometrial destruction.

### Etamsylate

We found insufficient evidence from one systematic review about effects of etamsylate compared with placebo, mefenamic acid, aminocaproic acid, or tranexamic acid.

### Intrauterine progestogens

We found no systematic review or RCTs comparing intrauterine progestogens versus placebo. Two systematic reviews and three subsequent RCTs found conflicting evidence about menstrual blood loss, satisfaction rates, and quality of life scores with levonorgestrel releasing intrauterine devices compared with other treatments (endometrial resection, thermal balloon ablation🅖, norethisterone, medical treatment, non-steroidal anti-inflammatory drugs, and hysterectomy).

### Dilatation and curettage after medical failure; gonadorelin (gonadotrophin releasing hormone) analogues; myomectomy after medical failure

We found no RCTs on the effects of these interventions.

## UNLIKELY TO BE BENEFICIAL

### Oral progestogens (longer cycle)

We found no RCTs comparing oral progestogens versus placebo. One RCT identified by a systematic review found no significant difference in menstrual blood loss between a longer treatment cycle of oral progestogen and a levonorgestrel releasing intrauterine device.

## LIKELY TO BE INEFFECTIVE OR HARMFUL

### Oral progestogens in luteal phase only

We found no RCTs comparing oral progestogens versus placebo. One systematic review has found that luteal phase oral progestogens increase mean menstrual blood loss compared with danazol, tranexamic acid, or a progesterone releasing intrauterine device.

**DEFINITION**   Menorrhagia is defined as heavy but regular menstrual bleeding. Idiopathic ovulatory menorrhagia is regular heavy bleeding in the absence of recognisable pelvic pathology or a general bleeding disorder. Objective menorrhagia is taken to be a total menstrual blood loss of 80 mL or more in each menstruation.[1] Subjectively, menorrhagia may be defined as a complaint of regular excessive menstrual blood loss occurring over several consecutive cycles in a woman of reproductive years.

**INCIDENCE/**
**PREVALENCE**   In the UK, 5% of women (aged 30–49 years) consult their general practitioner each year with menorrhagia.[2] In New Zealand, 2–4% of primary care consultations by premenopausal women are for menstrual problems.[3]

# Menorrhagia

**AETIOLOGY/ RISK FACTORS**   Idiopathic ovulatory menorrhagia is thought to be caused by disordered prostaglandin production within the endometrium.[4] Prostaglandins may also be implicated in menorrhagia associated with uterine fibroids, adenomyosis, or the presence of an intrauterine device. Fibroids have been reported in 10% of women with menorrhagia (80–100 mL/cycle) and 40% of those with severe menorrhagia (≥ 200 mL/cycle).[5]

**PROGNOSIS**   Menorrhagia limits normal activities and causes iron deficiency anaemia in two thirds of women proved to have objective menorrhagia.[1,6,7] One in five of all women in the UK and one in three women in the USA have a hysterectomy before the age of 60 years; menorrhagia is the main presenting problem in at least 50% of these women.[8–10] About 50% of the women who have a hysterectomy for menorrhagia are found to have a normal uterus.[11]

Please refer to CD-ROM for full text and references.

*Hani Gabra, Charles Redman, and Jennifer Byrom*

## What are the effects of treatments for ovarian cancer that is advanced at first presentation?

We found insufficient evidence on the effects of any treatments on quality of life.

### BENEFICIAL

**Adding platinum to chemotherapy regimens**

One systematic review has found that adding platinum to any non-platinum regimen significantly improves survival, particularly if platinum is added to a combination regimen.

### LIKELY TO BE BENEFICIAL

**Adding paclitaxel to platinum regimens**

One systematic review and one additional RCT have found that adding paclitaxel to platinum based chemotherapy improves progression free survival and overall survival after primary surgery for advanced ovarian cancer.

**Combination platinum regimens versus combination non-platinum regimens**

Seven RCTs have compared combination platinum regimens versus many different non-platinum combination regimens. Most RCTs have found that platinum regimens improve outcomes, although benefits and harms depend on the regimens being compared. None have found that platinum significantly decreased progression free survival or overall survival.

### TRADE OFF BETWEEN BENEFITS AND HARMS

**Combination platinum regimens versus single agent platinum regimens**

One systematic review and three additional RCTs found no evidence that combination platinum based regimens improved progression free survival or overall survival compared with single agent platinum regimens.

### UNKNOWN EFFECTIVENESS

**Carboplatin plus paclitaxel versus carboplatin plus docetaxel**

We found no reliable RCTs comparing the effects of carboplatin plus paclitaxel versus carboplatin plus docetaxel.

**Paclitaxel plus cisplatin versus paclitaxel plus carboplatin**

One RCT found no significant difference in progression free survival or overall survival between paclitaxel plus cisplatin versus paclitaxel plus carboplatin, although it may have lacked power to exclude clinically important effects.

**Routine interval debulking after primary surgery plus chemotherapy**

One RCT found that interval debulking❻ after primary surgery plus chemotherapy improved overall survival over about 3.5 years. A second RCT found that interval debaulking had no significant effect on survival, but it was was probably underpowered to detect a clinically important effect.

**Primary surgery versus no surgery; primary surgery plus chemotherapy versus chemotherapy alone**

We found no RCTs.

# Ovarian cancer

◄ **UNLIKELY TO BE BENEFICIAL**

### Routine second look surgery

Two RCTs found no evidence that routine second look surgery⊙ improves overall survival compared with watchful waiting in women undergoing chemotherapy after primary surgery for advanced ovarian cancer.

**DEFINITION**    Ovarian tumours are classified according to the assumed cell type of origin (surface epithelium, stroma, or germ cells). Most malignant ovarian tumours (85–95%) are derived from the epithelium of the ovarian surface, and are thus termed epithelial.[1] These can be further grouped into histological types (serous, mucinous, endometroid, and clear cell). Epithelial ovarian cancer is staged using the FIGO classification (see table A on web extra). This review concerns only advanced epithelial ovarian cancer, which is regarded as FIGO stages II–IV.

**INCIDENCE/**    The worldwide annual incidence of ovarian cancer exceeds 140 000.[2] Rates
**PREVALENCE**    vary between countries. Differences in reproductive patterns, including age of menarche and menopause, gravidity, breast feeding, and use of the oral contraceptive pill may contribute to this variation. Rates are highest in Scandinavia, northern America, and the UK and lowest for Africa, India, China, and Japan.[3] In the UK, ovarian cancer is the fourth most common malignancy in women and is the leading cause of death from gynaecological cancers, with a lifetime risk of about 2%.[4] In the UK, the incidence was 5174 in 1988[5] and 6880 in 1998.[6] The incidence of ovarian cancer seems to be stabilising in some other countries, and in more affluent countries (Finland, Denmark, New Zealand, and the USA) rates are declining.

**AETIOLOGY/**    Risk factors include increasing age, family history of ovarian cancer, low fertility,
**RISK FACTORS** use of fertility drugs, and low parity.[7–11] Case control studies found that using the combined oral contraceptive pill for more than 5 years was associated with a 40% reduction in the risk of ovarian cancer.[3,7,12,13]

**PROGNOSIS**    Over 80% of women present with advanced disease, and the overall 5 year survival rates are poor (< 30%).[14] For advanced disease the major independent prognostic factors seem to be stage, and residual tumour mass after surgery.

---

Please refer to CD-ROM for full text and references.

# Premenstrual syndrome 405

### Search date October 2002

*Katrina Wyatt*

## What are the effects of treatments?

### BENEFICIAL

#### Diuretics
RCTs have found that spironolactone improves symptoms of premenstrual syndrome including breast tenderness and bloating, compared to placebo. Two RCTs have found that metolazone or ammonium chloride versus placebo reduce premenstrual swelling and weight gain.

#### Non-steroidal anti-inflammatory drugs
RCTs found that prostaglandin inhibitors significantly improved a range of premenstrual symptoms but did not reduce premenstrual breast pain, compared to placebo.

#### Selective serotonin reuptake inhibitors
One systematic review and subsequent RCTs have found that selective serotonin reuptake inhibitors significantly improve premenstrual symptoms, but cause frequent adverse events compared to placebo.

### LIKELY TO BE BENEFICIAL

#### Cognitive behavioural therapy
RCTs found that cognitive behavioural therapy significantly reduced premenstrual symptoms compared to control treatments, but the evidence is insufficient to define the size of an effect.

#### Exercise
One RCT has found that aerobic exercise significantly improves premenstrual symptoms compared to placebo. Another RCT has found that high intensity aerobic exercise improves symptoms significantly more than low intensity.

#### Oestrogens
Limited evidence from small RCTs suggests that oestradiol improves symptoms compared to placebo, but the magnitude of any effect remains unclear.

#### Oral contraceptives
RCTs found limited evidence that oral contraceptives improved premenstrual symptoms compared to placebo.

### TRADE OFF BETWEEN BENEFITS AND HARMS

#### Bromocriptine (breast symptoms only)
RCTs have found limited evidence that bromocriptine relieves breast tenderness compared to placebo, although adverse effects are common.

#### Danazol
RCTs have found that danazol significantly reduces premenstrual symptoms compared to placebo, but has important adverse effects associated with masculinisation when used continuously in the long term.

#### Gonadorelin analogues
RCTs have found that gonadorelin analogues (GnRH in previous nomenclatrues) significantly reduce premenstrual symptoms compared to placebo. RCTs have found that gonadorelin plus oestrogen plus progestogen (addback treatment) improves symptom scores less than that gonadorelin analogue alone but more ▶

than placebo. One small RCT found a similar reduction in symptom scores with gonadorelin analogue plus tibolone compared to gonadorelin analogue plus placebo. Treatment with gonadorelin analogues for more than 6 months carries a significant risk of osteoporosis, limiting their usefulness for long term treatment.

### Non-selective serotonin reuptake inhibitor antidepressants/anxiolytics

RCTs have found that non-selective serotonin reuptake inhibitor antidepressants and anxiolytic drugs significantly improve at least one symptom of premenstrual syndrome compared to placebo, but a proportion of women stop treatment because of adverse effects. We found insufficient evidence from small RCTs about effects of β blockers and lithium.

**UNKNOWN EFFECTIVENESS**

### Hysterectomy with or without bilateral oophorectomy

We found no RCTs. Observational studies have found that hysterectomy plus bilateral oophorectomy is curative. Hysterectomy alone may reduce symptoms, but evidence is limited because of the difficulty in providing controls. The risks are those of major surgery. Infertility is an irreversible consequence of bilateral oophorectomy.

### Progestogens

We found insufficient evidence from one small RCT about the effects of progestogens compared to placebo.

### Pyridoxine

One systematic review of poor quality RCTs found insufficient evidence about the effects of pyridoxine (vitamin $B_6$). In the review, an analysis of weak RCTs suggested that pyridoxine significantly reduced symptoms compared to placebo. Additional RCTs with weak methods found conflicting evidence on the effects of pyridoxine.

### Tibolone

One small RCT found limited evidence that tibolone improved premenstrual symptom score compared to placebo (multivitamins).

### Chiropractic treatment; dietary supplements; endometrial ablation; evening primrose oil; laparoscopic bilateral oophorectomy; reflexology; relaxation treatment

We found insufficient evidence about the effects of these interventions.

**LIKELY TO BE INEFFECTIVE OR HARMFUL**

### Progesterone

One systematic review of progesterone has found a small but significant improvement in overall premenstrual symptoms and no increase in the frequency of withdrawals caused by adverse effects, compared to placebo. However, the improvement is unlikely to be clinically important. It remains unclear whether the route or timing of administration of progesterone is important.

**DEFINITION** A woman has premenstrual syndrome if she complains of recurrent psychological or somatic symptoms (or both) occurring specifically during the luteal phase of the menstrual cycle and resolving by the end of menstruation❶.[1]

**INCIDENCE/** Premenstrual symptoms occur in 95% of all women of reproductive age;
**PREVALENCE** severe, debilitating symptoms (premenstrual syndrome)❻ occur in about 5% of those women.[1]

◀ **AETIOLOGY/**   The aetiology is unknown, but hormonal and other (possibly neuroendocrine)
**RISK FACTORS** factors probably contribute.[2,3] There may be enhanced sensitivity to progesterone, possibly caused by a deficiency of serotonin.[2]

**PROGNOSIS**   Except after oophorectomy, symptoms usually recur when treatment is
stopped.

Please refer to CD-ROM for full text and references.

# Pyelonephritis in non-pregnant women

**Search date November 2002**

*Bazian Ltd*

## What are the effects of treatments?

### LIKELY TO BE BENEFICIAL

**Intravenous antibiotics (ampicillin, co-trimoxazole) in women admitted to hospital with uncomplicated infection***

We found no RCTs comparing intravenous antibiotics versus no antibiotics. However, consensus holds that these drugs are effective, and it is unlikely that such an RCT would now be performed. We found insufficient evidence to compare clinical effects of different intravenous regimens.

**Oral antibiotics (co-trimoxazole, co-amoxiclav, or a fluoroquinolone) for women with uncomplicated infection***

We found no RCTs comparing oral antibiotics versus no antibiotics. However, consensus holds that these drugs are effective, and it is unlikely that such an RCT would now be performed. One systematic review❶ and one subsequent RCT in women with uncomplicated pyelonephritis have found no consistent differences among oral co-trimoxazole, co-amoxiclav, or fluoroquinolones (ciprofloxacin, norfloxacin, levofloxacin, or lomefloxacin) in bacteriological or clinical cure rates.

### UNKNOWN EFFECTIVENESS

**Inpatient versus outpatient management**

We found no RCTs comparing inpatient versus outpatient management of women with acute uncomplicated pyelonephritis.

*Not based on placebo controlled RCTs. Such studies are likely to be considered unethical.

**DEFINITION**    Acute pyelonephritis, or upper urinary tract infection, is an infection of the kidney characterised by pain when passing urine, fever, flank pain, nausea, and vomiting. White blood cells are almost always present in the urine and occasionally white blood cell casts are also seen on urine microscopy. Uncomplicated infection occurs in an otherwise healthy person without any other underlying disease. Complicated pyelonephritis occurs in people with structural or functional urinary tract abnormalities or additional diseases. People with acute pyelonephritis may also be divided into those able to take oral antibiotics and without signs of sepsis who may be managed at home, and those requiring treatment delivered by injection whilst in hospital.

**INCIDENCE/ PREVALENCE**    In the USA, there are 250 000 cases of acute pyelonephritis a year.[1] Worldwide prevalence and incidence are unknown.

**AETIOLOGY/ RISK FACTORS**    Pyelonephritis is most commonly caused when bacteria in the bladder ascend the ureters and invade the kidneys. In some cases, this may result in bacteria entering and multiplying in the bloodstream.

**PROGNOSIS**    Complications include sepsis, infection that spreads to other organs, renal impairment, and renal abscess. Conditions such as underlying renal disease, diabetes mellitus, and immunosuppression may worsen prognosis, but we found no good long term evidence about rates of sepsis or death among such people.

Please refer to CD-ROM for full text and references.

# Recurrent cystitis in non-pregnant women

Search date April 2003

*Adriana Wechsler*

## What are the effects of interventions to prevent further recurrence of cystitis?

### BENEFICIAL

**Continuous antibiotic prophylaxis (trimethoprim, co-trimoxazole, nitrofurantoin, cefaclor, or a quinolone)**

RCTs have found that continuous antibiotic prophylaxis for 6–12 months with trimethoprim, co-trimoxazole, nitrofurantoin, cefaclor, or a quinolone reduces rates of recurrent cystitis compared with placebo❶, and have found no consistent difference in recurrence rates among different continuous regimens. One RCT comparing continuous daily antibiotic prophylaxis versus postcoital antibiotic prophylaxis found no significant difference in rates of positive urine culture after 1 year.

**Postcoital antibiotic prophylaxis (co-trimoxazole, nitrofurantoin, or a quinolone)**

Four RCTs have found that co-trimoxazole, nitrofurantoin, or a quinolone up to 2 hours after sexual intercourse reduces the rates of cystitis compared with placebo❶. One RCT comparing continuous daily antibiotic prophylaxis versus postcoital antibiotic prophylaxis found no significant difference in rates of positive urine culture after 1 year.

### UNKNOWN EFFECTIVENESS

**Cranberry juice and cranberry products**

One systematic review of two weak RCTs provided insufficient evidence on the effects of cranberry juice and other cranberry products in women with recurrent cystitis.

**Prophylaxis with methenamine hippurate**

One systematic review of weak RCTs provided insufficient evidence to assess methenamine hippurate (hexamine hippurate) in women with recurrent cystitis.

**Single dose self administered co-trimoxazole**

One small RCT found single dose, self administered co-trimoxazole started at the onset of cystitis symptoms was less effective in reducing recurrence rates over 1 year than continuous co-trimoxazole prophylaxis. However, evidence was too limited to draw firm conclusions.

**DEFINITION**  Cystitis is an infection of the lower urinary tract, which causes pain when passing urine, and causes frequency, urgency, haematuria, or suprapubic pain not associated with passing urine. White blood cells and bacteria are almost always present in the urine. The presence of fever, flank pain, nausea, or vomiting suggests pyelonephritis (upper urinary tract infection) (see pyelonephritis in non-pregnant women, p 408). Recurrent cystitis may be either a reinfection (after successful eradication of infection) or a relapse after inadequate treatment.

**INCIDENCE/ PREVALENCE**  The incidence of cystitis among premenopausal sexually active women is 0.5–0.7 infections per person year,[1] and 20–40% of women will experience cystitis during their lifetime. Of those, 20% will develop recurrence, almost always (90% of cases) because of reinfection rather than relapse. Rates of infection fall during the winter months.[2] ▶

© BMJ Publishing Group Ltd 2003

# Recurrent cystitis in non-pregnant women

**AETIOLOGY/ RISK FACTORS** Cystitis is caused by uropathogenic bacteria in the faecal flora that colonise the vaginal and periurethral openings, and ascend the urethra into the bladder. Prior infection, sexual intercourse, and exposure to vaginal spermicide are risk factors for developing cystitis.[3,4]

**PROGNOSIS** We found little evidence on the long term effects of untreated cystitis. One study found that progression to pyelonephritis was infrequent, and that most cases of cystitis regressed spontaneously, although symptoms sometimes persisted for several months.[5] Women with a baseline rate of more than two infections a year, over many years, are likely to have ongoing recurrent infections.[6]

Please refer to CD-ROM for full text and references.

## What are the effects of interventions to prevent and treat mammalian bites?

### LIKELY TO BE BENEFICIAL

**Antibiotics for treatment of infected mammalian bites***

We found no RCTs of antibiotics versus placebo for infected mammalian bites. However, there is consensus that antibiotics are likely to be beneficial

**Antibiotic prophylaxis**

Limited evidence from one systematic review found no significant difference with antibiotics versus control in the infection rate in people bitten by a dog, cat, or human in the preceding 24 hours. Meta-analysis according to the site of the wound found that antibiotics significantly reduced infections of the hand. One small RCT in the review found that in people with human bites, antibiotics versus control significantly reduced the rate of infection.

**Debridement, irrigation, and decontamination***

We found no reliable studies assessing debridement, irrigation, decontamination measures, or serum infiltration in the wound. However, there is consensus that such measures are likely to be beneficial.

**Education to prevent bites**

We found no RCTs of the effect of education programmes on the incidence of mammalian bites. One RCT found that an educational programme versus no education in school children significantly increased precautionary behaviour around dogs.

*No RCT evidence, but there is consensus that treatment is likely to be beneficial.

### UNKNOWN EFFECTIVENESS

**Comparative effectiveness of different antibiotics for treatment of infected mammalian bites**

One RCT in people with infected and uninfected animal and human bites comparing penicillin with or without dicloxacillin versus amoxicillin/clavulanic acid found no significant difference in failure rate (which was undefined).

**Education to prevent bites in specific occupational groups**

We found no RCTs of education to prevent bites in specific occupational groups.

**Primary wound closure**

One poor quality RCT comparing primary wound closure versus no closure in people with dog bites found no significant difference in the incidence of infection, but the RCT was too small to exclude clinically important effects.

**Tetanus toxoid after mammalian bites**

We found no evidence on the effects of tetanus toxoid in preventing tetanus after human or animal bites.

**DEFINITION**  Bite wounds are mainly caused by humans, dogs, or cats. They include superficial abrasions🄖 (30–43%), lacerations🄖 (31–45%), and puncture🄖 wounds (13–34%).[1]  ▶

# Bites (mammalian)

**INCIDENCE/ PREVALENCE** In areas where rabies is poorly controlled among domestic animals, dogs account for 90% of reported mammalian bites compared with less than 5% in areas where rabies is well controlled. In the USA, an estimated 3.5–4.7 million dog bites occur each year.[2] About one in five people bitten by a dog seek medical attention, and 1% of those require admission to hospital.[3,4] Between a third and half of all mammalian bites occur in children.[5]

**AETIOLOGY/ RISK FACTORS** In over 70% of cases, people are bitten by their own pets or by an animal known to them. Males are more likely to be bitten than females, and are more likely to be bitten by dogs, whereas females are more likely to be bitten by cats.[2] One study found that children under 5 years old were significantly more likely than older children to provoke animals before being bitten.[6] One study of infected dog and cat bites found that the most commonly isolated bacteria was *Pasteurella*, followed by *Streptococci, Staphylococci, Moraxella, Corynebacterium*, and *Neisseria*.[7] Mixed aerobic and anaerobic infection was more common than anaerobic infection alone.

**PROGNOSIS** In the USA, dog bites cause about 20 deaths a year.[8] In children, dog bites frequently involve the face, potentially resulting in severe lacerations and scarring.[9] Rabies, a life threatening viral encephalitis, may be contracted as a consequence of being bitten or scratched by a rabid animal. More than 99% of human rabies is in developing countries where canine rabies is endemic.[10]

---

Please refer to CD-ROM for full text and references.

*E Andrea Nelson, Nicky Cullum, and June Jones*

## What are the effects of treatments?

### BENEFICIAL

**Compression**

One systematic review has found that compression heals more venous leg ulcers than no compression. We found insufficient evidence from RCTs to compare the effects of different types of multilayer compression, or multilayer high compression versus short stretch bandages. One systematic review found that multilayer compression increased ulcer healing compared with single layer bandages.

**Pentoxifylline**

One systematic review and two subsequent RCTs have found that oral pentoxifylline increases the proportion of ulcers healed over 6–12 months compared with placebo.

### LIKELY TO BE BENEFICIAL

**Cultured allogenic bilayer skin replacement**

One RCT found that cultured allogenic bilayer skin replacement increased the proportion of ulcers healed after 6 months compared with a non-adherent dressing.

**Flavonoids**

Two RCTs found that flavonoids increased ulcer healing compared with placebo or standard care.

**Peri-ulcer injection of granulocyte–macrophage colony stimulating factor (GM-CSF)**

One RCT found that peri-ulcer injection of GM-CSF increased the proportion of ulcers healed after 13 weeks' treatment compared with placebo.

**Sulodexide**

Two RCTs found that sulodexide plus compression increased the proportion of ulcers healed after 60–90 days' treatment compared with compression alone.

**Systemic mesoglycan**

One RCT found that systemic mesoglycan plus compression increased the proportion of ulcers healed after 24 weeks' treatment compared with compression alone.

### UNKNOWN EFFECTIVENESS

**Antimicrobial agents; aspirin; debriding agents; foam, film, or alginate (semi-occlusive) dressings versus simple dressings in the presence of compression; intermittent pneumatic compression; low level laser treatment; oral rutosides; oral zinc; skin grafting; thromboxane α2 antagonists; topical calcitonin gene related peptide plus vasoactive intestinal polypeptide; topical keratinocyte growth factor 2; topical mesoglycan; topical negative pressure; ultrasound; vein surgery**

We found insufficient evidence about the effects of these interventions on ulcer healing.

# Venous leg ulcers

## UNLIKELY TO BE BENEFICIAL

### Hydrocolloid dressings versus simple low adherent dressings in the presence of compression

One systematic review found that, in the presence of compression, hydrocolloid dressings did not heal more venous leg ulcers than simple, low adherent dressings.

### Topically applied autologous platelet lysate

One RCT found no significant difference in time to healing of ulcers after 9 months between topically applied autologous platelet lysate and placebo.

## What are the effects of interventions to prevent recurrence?

## BENEFICIAL

### Compression

We found limited evidence that compression reduced recurrence, and that non-compliance with compression is a risk factor for recurrence.

## UNKNOWN EFFECTIVENESS

### Rutoside; stanozolol; vein surgery

We found insufficient evidence about the effects of these interventions on ulcer recurrence.

| | |
|---|---|
| **DEFINITION** | Definitions of leg ulcers vary, but the following is widely used: loss of skin on the leg or foot that takes more than 6 weeks to heal. Some definitions exclude ulcers confined to the foot, whereas others include ulcers on the whole of the lower limb. This review deals with ulcers of venous origin in people without concurrent diabetes mellitus, arterial insufficiency, or rheumatoid arthritis. |
| **INCIDENCE/ PREVALENCE** | Between 1.5 and 3/1000 people have active leg ulcers. Prevalence increases with age to about 20/1000 in people aged over 80 years.[1] |
| **AETIOLOGY/ RISK FACTORS** | Leg ulceration is strongly associated with venous disease. However, about a fifth of people with leg ulceration have arterial disease, either alone or in combination with venous problems, which may require specialist referral.[1] Venous ulcers (also known as varicose or stasis ulcers) are caused by venous reflux or obstruction, both of which lead to poor venous return and venous hypertension. |
| **PROGNOSIS** | People with leg ulcers have a poorer quality of life than age matched controls because of pain, odour, and reduced mobility.[2] In the UK, audits have found wide variation in the types of care (hospital inpatient care, hospital clinics, outpatient clinics, home visits), in the treatments used (topical agents, dressings, bandages, stockings), in healing rates, and in recurrence rates (26–69% in 1 year).[3,4] |

Please refer to CD-ROM for full text and references.

**Note**

When looking up a class of drug, the reader is advised to also look up specific examples of that class of drug where additional entries may be found. The reverse situation also applies. Abbreviations used: CVD, cardiovascular disease; HRT, hormone replacement therapy; IVF, in vitro fertilisation; MI, myocardial infarction; NSAIDs, non-steroidal anti-inflammatory drugs; STD, sexually transmitted disease.

Subject index

see also Alzheimer's disease
Denture stomatitis treatment 302
  antifungal drugs 302
  denture hygiene 302
Deoxyribonuclease
  bronchiectasis treatment 331
  chronic obstructive pulmonary
    disease treatment 334
Depression 220–3
  aetiology/risk factors 63, 223
  antidepressant treatment 220–1
    continuation/maintenance
      treatment 220
    in children/adolescents 62–3
  befriending therapy 222
  bibliotherapy 222
  care pathways 221, 222
  children and adolescents 62–4
  cognitive therapy 220, 222
    in children/adolescents 62
    with drug treatment 221
  definition 63, 222–3
  electroconvulsive therapy 220
    in children/adolescents 62
  exercise and 222
  family therapy 63
  group therapy 63
  incidence/prevalence 223
    in children/adolescents 63
  interpersonal therapy 220, 222
    in children/adolescents 62
    with drug treatment 221
  non-directive counselling 221
  problem solving therapy 221,
    222
  prognosis 63–4, 223
  psychological treatments 220,
    221, 222
    in children/adolescents 62,
      63
    with drug treatment 221
  St John's wort benefits 221–2
    in children/adolescents 63
  see also Bipolar disorder
Dermabrasion, wrinkle treatment
  366

Desferrioxamine mesylate, malaria
  treatment 178
Desipramine, depression treatment
  in children/adolescents 63
Dexamethasone
  childhood asthma treatment 50
  heel pain management 270,
    271
  malaria treatment 179
Dexfenfluramine, obesity
  management 127
Dextromethorphan
  cough treatment 319
  postherpetic neuralgia treatment
    186
Diabetes
  aetiology/risk factors 125
  cardiovascular disease in
    129–33
    aetiology/risk factors 132–3
    antiplatelet drug effects
      130–1
    blood glucose control 131
    blood pressure control 129
    incidence/prevalence 132
    lipid regulation 129–30
    prognosis 133
    smoking cessation and 129
    surgical treatment 131–2
  definition 124
  incidence/prevalence 124
  oropharyngeal candidiasis and
    301, 302
  prognosis 125
  see also Diabetic foot ulcers;
    Diabetic retinopathy;
    Glycaemic control
Diabetic foot ulcers 122–3
  aetiology/risk factors 123
  definition 123
  incidence/prevalence 123
  prevention 122
    patient education 122
    referral to foot care clinics
      122
    screening benefits 122
    therapeutic footwear 122

# Clinical evidence
## *concise* comments

*Clinical Evidence* is an evolving resource and we welcome any
feedback on the content of this issue and suggestions for future issues.

Please photocopy and complete this form, then return it to us.

For UK and rest of world - Fax: + 44 (0) 20 7383 6242, mail: BMJ Clinical Evidence,
BMJ Publishing Group, BMA House, Tavistock Square, London WC1H 9JR, UK

For North and South America - Fax: 1-240-646-7005, mail: BMJ Clinical Evidence,
PO Box 512, Annapolis Jct, MD20701-0512, USA

## Alternatively, email us at CEfeedback@bmjgroup.com

Name: ...................................................................................................................

Address: ...............................................................................................................

..............................................................................................................................

...........................................................Email: ..............................................

### Position

- [ ] GP/Primary Care Physician
- [ ] Hospital Doctor/ Specialist Physician
- [ ] Pharmacist
- [ ] Resident/Registrar

- [ ] Nurse
- [ ] PAM
- [ ] Manager
- [ ] Press
- [ ] Researcher
- [ ] Administrator

- [ ] Librarian
- [ ] Medical Student
- [ ] Member of Public/ Patient Support Group
- [ ] Other......................

### 1. Comments concerning the selection of studies

Section.................................................................................................................

Topic ....................................................................................................................

Reference ............................................................................................................

Comment...............................................................................................................

..............................................................................................................................

..............................................................................................................................

### 2. Suggestions for future issues

..............................................................................................................................

..............................................................................................................................

..............................................................................................................................

### 3. Other comments/questions

..............................................................................................................................

..............................................................................................................................

..............................................................................................................................

# Estimating cardiovascular risk and treatment benefit

*Adapted from the New Zealand guidelines on management of dyslipidaemia[1] and raised blood pressure[2] by Rod Jackson*

**Appendix 1**

## How to use these colour charts

The charts help the estimation of a person's absolute risk of a cardiovascular event and the likely benefit of drug treatment to lower cholesterol or blood pressure. For these charts, cardiovascular events include: new angina, myocardial infarction, coronary death, stroke or transient ischaemic attack (TIA), onset of congestive cardiac failure, or peripheral vascular syndrome.

There is a group of patients in whom risk can be assumed to be high (>20% in 5 years) without using the charts. They include those with symptomatic cardiovascular disease (angina, myocardial infarction, congestive heart failure, stroke, TIA, and peripheral vascular disease), or left ventricular hypertrophy on ECG.

To estimate a person's absolute 5 year risk:
■ Find the table relating to their sex, diabetic status (on insulin, oral hypoglycaemics, or fasting blood glucose over 8 mmol/L), smoking status, and age. The age shown in the charts is the mean for that category, i.e. age 60 = 55 to 65 years.
■ Within the table find the cell nearest to the person's blood pressure and total cholesterol : HDL ratio. For risk assessment it is enough to use a mean blood pressure based on two readings on each of two occasions, and cholesterol measurements based on one laboratory or two non-fasting Reflotron measurements. More readings are needed to establish the pre-treatment baseline.
■ The colour of the box indicates the person's 5 year cardiovascular disease risk (see below).

Notes: (1) People with a strong history of CVD (first degree male relatives with CVD before 55 years, female relatives before 65 years) or obesity (body mass index above 30 kg/m$^2$) are likely to be at greater risk than the tables indicate. The magnitude of the independent predictive value of these risk factors remains unclear — their presence should influence treatment decisions for patients at borderline treatment levels. (2) If total cholesterol or total cholesterol : HDL ratio is greater than 8 then the risk is at least 15%. (3) Nearly all people aged 75 years or over also have an absolute cardiovascular risk over 15%.

Charts reproduced with permission from The National Heart Foundation of New Zealand. Also available on http://www.nzgg.org.nz/library/gl_complete/bloodpressure/table1.cfm.

## REFERENCES

1. Dyslipidaemia Advisory Group. 1996 National Heart Foundation clinical guidelines for the assessment and management of dyslipidaemia. *NZ Med J* 1996;109:224–232.
2. National Health Committee. Guidelines for the management of mildly raised blood pressure in New Zealand: Ministry of Health National Health Committee Report, Wellington, 1995.

| RISK LEVEL 5 year CVD risk (non-fatal and fatal) | | BENEFIT (1) CVD events prevented per 100 treated for 5 years* | BENEFIT (2) Number needed to treat for 5 years to prevent one event* |
|---|---|---|---|
| Very High | >30% | >10 per 100 | <10 |
| | 25–30% | 9 per 100 | 11 |
| | 20–25% | 7.5 per 100 | 13 |
| High | 15–20% | 6 per 100 | 16 |
| Moderate | 10–15% | 4 per 100 | 25 |
| Mild | 5–10% | 2.5 per 100 | 40 |
| | 2.5–5% | 1.25 per 100 | 80 |
| | <2.5% | <0.8 per 100 | >120 |

*Based on a 20% reduction in total cholesterol or a reduction in blood pressure of 10–15 mm Hg systolic or 5–10 mm Hg diastolic, which is estimated to reduce CVD risk by about a third over 5 years.

**RISK LEVEL: MEN**

## NO DIABETES

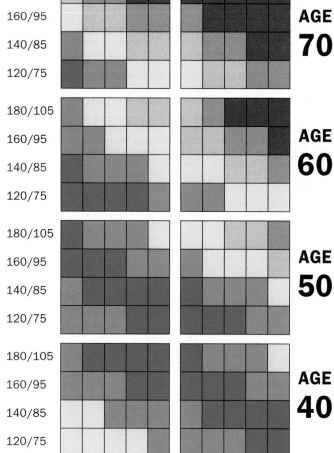

Nonsmoker — Smoker

Ratio of Total Cholesterol:HDL

Blood Pressure

AGE **70**
AGE **60**
AGE **50**
AGE **40**

Ratio of Total Cholesterol:HDL

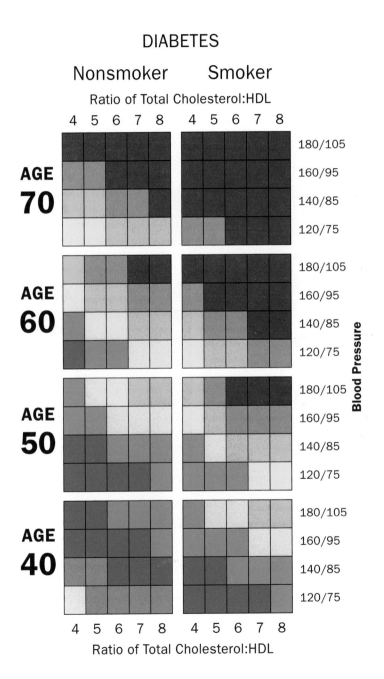

DIABETES

Nonsmoker     Smoker

Ratio of Total Cholesterol:HDL

Ratio of Total Cholesterol:HDL

Blood Pressure

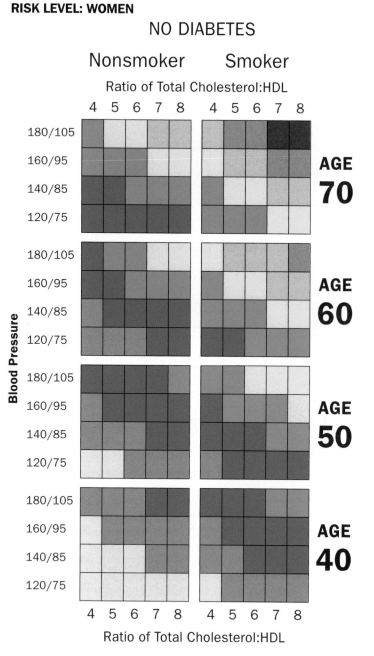

**Estimating cardiovascular risk and treatment benefit**

**Appendix 1**

**RISK LEVEL: WOMEN**

## NO DIABETES

Nonsmoker          Smoker

Ratio of Total Cholesterol:HDL

AGE **70**

AGE **60**

AGE **50**

AGE **40**

Blood Pressure

Ratio of Total Cholesterol:HDL

# Estimating cardiovascular risk and treatment benefit

## DIABETES

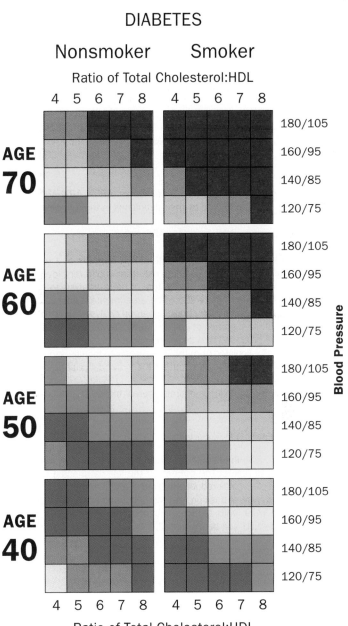

# The number needed to treat: adjusting for baseline risk

*Adapted with permission from Chatellier et al, 1996[1]*

## BACKGROUND

The number needed to treat (NNT) to avoid a single additional adverse outcome is a meaningful way of expressing the benefit of an active treatment over a control. It can be used both to summarise the results of a therapeutic trial or series of trials and to help medical decision making about an individual patient.

If the absolute risk of adverse outcomes in a therapeutic trial is ARC in the control group and ART in the treatment group, then the absolute risk reduction (ARR) is defined as (ARC − ART). The NNT is defined as the inverse of the ARR:

$$NNT = 1/(ARC - ART)$$

Since the Relative Risk Reduction (RRR) is defined as (ARC − ART)/ARC, it follows that NNT, RRR, and ARC are related by their definitions in the following way:

$$NNT \times RRR \times ARC = 1$$

This relationship can be used to estimate the likely benefits of a treatment in populations with different levels of baseline risk (that is different levels of ARC). This allows extrapolation of the results of a trial or meta-analysis to people with different baseline risks. Ideally, there should be experimental evidence of the RRR in each population. However, in many trials, subgroup analyses show that the RRR is approximately constant in groups of patients with different characteristics. Cook and Sackett therefore proposed that decisions about individual patients could be made by using the NNT calculated from the RRR measured in trials and the baseline risk in the absence of treatment estimated for the individual patient.[2]

The method may not apply to periods of time different to that studied in the original trials.

## USING THE NOMOGRAM

The nomogram shown on the next page allows the NNT to be found directly without any calculation: a straight line should be drawn from the point corresponding to the estimated absolute risk for the patient on the left hand scale to the point corresponding to the relative risk reduction stated in a trial or meta-analysis on the central scale. The intercept of this line with the right hand scale gives the NNT. By taking the upper and lower limits of the confidence interval of the RRR, the upper and lower limits of the NNT can be estimated.

## REFERENCES

1. Chatellier G, Zapletal E, Lemaitre D, *et al*. The number needed to treat: a clinically useful nomogram in its proper context. *BMJ* 1996;321:426–429.
2. Cook RJ, Sackett DL. The number needed to treat: a clinically useful measure of treatment effect. *BMJ* 1995;310:452–454.

# The number needed to treat

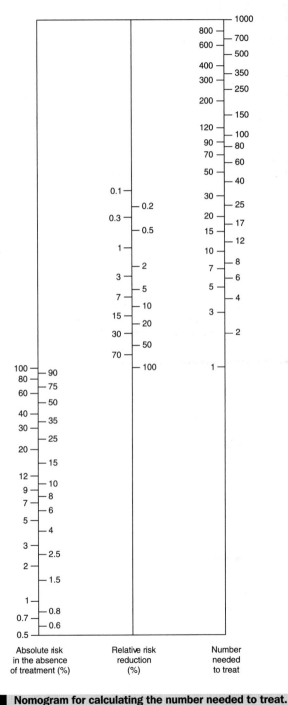

| | | |
|---|---|---|
| Absolute risk in the absence of treatment (%) | Relative risk reduction (%) | Number needed to treat |

# Clinical Evidence mini CD-ROM

The *Clinical Evidence* mini CD-ROM allows you to:
- Refer to the full *Clinical Evidence* content, including clinical questions, summary, and background information, evidence detail, figures, tables and appendices
- Choose the method of navigation you prefer, through the table of contents, topic sections, or the search engine
- Hyperlink references to abstracts where they appear on PubMed and Cochrane (Internet access required)
- Hyperlink to the glossary, figures, tables, and references
- Print the full text of the topics

**To access *Clinical Evidence* help:**
- From within the *Clinical Evidence* CD-ROM, simply click on the link at the top of the screen or from within Windows, select Programs > Clinical Evidence > Help (if you have already installed *Clinical Evidence*)
- For technical help, please go to the FAQs at www.clinicalevidence.com
- For damaged CD-ROMs please contact:
BMJ Publishing Group • Tel: +44(0) 207 383 6270 • subscriptions@bmjgroup.com (UK/ROW)
For individual subscriptions • Tel: +1 800 373 2897/+1 240 646 7000 • clinevid@pmds.com (USA)
For individuals receiving *Clinical Evidence* courtesy of United Health Foundation:
ce@unitedhealthfoundation.org

**To install *Clinical Evidence***
(i) Exit from any programs you have running.
(ii) Insert the *Clinical Evidence* Installation CD-ROM into the CD-ROM drive. The installation starts automatically (if it does not, select Run from the Start menu and enter d:\setup (where d: is your CD-ROM drive letter).
(iii) Follow the on-screen instructions. As part of this process, you can install Adobe Acrobat Reader so you can efficiently print *Clinical Evidence* topics — this can also be installed later by following the instructions below. An additional 20 Mbytes of hard disk space is required for this.

**Minimum system requirements**
An IBM compatible PC with at least this specification:
- 60 MBytes hard disk space
- 90 MHz processor
- 32 MBytes of RAM
- CD-ROM drive
- Modem, if you want to access the Internet for updates, etc.
- SVGA monitor recommended

**Operating systems**
This software has been tested with the following operating systems:
- Microsoft Windows 95
- Microsoft Windows 98
- Microsoft Windows 2000 Professional
- Microsoft Windows XP Professional
- Microsoft Windows NT SP6
- Microsoft Windows 2000 Server

*Please note*
Windows XP Home Edition may require special handling. Please refer to the appropriate section in the Readme file, or access the full text at www.clinicalevidence.com. The Readme file is located at:
Start > Programs > Clinical Evidence > Readme (if you have already installed *Clinical Evidence*) or contact technical help.

**Browsers**
Microsoft Internet Explorer 5.5 is the recommended browser, and should be your default browser when installing *Clinical Evidence*.
This software has been tested with the following browsers:
- Microsoft Internet Explorer 5.0 (English)
- Microsoft Internet Explorer 5.5 (English)
- Microsoft Internet Explorer 6.0 (English)
- Netscape 4.7 (English)
- Netscape 6.0 (English)

*Please note*
Microsoft Internet Explorer 4 is not a supported browser.
Microsoft Internet Explorer 6 is not compatible with Windows 95.
Internet Explorer 5.5 and 6.0 are available on the installation CD-ROM — see below for details.

**To install Microsoft Internet Explorer v5.5**
(i) With the *Clinical Evidence* Installation CD-ROM in the CD-ROM drive, select Run from the Start menu.
(ii) Type d:\other\ie5.5\ie5setup and click OK (where d: is your CD-ROM drive letter).
(iii) Follow the on-screen instructions. The typical installation requires approximately 17 Mbytes of hard disk space.

**To install Microsoft Internet Explorer v6.0**
(i) With the *Clinical Evidence* Installation CD-ROM in the CD-ROM drive, select Run from the Start menu.
(ii) Type d:\other\ie6.0\ie6setup and click OK (where d: is your CD-ROM drive letter).
(iii) Follow the on-screen instructions. The typical installation requires approximately 25 Mbytes of hard disk space.

**To install Adobe Acrobat Reader v5.0.5**
(i) With the *Clinical Evidence* Installation CD-ROM in the CD-ROM drive, select Run from the Start menu.
(ii) Type d:\Adobe\ar505enu and click OK (where d: is your CD-ROM drive letter).
(iii) Follow the on-screen instructions.